AUDIOMETRY IN INFANCY

SANFORD E. GERBER, Ph.D.

Professor of Audiology
Coordinator, Speech and Hearing Sciences
University of California, Santa Barbara

and

the staff of the
UCSB Speech and Hearing Center
Santa Barbara, California

GRUNE & STRATTON

A Subsidiary of Harcourt Brace Jovanovich, Publishers
New York San Francisco London

Library of Congress Cataloging in Publication Data
Main entry under title:

Audiometry in infancy.

Bibliography: p.
Includes indexes.
1. Audiometry. 2. Hearing disorders in children—Diagnosis. 3. Hearing disorders in children. I. Gerber, Sanford E. [DNLM: 1. Audiometry—In infancy and Childhood. 2. Hearing disorders—Diagnosis. 3. Hearing disorders—In infancy and Childhood. WV272 A902]
RF294.A834 617.8′07′5 77-23785

Grune & Stratton, Inc.
111 Fifth Avenue
New York, New York 10003

Distributed in the United Kingdom by
Academic Press, Inc. (London) Ltd.
24/28 Oval Road, London NW 1

Library of Congress Catalog Number 77-23785
International Standard Book Number 0-8089-1038-8

Printed in the United States of America

to my own children

for Howard, who might read this book
for Michael, who probably won't
for Naomi, who can't
for Shoshana, who never had the chance
for Sharon, who may

CONTENTS

List of Figures

List of Tables

CONTRIBUTORS

The contributors to AUDIOMETRY IN INFANCY are all on the staff of the Speech and Hearing Center of the University of California at Santa Barbara. They are:

ROBERT E. CARREL, M.D., Research Associate
BARBARA K. CONE, M.A.[1]
JANIS M. COSTELLO, Ph.D., Associate Professor of Speech Pathology
JOSEPH R. DiBARTOLOMEO, M.D., Research Associate
SUSAN FELSENFELD, B.A.
JOHN N. GARDI, Ph.C.[2]
DIANE B. GILCHRIST, M.A., Lecturer in Speech Pathology
THEODORE D. HANLEY, Ph.D. Professor of Speech Science
ROBERT J. HANSON, JR., Ph.D., Assistant Professor of Speech Science
ROBERTA A. JACKSON, M.A., Lecturer in Speech Pathology
BRONWYN L. JONES, M.A.
ROBERT L. KOEGEL, Ph.D., Associate Professor of Language Pathology
MAURICE I. MENDEL, Ph.D., Associate Professor of Audiology
ANTHONY MULAC, Ph.D., Associate Professor of Speech
CAROL A. PRUTTING, Ph.D., Assistant Professor of Language
ELIZABETH A. SKARAKIS, M.A.[3]

[1]Present address: University of Texas at Dallas
[2]Present address: University of California at San Francisco
[3]Present address: Los Angeles Children's Hospital

FOREWORD

Having made, in recent weeks, a broad and comprehensive study of forewords, I conclude that the genre, in all but a few isolated cases, consists of encomia describing the author (editor) as a direct scholarly descendant of and a quantum intellectual leap beyond Darwin or Freud, Adam Smith, or Marie Curie. Casual mention is made of the subject of the book and the unique qualifications of the writer to prepare the material for the hungry eyes of a breathlessly anticipatory leadership.

Fearlessly, I shall eschew this pattern. Encomia bestowed upon Sanford Gerber would be wasted on those who know him and his work, ignored by the few readers who do not. Instead of adulatory words about the editor and extraordinarily accomplished scholars who have contributed to this volume, I should like to concentrate upon the significance and timeliness of this work.

Jonathan Spivak, in the April 12, 1976, issue of the *Wall Street Journal* writes,

> Today—during this one day—the world's population will increase by some 200,000, the size of a Des Moines or a Salt Lake City or a Grand Rapids.
>
> Tomorrow there'll be a similar increase, and the next day. And the next. And the next, for many years to come.
>
> So goes the grim progression that threatens to overcrowd the globe and strain its ability to feed, clothe and shelter its inhabitants. "The magnitude of the new population boom surpasses all earlier expectations," warns a United Nations report on the long-range implications of world population growth. "The longer the high tempo persists . . . the more precarious will be prospects for a healthy life on this planet."

Let me underscore that last line, "the more precarious will be prospects for a healthy life on this planet," and continue with a quotation by Bernard Z. Friedlander from the 1975 book, *Exceptional Infant:* "Systematic early identification of children who are known to suffer developmental disability, or who have a high risk of doing so, is potentially the single most powerful means at hand for reducing the impact of exceptionality—on the individual child, on the family, and on the community and society at large."

As we proceed from the general toward the specific, the pattern becomes even clearer—mind-boggling population growth, life-threatening by its sheer magnitude, then the hopeful prospects afforded by systematic early identification of the high-risk infant. And so we come to the subject of this important book, *Audiometry in Infancy,* written and edited by my good friends and colleagues.

Exceptionality is hydra-headed; thus it is appropriate that its foes should draw swords against individual manifestations of congenital and early-childhood disorders. Not least among these certainly is impairment of the sense of hearing and early detection is a desideratum recognized more than a decade ago by Mrs. Marion Downs of the University of Colorado Medical Center, who devised and published reports on techniques for infant screening. More recently, in 1971, Dr. Aram Glorig wrote in *Hearing and Speech News*,

> If we in medicine, rehabilitation, and other health-related fields have learned anything from our years of experience and effort, it is that early education of the handicapped child is of prime importance. This educational need applies to any handicap, but it is especially true for the congenitally deaf child.
>
> However, there is a second axiom of equal importance in dealing with the handicapped child. The first step in making early education possible is the immediate diagnosis of the handicap.
>
> It would seem then, that tests for detecting deafness at birth would be the optimal solution. The newborn child offers a distinct advantage for screening procedures, because he is a captive subject for at least the first three days of life. This is probably the only real advantage afforded by testing in the nursery, but it makes neotate testing a very attractive alternative.

Downs and Glorig, as the sophisticated reader will recognize, are only two of a score or more who have commented on the theory, philosophy and technology of neonatal hearing screening. However, it has been left to Gerber and his co-authors to put it all together, to explore the subject in its many dimensions and to summarize the present state of the art for a wide spectrum of readership, from its primary target, the practicing clinical audiologist, through many other specialists, not the least of which is the educator.

I commend this book to all who join me in believing that no effort directed toward enhancement of the communication abilities of the aurally impaired child—in which identification is the first and critical step—is wasted.

Theordore D. Hanley, Ph.D.

Speech and Hearing Center
University of California
Santa Barbara, California 93106

PREFACE

For about the past dozen years I have been involved with increasing time and frequency in the study of the newborn. Most of my research, most of my clinical activities, and most of my teaching are now centered on the infant. There are several reasons why this population is interesting. For one thing, babies tend to be really very nice people and I enjoy their company. Second, the miracle of life is always very evident in the newborn nursery. Third, development in the first few days or weeks of life is fascinatingly rapid. Finally, and of most significance, has been my firm belief that early intervention is the best form of prevention. We cannot usually keep a child from being deaf; we can minimize the handicap produced by his hearing loss if we identify and intervene as early as possible. It is my personal clinical philosophy that there is no time which is too soon to begin habilitation.

It turns out, also, that many other people think so too. There are more and more programs in hospitals, medical schools, and university Speech and Hearing Clinics directed at the very youngest children. We now know from the work of our colleagues in neurophysiology and in early education that it does matter if one examines and habilitates at the youngest ages. There are, however, rather few books to guide us on what to do; although, the few books which exist in the field are very good. It was our purpose here not to duplicate them, but to produce a volume which would lead one to and through some evaluative methods.

The book divides itself into three natural parts. The first of these defines the nature and the scope of the problem. It attempts to deal with causes of congenital or early acquired hearing loss, the concomitant pathologies, and the predictability of hearing loss. The second part of the book deals with the diagnostic methods. The distribution of the chapters is intended to be a relatively accurate reflection of their importance, so that each of the methods merits a single chapter with the exception of those methods attempting to assess the central nervous system directly. The third part deals with communication development, phonological development, sensory and educational development. It attempts to deal with the question, "Does it matter if we intervene early?"

At first I had thought to write the entire book myself. I very early recognized both my temporal and intellectual limitations with respect to the book that I thought I wanted. Then I decided to solicit contributors and looked about for the most qualified people. I am very proud that these most qualified people turn out to be my own colleagues at the UCSB Speech and Hearing Center. I think that their contributions attest to my good sense in selecting them as contributors. I am very grateful to them for their efforts on behalf of these babies.

Some acknowledgements, of course, are in order. My good friend and assistant, Ms. Bronwyn Jones, was largely a co-editor. She read and commented on each and every contribution, especially mine; she checked all the references; and she co-authored one chapter. Another graduate student, Ms. Susan Wyant, co-ordinated all the figures and handled solicitation of permissions. Still another of our graduate students, Ms. Dolores Crummett, did much of the typing along with our secretaries, Sandra Nicassio and Elizabeth Norton. In addition, I am delighted to acknowledge Dr. Larry Bradford of the Menninger Foundation who first proposed the project to me.

I am necessarily grateful to all those babies for whose benefit the book is intended. Last, and never least, I acknowledge my wife Louise, because she loves me.

Sanford E. Gerber

I

The Problem

Robert E. Carrel

1
Epidemiology of Hearing Loss

More than 1 in 1000 births with hearing loss have been detected worldwide (Fraser, 1971; Stewart, 1974). These are reports of screening only for severe hearing loss with residual hearing; the true incidence of congenital hearing loss would be more accurately projected to be 1 in 200. In this country 6% of four-year-olds show evidence of hearing loss, and 3–4% of seven-year-olds have abnormal audiologic findings (Newman, 1975); this is related in part to the high incidence of middle ear infections in the younger age group.

The problems of understanding epidemiology of hearing loss are compounded by the varying terminologies in use. For the sake of simplification and better understanding of the epidemiology, hearing loss is considered here as being either congenital (present at the time of birth) or noncongenital (presumed to have its onset after birth); these two major subgroups are divided according to etiologies. Classification according to degree of hearing loss, audiometric findings, and pathology is covered in Chapters 2 and 3.

Despite our attempt to simplify the classifications, there are limitations in knowing for certain that a hearing loss was not present at birth, since the loss may be partial, unilateral, and/or limited to a narrow frequency range, making it undetectable utilizing the methodology currently available for newborn screening. In addition, factors present at the time of birth, which might eventually result in hearing loss, may not manifest themselves until later, after birth (see Chap. 3).

Hearing loss, like any other biologic symptom or sign, may have multiple causes. Considerations of cause, as in any disease entity, are included in a differential diagnosis. The causes may be inherited or sporadic (noninherited), intrinsic (related to factors within the organism such as malformation), or extrinsic (related to external factors).

Differential diagnoses of congenital hearing loss may be comprised of the following: infection; trauma; maldevelopment; prematurity; metabolism; toxic; genetic (etiology of pathology unknown); and/or environmental.

CONGENITAL LOSSES

Infection

Any infectious agent—whether it be viral, bacterial, protozoal, etc.—which can damage the central nervous system prenatally, either by direct involvement or by influencing maldevelopment later in prenatal life (teratogenesis), can cause congenital deafness. Prenatal rubella, for example, is well known for its teratogenic effects. Ten to 40% of infants born to mothers whose pregnancy was complicated by rubella show varying degrees and incidences of hearing loss, depending on when in the pregnancy the mother was infected, the population studied, the intensity of follow-up, etc. The virus may still be present at the time of birth and the hearing loss may not be present for many months after birth. Fisch (1964) observed that 24% of all congenital deafness observed after a major rubella epidemic was caused by maternal rubella, and almost 6% in the absence of a major epidemic. Although rubella is now a preventable disease through immunizations, our decreasing concern about this potentially severely damaging disease has resulted in increasing populations of unimmunized children (Chap. 3).

Cytomegalovirus (CMV), although far less known than rubella, can result in hearing loss as a complication of prenatal infection. Two to 3% of pregnant women excrete the virus, and up to 1% of newborns do similarly. Although the incidence of hearing loss as a result of prenatal CMV infection is not known, it has been definitely demonstrated congenitally in newborns as a complication of the mother's CMV infection. Aural pathology can be a result (Myers and Stool, 1968). Efforts are currently in progress to develop an appropriate immunization.

Toxoplasmosis, a protozoan organism, can cause disease and complications in a fashion similar to the previous two viral agents. It is transmitted through ingestion of raw meat, and is estimated to be present in 0.25% of live births. Data are not available relative to the number of cases of hearing loss that result.

Herpes simplex, a common virus, can also produce congenital hearing loss.

Congenital syphilis, a disease only recently thought to be controlled, is again presenting in the newborn. This spirochetal agent can have protean manifestations, including involvement of the central nervous system, with auditory nerve deafness appearing after birth.

Although rubella has long been considered the primary cause of congenital hearing loss due to prenatal infection, other microbial agents, including some not discussed in the preceding material, may play an important role in determining causes where the etiology has been previously unknown. Immunologic studies suggest that 1–2% of all newborns show serologic evidence of prenatal infection. Combined immunoglobin and hearing screening in the newborn period may eventually reveal the true incidence of hearing loss associated with various forms of prenatal infection.

Trauma

Trauma can cause congenital hearing loss. For the sake of simplicity, direct mechanical trauma as well as perinatal hypoxia are included under the concept of trauma. Understanding the effects of trauma is most complex since the complications, including hearing loss, are related to multiple factors, including, but not limited to, temperature, blood pressure, and metabolism. Thirteen to 14% of congenital hearing loss is related to trauma.

Maldevelopment

Maldevelopment includes all prenatal malformations, whether they be limited to the hearing mechanism or the brain, or involve the whole organism. They may be inherited with or without a chromosomal abnormality or they may be sporadic, again with or without a chromosomal abnormality. Tables of these conditions, associated with hearing loss, are found in Chapter 2. The incidence of congenital hearing loss in association with some types of maldevelopment is well documented.

In Down's syndrome (mongolism)—which occurs in 1 in 600 births—1% of the cases is inherited. It is estimated that Down's syndrome individuals have no evidence of congenital hearing loss, but are unusually subject to middle ear disease.

Treacher-Collins Disease, which is inherited as an autosomal dominant trait with variable penetrance, constitutes many cases of congenital hearing loss (Chap. 2). A chromosomal abnormality is not associated.

Almost 100 cases of congenital hearing loss have been reported where the organism malformation has been relatively minor, including preauricular pits, prominent auricles, thick auricles, low-set ears, hypertrophic and thickened ear lobes, etc. (DiBartolomeo, 1974; Jaffe, 1976). These cases have demonstrated the importance of looking for congenital hearing problems in the presence of minor malformations about the ear (Chap. 3). They are grouped as otofacial cervical abnormalities and are inherited usually as autosomal dominant.

Gestational Disorders Including Prematurity

Under this etiologic classification are included prematurity, low birth weight for gestational age, and postmature infants. This group of infants demonstrates a higher incidence of neurologic deficits including hearing loss than seen in the normal full-term population. This is probably contributed to by multiple factors including increased incidence of susceptibility of the brain to trauma, as well as higher incidences of malformation, hyperbilirubinemia, and other metabolic disorders such as hypocalcemia and hypoglycemia. Approximately 10% of infants screened for hearing loss because of prior high-risk factors were low birth weight infants.

Metabolism

Diseases associated with metabolic disorders may have associated hearing loss. Many of these may be inherited as an autosomal recessive disorder. They are considered here as separate from the other major categories of genetically determined hearing loss, since the pathology is related to the metabolic abnormality.

Metabolic diseases can be related to disorders of neuronal lipid, carbohydrates, and amino-acid metabolism, as well as endocrinologic disorders such as thyroid dysfunction. In some areas of the world, nerve deafness may be the sole neurologic abnormality of endemic goiterus cretinism (Fig. 1-1). Hearing loss is also seen in the various forms of gargoylism (Hunter–Hurler syndrome, Fig. 1-2), as well as closely related forms of the so-called mucolipidoses.

Although the incidence of hearing loss associated with metabolic abnormality is not known, this probably represents a small but very significant group. Deafness associated with endemic cretinism is not correctible by thyroid treatment after birth, pointing to a congenital origin. The hearing impairment associated with the various forms of gargoylism (Hurler's disease, Hunter's disease, etc.) are usually progressive and detected postnatally, although the basic metabolic abnormality occurred at the time of conception. On the other hand, Pendred's disease (Fig. 1-3) accounts for about 7% of congenital deafness and, according to Fraser (1971) is"the most common autosomal recessive syndrome involving deafness . . ."

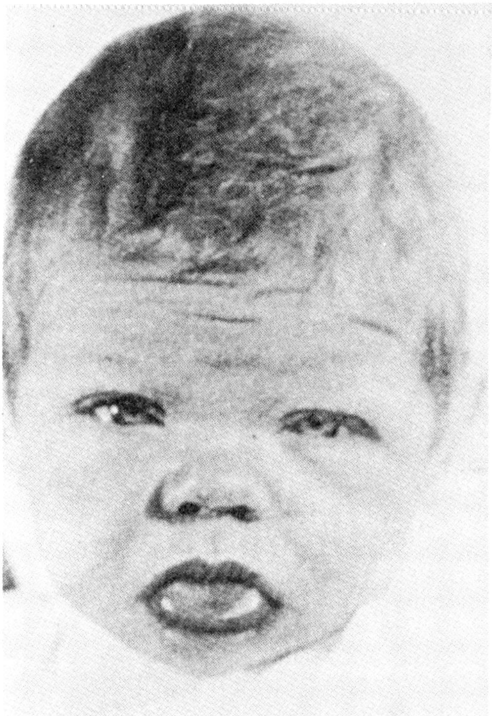

Fig. 1-1. Cretinism. From Nelson WE: Pediatrics, 6th ed. Saunders.

Intoxication

Toxins, whether they be of extrinsic or intrinsic origin, are included in the concept of intoxication as an etiology. Streptomycin and chloroquine taken prenatally can result in congenital hearing loss; while kanamycin, for example, does not cross the placental barrier. There is suggestive evidence that similar effects may be seen with quinine, excessive amounts of salicylates, and thalidomide.

Kernicterus is considered a manifestation of intoxication, the damage being related primarily to an elevated blood level of indirect bilirubin of approximately 20 mg/100 ml (however, see Chap. 3). This may be related to Rh incompatibility, prematurity, or any other condition that might cause a marked rise in the indirect serum bilirubin levels. Although most cases of kernicterus are related to the postnatal rise in bilirubin, a few have been

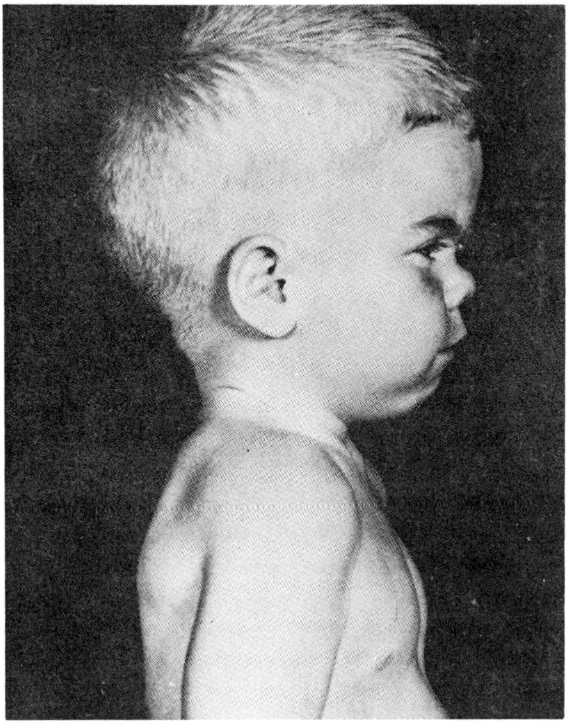

Fig. 1-2. Hunter–Hurler syndrome. Patient showing stigmata of Hunter form of mucopolysaccharidosis (gargoylism). Note hirsutism, heavy eyebrows, depressed nasal bridge, thick lips, and protruding abdomen. (From FO Black et al: Congenital Deafness. Colorado Associated Univ Pr, 1971)

speculated to be associated with a prenatal toxic effect. Approximately 43% of individuals with kernicterus show varying degrees of auditory imperception; 10–12% of congenital deafness is thought to be associated with kernicterus.

Genetic—Without Evidence of Other Malformation

Approximately 50% of all cases of congenital deafness are inherited (Fraser, 1971). In most of these cases, there is no evidence of abnormality other than the deafness. In school populations of deaf children, up to 57% have had their hearing loss determined on a genetic basis. These cases may be determined as autosomal recessive (approximately two-thirds of congenital

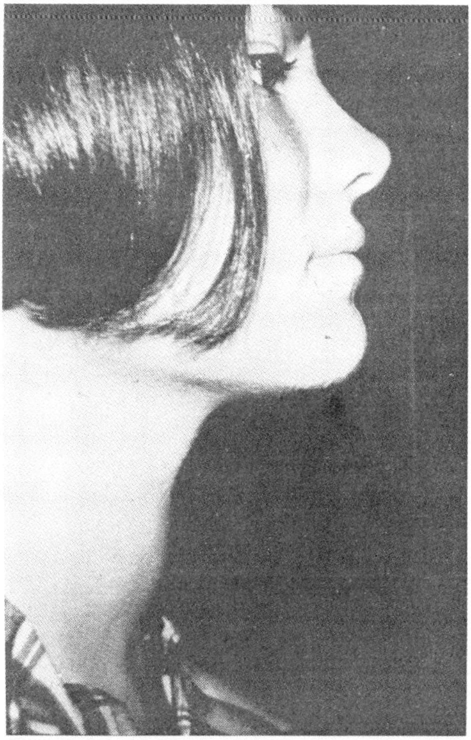

Fig. 1-3. Pendred's disease. (From Black FO et al: Congenital Deafness. Colorado Associated Univ Pr, 1971.)

deafness), autosomal dominant (a little less than one-third) and as X-linked recessive (approximately 3–4%).

AUTOSOMAL RECESSIVE

Autosomal recessive congenital deafness is usually severe. The basic units of genetic information, the genes, are arranged in pairs on chromosomes and their position is called a locus. Every individual is suspected of having at least five so-called abnormal genes that do not manifest themselves as a disease entity and hence are considered recessive. When their locus is on a nonsex chromosome, they are called autosomal; hence the concept autosomal recessive. When two individuals carrying the same autosomal recessive abnormal gene mate and have children, their risk for producing a child carrying the same abnormal gene from both parents and thus having evidence of the disease, such as deafness, is one in four, or 25%. A hypothetical pedigree for such genetic transmission is shown in Fig. 1–4.

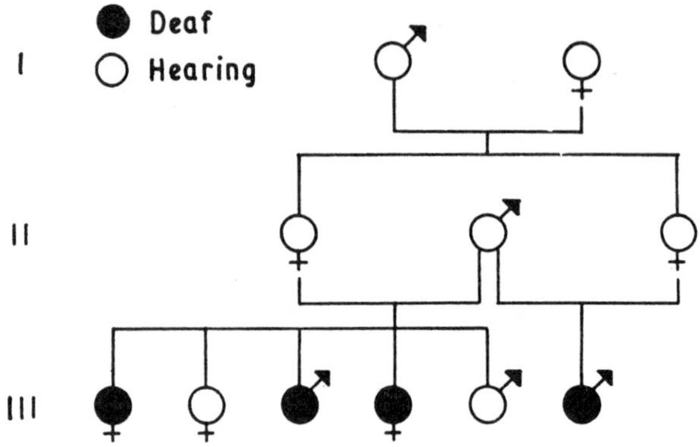

Fig. 1-4. Recessive deafness. Recessive inheritance of the syndrome of deafness with retinitis pigmentosa among the offspring of both unions between a man and two sisters after the data of Liebreich (1861). (From Fraser GR: J Med Gen, 1964.)

If two congenitally deaf individuals, whose congenital deafness was caused by the same abnormal autosomal recessive genes mate, their risk for having deaf children would be 100%. Numerous families, where both parents were indeed deaf, and the deafness was thought to be determined as an autosomal recessive condition, have been followed. Since most of the children born to these families are not deaf, studies have suggested that there are five to ten different loci for determining autosomal recessive disease; that is, there are five to ten different gene pairs for determining autosomal recessive deafness. The risk for two parents, whose deafness is related to inherited factors, is discussed at the end of this section.

AUTOSOMAL DOMINANT DEAFNESS

Autosomal dominant congenital deafness is also typically severe. In autosomal dominant disease, the genetic information from one gene is enough to determine disease. In autosomal dominant conditions, the risk for having an effected child is 50%. If both parents carry the same autosomal dominant disorder, the risk is 75%. In some autosomal dominant conditions, the offspring may receive the abnormal gene but might not manifest the disease including deafness. This may be true in a condition called Waardenburg's syndrome (see Chap. 3). In such a situation, the condition is still considered autosomal dominant, but with incomplete penetrance. Although these individuals might not be deaf, they still carry the autosomal dominant gene, and their risk for having a deaf child themselves still remains at 50%. A hypothetical pedigree for an autosomal dominant condition is shown in Fig. 1-5.

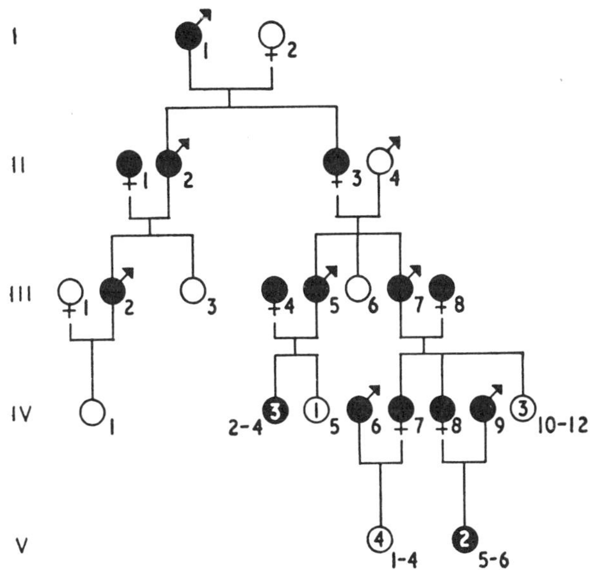

Fig. 1-5. Dominant deafness. Pedigree of dominant deafness in five generations after Fay (1898): I.i is number 507 of that report. Recessive deafness is likely in the case of the deaf persons who married into the family (II.i; III.4; IV.6; IV.9.) (From Fraser GR: J Med Gen, 1964.)

X-LINKED RECESSIVE CONGENITAL DEAFNESS

X-linked recessive cases of congenital deafness constitute approximately 3–4% of all cases of congenital deafness. In X-linked recessive disease, the locus for the gene determining the condition is on the X chromosome, one of the sex chromosomes. Females have two X chromosomes and males have an X and a Y chromosome. When a female has one abnormal gene on an X chromosome, the condition does not manifest itself. In the male, however, where there is only one X chromosome, the presence of the abnormal gene on that chromosome results in disease. In these conditions, the female carrier is normal. It is presumed that she has inherited her carrier state from her normal carrier mother. Half of her brothers would show disease and half of her sisters would be carriers. She has a 50% chance of producing a son with disease and half of her daughters would be carriers. A hypothetical pedigree for X-linked recessive disease is shown in Fig. 1-6.

Nance et al. (1971), for example, have described X-linked mixed hearing losses. In those same proceedings, Fraser reminded us of the Hartness

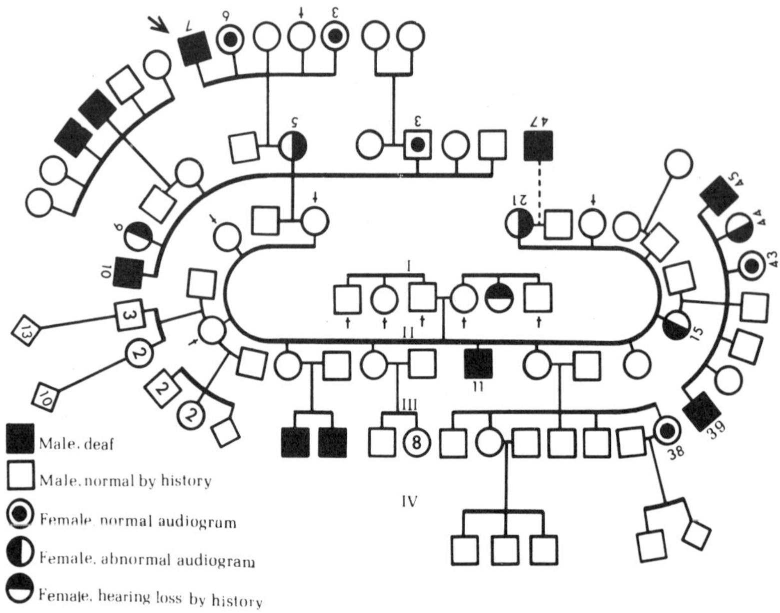

Fig. 1-6. X-linked deafness. Pedigree of family. Numbers under figures indicate subjects who were studied. (From Nance WE et al: in Bergsma D (ed): The Clinical Delineation of Birth Defects: Part IX, Ear. Williams and Wilkins, 1971.)

family, described by Kramer in 1835, whose six sons were deaf and five daughters normal.

Risk for Parents Having a Deaf Child

The risk, for any couple who have normal hearing, of having a child who will be diagnosed as being congenitally deaf is approximately 1 in 1000 to 1 in 2000. If one parent is deaf, and the deafness is known to be related to factors other than genetic, the risk just stated is not increased. If both parents are deaf, and the deafness in both cases is proven to be related to nongenetic factors, the risk is not increased.

If both parents are deaf and the deafness in both cases is determined as autosomal recessive, the risk for having a deaf child is 100% when both parents' autosomal recessive deafness is related to the same autosomal recessive gene abnormality. Since, however, there are thought to be a number of different genes determining autosomal recessive deafness, the risk may be as low as 1 in 200. Unfortunately, at this time it is impossible to determine biomedically whether the autosomal recessive deafness is related to the same or different loci in most cases.

When one parent is deaf as a result of an autosomal dominant condition, approximately 50% of their children may be expected to be deaf. When both are deaf due to either the same or different autosomal dominant conditions, the risk for having a deaf child is 75%. If a father is deaf as a result of an X-linked recessively determined deafness and the mother is normal, the risk for having a congenitally deaf child is not increased. Any daughter born of such a marriage, however, has a 50% risk of being a carrier and of producing congenital deafness in 50% of her sons and a similar carrier state in 50% of her daughters.

As can be seen, although the risks for progeny can be determined when the exact genetic mechanism of deafness is known, there are many cases of genetic deafness where this is not known. Since over 80% of deaf people marry deaf mates, genetic counseling (presenting risk figures as previously stated) is considered essential. When the exact etiology of the deafness is known, the material previously stated is appropriate. Again, however, since the etiology is not known in many cases, empiric risk figures can be offered. It has been observed that the average risk for deaf parents having a deaf child is approximately 10% prior to the birth of the first child and drops to 1% after at least three normal hearing children have been born. When there is one normal hearing child and one deaf, the risk for each subsequent pregnancy is 50%. If the first child is born deaf, the risk of a subsequent child being deaf is approximately 80%.

NONCONGENITAL LOSSES

The differential diagnosis in determining the etiology of deafness determined following birth is similar to that of congenital hearing loss.

Infection

Infection is a major cause of postnatal acquired deafness. A number of the childhood illnesses, which can now be prevented, can result in hearing loss. One percent of all children who develop rubeola (red measles) during an epidemic will show frank clinical evidence of encephalitis. One-third of them die, and another third show significant neurologic impairment, including deafness. In fact, any organism that effects the brain directly or its covering, as in an encephalitis or meningitis, can result in varying degrees of hearing impairment. In the younger child, where there is an increased incidence of upper respiratory tract infection and subsequent middle ear infection, there is increased incidence of conductive loss. Most of the 6% of four-year-olds with evidence of hearing loss have this in association with transient middle ear infection.

Trauma

Trauma is used here to include direct trauma to the ear, damage to the hearing mechanism as a result of head injury, particularly basilar skull fracture, and damage to the hearing mechanism as a result of high intensity noise. The exact incidence of traumatic causes of hearing loss is not known, although it is suspected that it might be significant since the incidence of sensory-neural loss progressively increases after the age of four years, this increase in many cases is not explained solely by genetic mechanisms such as X-linked recessive determination.

Maldevelopment

There is an increased incidence of hearing loss in association with cranial-facial maldevelopments and other generalized maldevelopment disorders such as Down's syndrome. In many of these cases, the hearing loss is of a conductive type, and presumed to be related to an increased incidence of middle ear infection due both to malformation of the middle ear structures as well as, more commonly, abnormalities in middle ear drainage.

Intoxication

The same aspects of intoxication previously discussed are applicable here. Postnatal use of streptomycin, chloroquine, quinine, and salicylates have been implicated in causing hearing loss. The increasingly common use of kanamycin and gentamycin is cause for concern. Although cases of hearing impairment related to kernicterus are considered congenital, most cases of such damage associated with increased levels of bilirubin probably arise shortly after birth.

Genetic (Etiology of Pathology Unknown)

Many cases of genetically determined hearing loss have their onset following birth. These include recessive early onset deafness, sex-linked early onset deafness, dominant low frequency hearing loss, dominant midfrequency hearing loss, and dominant progressive hearing loss. Autosomal recessive early onset deafness, a progressive hearing loss, may occur at one year of age with severe hearing loss by six years of age. X-linked recessive deafness has a similar onset. Since there has been noted to be an increased incidence of sensory-neural hearing loss in childhood, it has been suggested that a number of these cases may well be related to X-linked transmission. Although pedigree information supports this consideration in some cases, many other family studies are negative and suggest other factors. Both dominant low and mid-frequency hearing loss begin either in early childhood or in early adult life. Eventually, all frequencies are effected in later life. Dominant progressive hearing loss is also characterized by childhood or early adult onset with progression. Furthermore, there are other types of genetically determined hearing loss that do not manifest themselves in childhood.

SUMMARY

The true incidence of hearing loss is probably higher than most of us would have anticipated. While the incidence of severe impairments is about 1 in 1000 births, it is likely that some measurable loss occurs in 1 infant of about every 200 born. Moreover, many children develop severe hearing losses in early childhood due to disease or to degnerative processes.

In this chapter we have considered both the genetic and acquired factors that may lead to the presence of severe hearing impairment at birth. In addition, we turned our attention to the causes of noncongenital losses, and we noted that some of the same etiologies that produce congenital impairment are operative after birth as well. Finally, there is a discussion of the least understood category of deafness, hearing losses of genetic origin that are not present at birth.

REFERENCES

DiBartolomeo JR: The auditory system: Pre and post natal development: Indices of dysfunction. Paper presented at Sensory and Perceptual Dysfunctioning in Infants: Identification, Diagnosis and Current Research. Los Angeles, University of Southern California, School of Medicine, Postgraduate Division, 1974

Fisch L (ed): Research in Deafness in Children. Oxford, Blackwell, 1964.

Fraser GR: Genetic approaches to the nosology of deafness, in Bergsma D (ed): The Clinical Delineation of Birth Defects: Part IX, Ear. Baltimore, Williams and Wilkins for the National Foundation March of Dimes, 1971

Jaffe BF: Pinna anomalies associated with congenital conductive hearing loss. Pediatrics 57:332–341, 1976

Myers EN, Stool S: Cytomegalic inclusion disease of the inner ear. Laryngoscope 78:1904–1915, 1968

Nance WE, Setleff R, McLeod A, et al: X-linked mixed deafness with congenital fixation of the stapedial footplate and perilymphatic gusher, in Bergsma D (ed): The Clinical Delineation of Birth Defects: Part IX, Ear. Baltimore, Williams and Wilkins for the National Foundation March of Dimes, 1971

Newman MH Jr: Hearing loss, in Strome M (ed): Differential Diagnosis in Pediatric Otolaryngology. Boston, Little, Brown, 1975

Stewart J: HRS screening. Paper presented to Western Society for Pediatric Research, Carmel, 1974

Joseph R. DiBartolomeo and
Sanford E. Gerber

2
Pathology of Hearing Loss

With the creation of Eve, the auditory organ of human beings was given a new and significant role. In primitive animals, the organ of hearing serves a basic protective function and aids in the localization of sound; but for man, there is a need to communicate his thoughts and desires, which can be accomplished effectively only through the use of language. This eternal need is best satisfied through the special sense of hearing. So strong is this desire of man to communicate that to deny him the auditory tools to help express his thoughts in terms of previous experiences is to afflict him with a most severe handicap. The intellect of man may not have reached its level of sophistication today were it not for the ability to relate previous auditory experiences to our present world of sound.

The miniature organ through which this complex information is processed lies within the temporal bone and the corridor through which the sound passes to stimulate this mechanism is the external auditory canal. Hippocrates (about 400 B.C.) was the first to inspect the tympanic membrane and recognize its significance as part of the organ of hearing. His records were the first to describe infections of the middle ear. Later, Aristotle (384–322 B.C.) suspected that the cochlea was the inner ear counterpart of the outer ear structure. The auditory–vestibular apparatus is the first organ of special sense to be completed during intra-uterine life. By the 26th week of pregnancy, the presence of a functioning auditory system can be demonstrated (Johansson, Wedenberg, and Westin, 1964). A normal child develops auditory orienting reflexes by the age of 3 or 4 months (Chap. 5). Usually, before a child is 7 or 8 months of age, he becomes sensitive to sound even at quiet levels and responds appropriately to such sounds. He learns to differentiate and recognize sounds and then to react to new auditory experiences in terms of memory and previous exposure. The ability to develop speech is most active during infancy, but is completely dependent on a functional auditory system for its source of stimulation.

The most difficult task any child has to learn is to express his thoughts in the form of speech. Unfortunately, for many centuries, individuals afflicted with congenital profound hearing loss were considered mentally retarded because of their failure to develop normal communicative faculties. Later, children suffering from deafness were recognized as intelligent, but were foolishly called deaf-mutes because it was falsely believed that there was a defective speech system as well as auditory apparatus. If a bilateral hearing loss develops during the prelingual years (at birth or in early infancy) the facility for speech will fail to develop well, and such individuals will be unable to achieve effective speech communication unless subjected to intense supportive educational procedures. Yet, severe hearing loss is not associated with intellectual deficit when alternative modes of communication are made available (Chaps. 12 and 13). The congenitally deaf child who tends to be very active and responsive during the early months of postpartum life does not show the characterologic deviation regularly observed in the environmentally deprived, and very frequently observed in the congenitally blind.

Despite our efforts to determine an auditory handicap at the earliest possible stage, there is great room for improvement. Throughout the world, approximately 1 infant in 900 is deaf (Stewart, 1974). In areas of general poor nutrition and medical care there is an increase of deaf males compared to females (Fraser, 1971).

Hearing loss today remains the most common physical disability in the United States—affecting more Americans than heart disease, cancer, blindness, tuberculosis, venereal disease, multiple sclerosis, and kidney disease put together. According to the U.S. Public Health Survey, there are approximately 236,000 deaf individuals of all ages and both sexes in the United States today. Among school aged children, there are approximately 38,000 in schools for the deaf, about 100,000 more requiring intensive special management, and circa 250,000 more who are aurally handicapped to an important degree in the regular school environment. In the U.S. and other parts of the world for which we have figures, between 3½ and 5% of school-aged children have a hearing loss. Over eight million of the American population today suffer a partial hearing impairment of handicapping degree. Six million of these Americans have involvement in both ears. Moreover, 700,000 persons suffer a combination of at least some degree of auditory deficit and some degree of visual handicap (Silverman, 1973). In the older age group, hearing handicaps become complicated by the development of visual disabilities.

CLASSIFICATION OF HEARING LOSS

Hearing loss may vary from mild to profound or even total. An individual with profound hearing loss may have an impairment from 81 to 100 dB or more. Such a patient would lack appreciation of sound within the intensity ranges usually associated with communication. This means at least an 80-dB increase compared with normal threshold over the range 500–8000 Hz. Anacusis or deafness is the total inability to hear sound which results in inability to develop speech through the use of the sense of hearing alone either unaided or aided. A hearing loss is congenital when the patient is born with it (Chap. 1). This condition develops in the uterus and may be the result of either hereditary or environmental factors. Congenital refers to the time of the appearance of the defect and not the mechanism by which the defect occurred. Adventitious hearing loss is that which develops after birth as a result of hereditary, environmental, or traumatic factors; hence, prelingual deafness is that hearing loss which occurs before the development of speech. Hereditary deafness is the result of inherited or genetic characteristics, that is, dominant or recessive genes. Environmental factors and trauma may be responsible for acquired (nongenetic) hearing loss. Familial hearing loss is that which appears in several members of the family but apparently is not hereditary; for example, it may be the result of blood incompatibility or endocrine system abnormality.

Our investigation of hearing loss is based on a clinical approach. We consider the age at which the handicap develops, the type of hearing loss involved, and other signs or symptoms that may be associated with the suspected hearing loss. We present a general classification based on whether the hearing loss appears at birth (congenital)—as a result of either hereditary (genetic) or environmental and traumatic influences (acquired)—or is delayed hearing loss, which occurs as early as the prelingual years (postnatal and infancy) or later in life, and may reflect either a genetic defect or an environmental insult which is responsible for such a handicap

Embryology

The human ear assumes its recognizable shape during the second month of intra-uterine life and has reached full development by the end of the sixth month. To prevent development of this special sense organ, a noxious or genetic influence must operate during the first 2 or 3 weeks of intra-uterine life. To arrest or interrupt embryologic development of the ear, factors must exert their influence between the fourth week, when the otic vesicle begins to show signs of cochlear and vestibular shape, and the end of the sixth month when the cochlear and acoustic sense organs have reached full development and are capable of function. The fully formed cochlear–vestibular structure may undergo degeneration caused by the action of noxious influences at any time between the second month of pregnancy and birth, and even the immediate postnatal period. The acoustic sensory epithelium and its associated structures must be specifically sensitive to such influences during the period of rapid development in the second and third and the beginning of the fourth month. Deafness can result from an initial failure of the development of the complex ear structures, a sudden change or arrest in the maturation of these structures, or a decrease in the function of these structures through degeneration (Ormerod, 1960).

Nosology

A nosology is a system of classification of diseases. A deafness nosology may be constructed in various ways. For example, a most familiar one classifies deafness by site of pathology as conductive, cochlear, or retrocochlear. Another may classify deafness according to time of onset as prenatal or postnatal, congenital or acquired, genetic or nongenetic. Yet another nosology may employ etiologic categories as shown in the previous chapter: infection, trauma, maldevelopment, intoxication, and genetic.

For diagnostic purposes, however, the nosology described by Konigsmark (1971) is very useful. He was concerned with extra-aural pathology as cues to the presence of deafness; hence, his nosology classifies deafness with associated handicaps. These include nervous system disorders, eye diseases, skeletal anomalies, integumentary system disorders, and several others. Konigsmark's nosology is so useful, in fact, and is such a thorough guide to the forms of deafness, that it is included here in its entirety (Tables 2-1–2-8). For the extensive supporting bibliography employed by Konigsmark, the reader is referred to his original paper. But notice also the quantitative information in the tables about the incidence of these disorders and the commentary on them.

CONGENITAL DEAFNESS

Profound hearing loss that is present at birth is congenital, whether it be the result of hereditary (genetically) determined factors or adverse environmental (acquired) influences that occur in the prenatal or perinatal period. Such a hearing loss seems to be a fairly common disease entity, possibly occurring in one in 2000 births. Of all cases of congenital deafness, including deafness associated with rubella, birth injury, and erythroblastosis fetalis, about one-half seem to be due to hereditary factors. Except in the rare case of conductive malformation combined with a sensory-neural hearing loss, treatment today is limited to diagnosis and educative habilitation rather than medical or surgical intervention.

Congenital deafness occurs as a result of pathology during prenatal development, which may result from a failure to develop: (1) the bony cochlea, (2) the membranous cochlea, (3) the organ of Corti and the tectorial membrane, or (4) the sound conducting mechanisms, middle ear and ossicles, and external auditory meatus. Such types of abnormalities are the result of inherited factors or might be due to toxic influences caused by certain forms of maternal illness during the first 3 weeks of pregnancy. Later, during pregnancy, the deafness might result from interruption in the development of: (1) the organ of Corti and tectorial membrane, (2) the ossicles of the middle ear, or (3) the external ear canal. These types of abnormality, the result of inherited factors or toxic influences during pregnancy, may also be due to endocrine insufficiency. According to Kroger and Freed (1956), the fetal and maternal systems are complementary, so that disturbances of a mother's biochemistry may be transferred to the fetal vascular system. Certainly those substances that cross the placental barrier (e.g., insulin) could affect fetal development. These changes may occur in any stage of development of the cochlear–vestibular apparatus. They are engendered by traumatic or toxic influences due to maternal injury, illness, or other abnormalities during this period. The defects in development that are enumerated and which are due to inherited factors or to the noxious influence of bacteria, viruses, toxemia, or other trauma are responsible for the majority of examples of congenital deafness.

The acquired causes of profound hearing loss in fetal life or in early childhood in which pathology has been demonstrated may also be the result of infection or drugs. Ototoxic drugs have caused a degeneration of the hair cells, the organ of Corti, and the peripheral cochlear neuron with preservation of the volume of the cochlear duct, saccule, the stria vascularis, and the tectorial membrane. Deafness due to known viral infection, maternal rubella, mumps, and measles occurring apparently as a complication of a viremia, have been associated with inflammatory and degenerative changes limited primarily to the endolymphatic system. Involvement may be limited to the cochlea, the pars superior, the pars inferior, or both.

Congenital malformations may present as anatomic abnormalities of the inner, middle, or outer ear. Since the embryologic development of the inner ear is different from that of the middle or external ear, the hearing deficit may occur as sensory–neural, conductive, or mixed. Congenital deafness implies aplasia or dysgenesis of the organ of Corti and related structures. Because of

Table 2-1.
Hereditary Deafness with No Associated Abnormalities

Type	No. of Cases	Transmission	Hearing Loss: *Onset*	Hearing Loss: *Progression*	Hearing Loss: *Severity*	Hearing Loss: *Type*	Vestibular Findings	Other Features
Dominant congenital severe deafness	Many	Dominant	Congenital	—	Severe	Neural	Normal	
Dominant progressive nerve deafness	100±	Dominant	Childhood	Slow	Mild to severe	Neural	Normal	Hearing loss includes high frequencies first, then all frequencies.
Dominant unilateral deafness	40±	Dominant	Congenital	—	Severe	Neural	Normal	Hearing loss usually unilateral, occasionally bilateral.
Dominant low frequency hearing loss	40±	Dominant	Childhood	Slow	Mild to severe	Neural	Normal	Low frequencies involved first, progressing to all frequencies.
Dominant mid-frequency hearing loss	60±	Dominant	Childhood	Slow	Mild to severe	Neural	Normal	Hearing loss generally begins in midfrequencies, progression to all frequencies.

Ostosclerosis	Many	Dominant	Adult	Slow	Mild to moderate	Conductive	Normal	
Recessive congenital severe deafness	Many	Recessive	Congenital	—	Severe	Neural	Normal	There are several genotypes.
Recessive early onset neural deafness	16	Recessive	Infant or childhood	Rapid	Severe	Neural	Normal	
Recessive congenital moderate hearing loss	6	Recessive	Congenital	None	Moderate	Neural	Normal	No progression of hearing loss has been found.
Sex-linked congenital deafness	40±	Sex-linked	Congenital	—	Severe	Neural	Normal	
Sex-linked early onset deafness	11	Sex-linked	Congenital	Rapid	Moderate to severe	Neural	Normal	
Sex-linked moderate hearing loss	5	Sex-linked	Childhood	Slow	Mild to moderate	Neural	Normal	Hearing loss involved the high frequencies.

From Konigsmark, BW: in Bergsma, D (ed): The Clinical Delineation of Birth Defects: Part IX, Ear. Baltimore, Williams and Wilkins for the National Foundation March of Dimes, 1971.

Table 2-2.
Hereditary Deafness with External Ear Malformations

Type	No. of Cases	Transmission	Hearing Loss: *Onset*	*Progression*	*Severity*	*Type*	Vestibular Findings	Other Features
Dominant preauricular pits and neural hearing loss	21	Dominant	First or second decade	Slow	Mild to severe	Neural	?	Hearing loss in about 90%. Uni- or bilateral preauricular pits in about 85%. Uni- or bilateral branchial fistula in about 20%.
Dominant thickened ears and incudostapedial joint abnormality	13	Dominant	Congenital	–	Moderate	Conductive	?	Hearing loss due to malformation of the incudostapedial joint. Hypertrophic ear lobes.
Dominant ear malformation and conductive hearing loss	24	Dominant	Congenital	–	Mild to moderate	Conductive	?	Hearing loss in about 80%. Uni- or bilateral preauricular pits in 60%. Uni- or bilateral deformed auricles in 60%.
Dominant faciocervical abnormalities	5	Dominant	Congenital	–	Moderate	Conductive	?	Hypoplasia of maxillo-zygomatic complex. Preauricular pits and fistulae. Hypoplasia of cervical muscles.
Recessive malformed low-set ears and conductive hearing loss	6	Recessive	Congenital	–	Mild to severe	Conductive	Normal	Uni- or bilateral malformed ears. Low-set ears in about half.

From Konigsmark, BW: in Bergsma, D (ed): The Clinical Delineation of Birth Defects: Part IX, Ear. Baltimore, Williams and Wilkins for the National Foundation March of Dimes, 1971.

Table 2-3.
Hereditary Deafness with Integumentary System Disease

Type	No. of Cases	Transmission	Hearing Loss				Vestibular Findings	Other Features
			Onset	*Progression*	*Severity*	*Type*		
Waardenburg's disease	About 2% of congenital deaf	Dominant	Congenital	None	Mild to severe	Neural	Abnormal	Lateral displacement of medial canthi. Broad high nasal root (75%). Hyperplasia of medial brows (50%). Heterochromia iridium (25%). Hearing loss (25%). White forelock (20%). Skin pigmentary change (10%).
Dominant albinism and congenital deafness	14	Dominant	Congenital	–	Severe	Neural	?	Albinism except for optic fundi and irides. Scanty eyebrows.
Leopard syndrome	10	Dominant	Congenital	None	Moderate to severe	Neural	Normal	Variable EKG abnormalities, hypertelorism, pulmonary stenosis, and growth retardation.
Hereditary piebaldness and congenital deafness	2	Recessive	Congenital	–	Severe	Neural	Normal	Depigmentation of head and arms containing hyperpigmented spots.

Table 2-3 — *Continued*

Type	No. of Cases	Transmission	Hearing Loss: *Onset*	*Progression*	*Severity*	*Type*	Vestibular Findings	Other Features
Sex-linked pigmentary abnormalities and congenital deafness	14	Sex-linked	Congenital	—	Severe	Neural	Abnormal	Spots of hypo- and hyperpigmentation over body.
Recessive atopic dermatitis and neural hearing loss	3	Recessive	Congenital	None	Moderate	Neural	Normal	Atypical atopic dermatitis, onset about 10 years of age.
Dominant anhidrosis and progressive hearing loss	14	Dominant	Adult	Slow	Mild to moderate	Neural	?	Congenital anhidrosis.
Dominant keratopachydermia, digital constrictions, and deafness	5	Dominant	Congenital	—	Severe	Neural	?	Hyperkeratosis of palms, soles, elbows, and knees. Soft tissue constrictions of fingers and toes.

Recessive pili torti and hearing loss	10	Recessive	Congenital	—	Moderate to severe	Neural	?	Congenital pili torti.
Dominant knuckle pads, leukonychia, and hearing loss	22	Dominant	Congenital	Slow	Moderate to severe	Neural or mixed	Abnormal (75%)	Congenital leukonychia. Childhood onset of knuckle pads. Disorganized middle ear bones.
Dominant onychodystrophy, coniform teeth, and hearing loss	5	Dominant	Congenital	None	Moderate to severe	Neural	?	Small coniform teeth with partial anodontia. Elevated sweat electrolyte concentration.
Recessive onychodystrophy and deafness	2	Recessive	Congenital	None	Severe	Neural	Hypoactive	Congenital onychodystophy.

From Konigsmark, BW: in Bergsma, D (ed): The Clinical Delineation of Birth Defects: Part IX, Ear. Baltimore, Williams and Wilkins for the National Foundation March of Dimes, 1971.

Table 2-4.
Hereditary Deafness Associated with Eye Disease

Type	No. of Cases	Transmission	Hearing Loss				Vestibular Findings	Other Features
			Onset	*Progression*	*Severity*	*Type*		
Dominant saddle nose, myopia, cataracts, and hearing loss	7	Dominant	Childhood	Slow	Moderate	Neural	?	Saddle nose defect. Severe myopia. Congenital and juvenile cataracts.
Dominant myopia, hearing loss, peripheral neuropathy, and skeletal abnormalities	15	Dominant	First or second decade	Slow to moderate	Moderate to severe	Neural	?	Eye defects including myopia, cataracts, retinitis pigmentosa. Peripheral neuropathy with shooting pains, weakness. Kyphoscoliosis, osteoporosis.
Recessive myopia and hearing loss	7	Recessive	Congenital	Nonprogression	Moderate to severe	Neural	None	Severe myopia. Mild intellectual impairment in some.

Recessive retinitis pigmentosa and congenital deafness (Usher's disease)	Many	Recessive	Congenital	–	Moderate or severe	Neural	Normal	Progressive visual loss with retinitis pigmentosa.
Recessive congenital deafness, ataxia, and retinitis pigmentosa (Hallgren's disease)	150	Recessive	Congenital	–	Severe	Neural	Abnormal	Vestibular ataxia. Mental deficiency and psychosis in some.
Heredopathia atactica, polyneuritiformis (Refsum's disease)	40	Recessive	First or second decade	Slow	Mild to severe	Neural	Normal	Progressive atypical retinitis pigmentosa. Hypertrophic peripheral neuropathy. Mild cerebellar ataxia and nystagmus. Increased plasma phytamic acid.
Recessive retinal degeneration, diabetes, obesity, and hearing loss (Alstrom's disease)	10	Recessive	Second decade	Slow	Moderate	Neural	?	Early onset of retinitis pigmentosa. Childhood onset of diabetes mellitus. Moderate obesity. Cataract.

Table 2-4 – *Continued*

Type	No. of Cases	Transmission	Hearing Loss				Vestibular Findings	Other Features
			Onset	*Progression*	*Severity*	*Type*		
Recessive retinitis pigmentosa, spastic diplegia, skeletal abnormalities, and hearing loss	2	Recessive	Congenital	–	Moderate to severe	–	–	Onset in infancy of spastic paraplegia. Atypical retinitis pigmentosa. Microcephaly. Brachydactyly.
Recessive retinal changes, deafness, muscular wasting, and mental retardation	4	Recessive	Childhood	?	Moderate	?	?	Retinal detachment and telangiectasias. Muscle wasting in face, limb, trunks. Marked intellectual defect.
Recessive optic atrophy, hearing loss, and juvenile diabetes	12	Recessive	Childhood	Slow	Moderate	Neural	Hypoactive	Childhood onset of progressive visual loss due to optic atrophy. Early onset of diabetes mellitus.

Familial hearing loss, polyneuropathy, and optic atrophy	3	Recessive or sex-linked	Infancy	Moderately rapid	Severe	Neural	?	Childhood onset of progressive peripheral neuropathy. Second decade onset of optic atrophy and visual loss.
Optico-cochleodentate degeneration	9	Recessive	Childhood	Slow	Moderate to severe	Neural	?	Early onset of progressive spastic quadriparesis, optic atrophy, and dementia.
Dominant corneal dystrophy and hearing loss	13	Dominant	Adult	Slow	Moderate		?	Late onset of variable ribbon-like corneal degeneration. Abnormal calcium metabolism.

From Konigsmark, BW: in Bergsma, D (ed): The Clinical Delineation of Birth Defects: Part IX, Ear. Baltimore, Williams and Wilkins for the National Foundation March of Dimes, 1971.

Table 2-5.
Hereditary Deafness Associated with Nervous System Disease

Type	No. of Cases	Transmission	Hearing Loss				Vestibular Findings	Other Features
			Onset	*Progression*	*Severity*	*Type*		
Dominant acoustic neurinomas	52	Dominant	Second or third decade	Slow	Moderate to severe	Neural	Hypoactive	Bilateral acoustic neurinomas develop.
Sensory radicular neuropathy	14	Dominant	Second or third decade	Moderate	Moderate to severe	Neural	?	Dorsal root ganglion involvement with shooting pains and sensory loss.
Dominant photomyoclonus, hearing loss, diabetes, and nephropathy	13	Dominant	Third decade	Moderate	Moderate	Neural	?	In cerebral and cerebellar cortex is neuronal loss and gliosis.
Recessive deafness, mental deficiency, ataxia, and hypogonadism (Richards-Rundle Disease)	5	Recessive	Infancy	Rapid	Moderate to severe	Neural	?	Onset in childhood of truncal ataxia, muscle wasting. Decreased estrogen and 17 ketosteroids.

Hurler's disease mucopolysaccharidosis type I	Many	Recessive	Infancy	Moderate	Mild to moderate	Neural	?	Progressive mental deterioration, bony deformities, corneal opacity.
Hunter's disease (MPS II)	Many	Sex-linked	Childhood	Slow	Mild to moderate	Neural	?	Slow mental retardation, dwarfing. Hepatosplenomegaly.
Sanfilippo disease (MPS III)	Many	Recessive	Childhood	Slow	Mild to moderate		?	Moderate mental deterioration. Bone deformities.
Scheie's disease (MPS V)	Few	Recessive	Adult	Slow	Mild to moderate	Neural	?	Normal intellect. Corneal opacities, mild bone changes.
Maroteaux-Lamy disease (MPS VI)	Few	Recessive	Childhood	Slow	Mild to moderate	Neural	Hypoactive	Normal intellect, moderate bone changes, marked corneal clouding.

From Konigsmark, BW: in Bergsma, D (ed): The Clinical Delineation of Birth Defects: Part IX, Ear. Baltimore, Williams and Wilkins for the National Foundation March of Dimes, 1971.

Table 2-6.
Hereditary Deafness Associated with Skeletal Disease

Type	No. of Cases	Transmission	Hearing Loss: *Onset*	Hearing Loss: *Progression*	Hearing Loss: *Severity*	Hearing Loss: *Type*	Vestibular Findings	Other Features
Dominant proximal symphalangism and hearing loss	360±	Dominant	Congenital	None	Mild to moderate	Conductive	?	Symphalangism more marked in lateral digits.
Cranio-facial dysostosis (Crouzon's disease)	Many	Dominant	Congenital	None	Mild to moderate	Mixed	?	Exophthalmos, hypoplastic mandible, craniostenosis, parrot beaked nose, external canal atresia.
Mandibulofacial dysostosis (Treacher-Collins disease)	Many	Dominant	Congenital	None	Moderate to severe	Conductive	?	Antimongoloid palpebral fissures, molar and mandibular hypoplasia, malformed ossicles.
Oral-facial digital II (Mohr syndrome)	7	Recessive	Congenital	None	Moderate	Conductive	?	Facial deformities. Digit abnormalities. Lobulated tongue.

Oto-palatal-digital syndrome	3	Recessive	Congenital	None	Mild to moderate	Conductive	?	Broad nasal root, hypertelorism, frontal bossing, mild dwarfism. Hands and feet: widely spaced and shortened first digits.
Recessive absence of tibia and deafness	4	Recessive	Congenital	—	Severe	?	?	Congenital absence of one or both tibias and malformed fibulas.
Recessive split-hand and foot syndrome	2	Recessive	Congenital	None	Moderate to severe	Neural	Hypoactive	Absent phalanges and syndactyly.
Progressive diaphyseal dysplasia (Englemann's disease)	50	Recessive	Second decade	Mild	Moderate	Neural	?	Thickening of diaphyseal cortex of limb bones. Occasional skull thickening and cranial nerve palsies.

From Konigsmark, BW: in Bergsma, D (ed): The Clinical Delineation of Birth Defects: Part IX, Ear. Baltimore, Williams and Wilkins for the National Foundation March of Dimes, 1971.

Table 2-6—*Continued*

Type	No. of Cases	Transmission	Hearing Loss				Vestibular Findings	Other Features
			Onset	*Progression*	*Severity*	*Type*		
Pagets disease of bones (osteitis deformans)	Many	Dominant	Adult	Slow	Mild to moderate	Neural	?	Skull involvement with narrowing of cranial nerve foramina and inner ear involvement.
Hyperostosis corticalis generalisata (van Buchem's disease)	8	Recessive	Adult	Slow	Mild to moderate	Neural	?	Osteosclerotic overgrowth of skeleton.
Osteopetrosis	Many	Recessive	Childhood	Slow	Mild to moderate	Mixed	?	Sclerotic, brittle bones, and anemia.
Craniometaphyseal dysplasia (Pyle's disease)	Many	Dominant	Childhood	Slow	Mild to moderate	Mixed	?	Metaphyseal dysplasia of long bones and skull.
Osteogenesis imperfecta (van der Hoeve's disease)	Many	Dominant	Third decade	Slow	Mild to moderate	Conductive	?	Frequent fractures. Blue sclerae.

From Konigsmark, BW: in Bergsma, D (ed): The Clinical Delineation of Birth Defects: Part IX, Ear. Baltimore, Williams and Wilkins for the National Foundation March of Dimes, 1971.

Table 2-7.
Hereditary Deafness with Renal Disease

Type	No. of Cases	Transmission	Hearing Loss: *Onset*	*Progression*	*Severity*	*Type*	Vestibular Findings	Other Features
Alport's disease	Many	Dominant	Second decade	Slow	Mild to moderate	Neural	Normal	Nephritis begins usually in 1st decade. Ocular lens abnormalities in some.
Dominant nephritis, ichthyosis, hearing loss and prolinuria	23	Dominant	Childhood	Slow	Mild to moderate	Neural	?	Variable degrees of nephritis, renal cysts, and ichthyosis.
Dominant urticaria, amyloidosis, nephritis, and hearing loss	9	Dominant	Second decade	Slow	Mild to moderate	Neural	?	Recurrent urticaria, amyloidosis with nephropathy and uremia.
Recessive renal, genital, and middle ear anomalies	4	Recessive	Congenital	—	Severe	Conductive	?	Uni- or bilateral renal agenesis; vaginal atresia, malformed incus.
Recessive renal acidosis and progressive hearing loss	2	Recessive	Second decade	Slow	Moderate	Neural	Normal	Childhood onset of progressive renal disease with calculi, acidosis.

From Konigsmark, BW: in Bergsma, D (ed): The Clinical Delineation of Birth Defects: Part IX, Ear. Baltimore, Williams and Wilkins for the National Foundation March of Dimes, 1971.

Table 2-8.
Hereditary Deafness with Other Abnormalities

Type	No. of Cases	Transmission	Hearing Loss				Vestibular Findings	Other Features
			Onset	*Progression*	*Severity*	*Type*		
Pendred's disease	Many	Recessive	Congenital	—	Moderate to severe	Neural	Depressed	Goiter develops in adolescence.
Recessive goiter, increased PBI stippled epiphyses, and deafness	2	Recessive	Congenital	—	Moderate to severe	Neural	?	Stippled epiphyses, goiter with high PBI.
Recessive heart disease and deafness	14	Recessive	Congenital	—	Severe	Neural	?	Prolonged QT intervals, recurrent Stokes-Adams attacks with sudden death.
Dominant mitral insufficiency, joint fusion, and hearing loss	3	Dominant	Congenital	—	Moderate to severe	Conductive	?	Fusion of cervical vertebrae, carpal, and tarsal bones. Mitral insufficiency.

From Konigsmark, BW: in Bergsma, D (ed): The Clinical Delineation of Birth Defects: Part IX, Ear. Baltimore, Williams and Wilkins for the National Foundation March of Dimes, 1971.

this, such deafness should not be progressive. Delayed deafness relates to the degenerative changes of the sense organ after its complete development and may be progressive.

The classical anomalies have recently been reviewed by Bergstrom (1976). We normally consider the major categories as the anomalies of Michel, Mondini, and Scheibe. In the case of a Michel anomaly (Fig. 2-1) there is no inner ear and there may also be no acoustic nerve, although the facial nerve is present. This occurs in only about 1% of those who are profoundly deaf. The Mondini anomaly (Fig. 2-2) is rather variable, according to Bergstrom, but generally one finds dysplasia and hypoplasia of the cochlear duct and its contents. In fact, Wright (1971) quoted Mondini himself (1791) as reporting normal semicircular canals, but with only the first 1½ coils of the cochlea being normal. The vast majority of congenital hearing losses (according to Bergstrom, about 70%) are of the Scheibe type. Scheibe anomalies may be genetic or may be the result of prenatal intoxication (Chap. 1). In general, the Scheibe malformation is characterized by an intact bony labyrinth but with collapse of the saccule, and atrophy of the stria vascularis

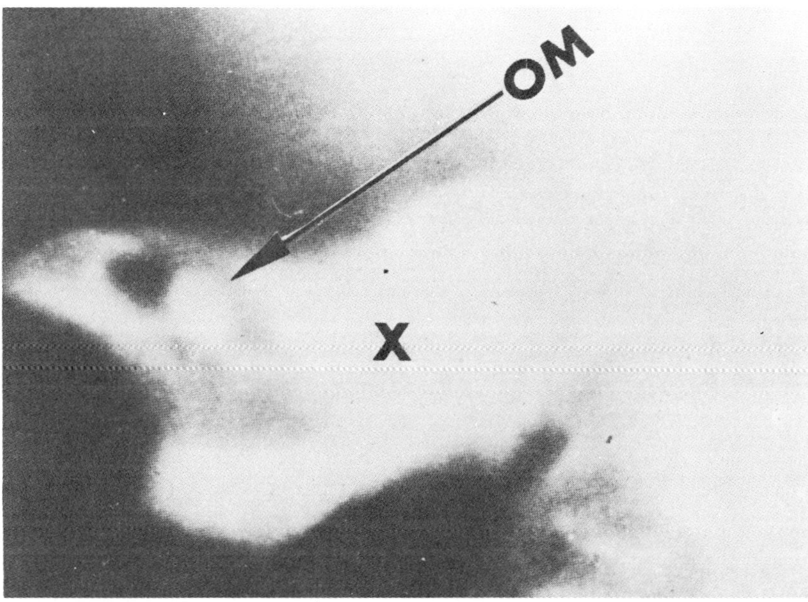

Fig. 2-1. Michel anomaly. Petrous pyramid polytomogram, right ear. Michel deformity of inner ear. OM is ossicular mass. Solid radiopaque area marked with an X is that of underveloped inner ear. (From FO Black et al: Congenital Deafness. Colorado Associated Univ Press, 1971.)

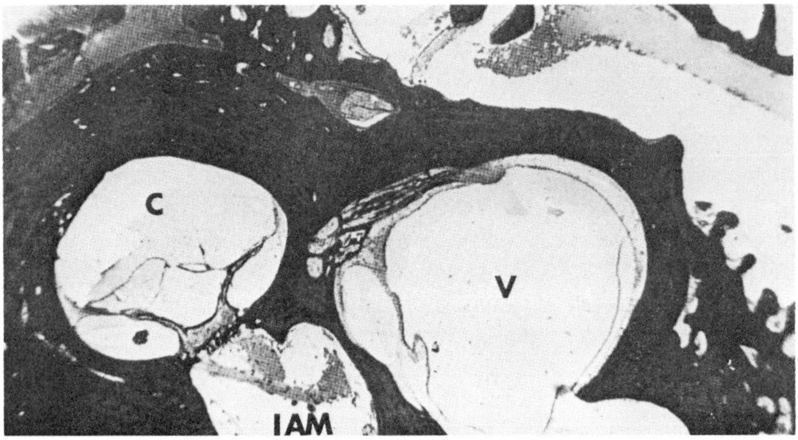

Fig. 2-2. Mondini anomaly. Histopathologic section of inner ear showing Mondini-type deformity. C is rudimentary cochlea. The internal auditory meatus (IAM) contains normal appearing cochlear, vestibular and facial nerves. The vestibule (V) contains a large, deformed utricle. (From Schuknecht H: in F McConnell and PH Ward, (eds): Deafness in Childhood. Vanderbilt Univ Pr, 1967.)

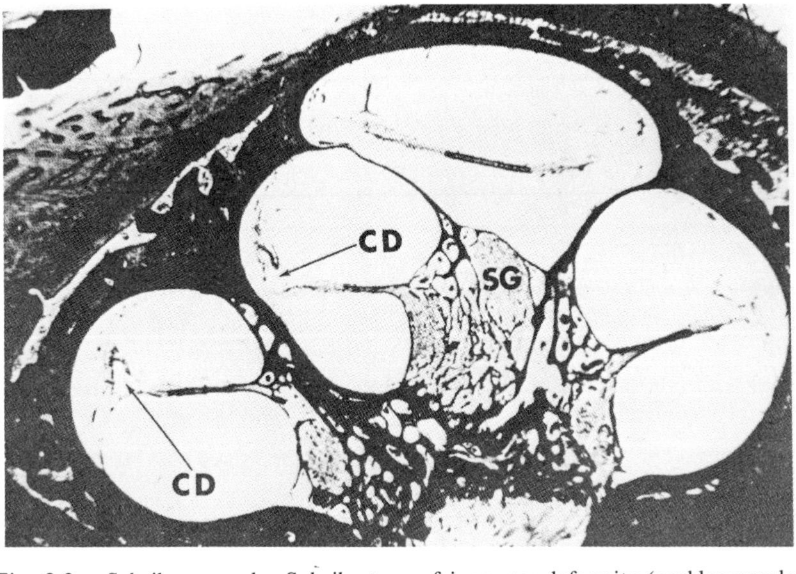

Fig. 2-3. Scheibe anomaly. Scheibe type of inner ear deformity (cochleosaccular aplasia). Note the poorly developed cochlear duct (CD) and the normal spiral ganglion (SG). The abnormal saccule is not shown. (From Schuknecht H: in F McConnell and PH Ward (eds): Deafness in Childhood, Vanderbilt University Press, 1967.)

and organ of Corti. An example of a Scheibe type anomaly is shown in Fig. 2-3. Bergstrom also refers to the rather poorly understood Alexander anomaly and the peculiar Bing-Siebenmann anomaly.

DELAYED HEARING LOSS

In the neonatal period, or any time after birth, hereditary or environmental factors may cause degeneration in part of the auditory apparatus that may have already developed to some degree or even reached complete maturity. This degeneration may affect: (1) the canal of the cochlea or scala media, (2) the sensory end organ including the tectorial membrane, or (3) the nerve elements, including the spiral ganglion and the basal nuclei.

In delayed hearing loss, genetic factors are much less common, except for early onset neural deafness. Environmental factors such as trauma, infection, and our increasing problem with noise, become of major significance. The degenerative changes associated with aging become obvious as our longevity increases.

GENETIC REVIEW

Approximately 50% of profound childhood hearing loss is hereditary or genetic in origin. Genetic hearing loss may be dominant, recessive, or X-linked (Chap. 1). The messengers which carry our hereditary characteristics are the chromosomes. In the human somatic or body cells, there are 23 pairs of chromosomes. Twenty-two of these pairs are called autosomes because they are equally represented in both sexes, and the members of each pair are morphologically indistinguishable. The twenty-third pair of chromosomes, called a sex chromosome, is different from the other pairs. The members of this pair, called the X and the Y, have different morphology. The X chromosome is morphologically similar to some of the autosomes and is the site of many known genes. The Y chromosome appears in each gamete. So far, the only human chromosome demonstrated to have a series of linked genes is the X chromosome. We now realize that there is more than one type of recessive deafness, and geneticists now believe that there are at least ten gene loci contributing to the condition. According to Nance and Sweeney (1975), in the families of congenitally deaf children about 90% have no history of deafness at all, and yet an estimated 35% of the children have inherited it. Physicians may be unaware of the pattern of their patients' families because 86–90% of these cases are of a recessive type of genetic deafness. Hereditary deafness is usually a bilateral disease entity. In unilateral deafness, hereditary factors are important in only 10% of cases. A great majority of human inherited deafness (90%) is of a recessive nature, and appears as deafness without other handicaps.

Dominant nerve deafness is frequently associated with a large number of syndromes. Given a deaf child with normal parents with no positive family history of deafness, in 65% of such cases that child's hearing loss etiology is environmental while the remaining 35% are recessively inherited. Many people have erroneous ideas about hereditary defects. In the case of dominant inherited deafness, it is impossible for the normal children of deaf parents to transmit it to their offspring. In the case of a recessively inherited deafness, it is necessary to have both parents as carriers of the particular gene, in which event the chance of offspring being affected is only 25%. Most of these cases, therefore, have no family history of deafness, making diagnosis of a hereditary condition very difficult. They are often erroneously termed congenital, sporadic recessive deafness. Usually, in consanguineous matings, the hereditary transmission of these recessive disorders becomes apparent. It is estimated by Proctor and Proctor (1967) that 7% of recessive deafness cases were offspring of consanguineous marriages. Similar results have been reported by Feinmesser and Tell (1976).

Despite a detailed family history looking for such factors as consanguinity, genetic dominance, and X-linked inheritance, 60–70% of the genetic cases are still unidentifiable (Nance et al., 1971). The causes of congenital malformations and disorders are manifold. A specific type of abnormality may be attributed to a variety of etiologic factors, both hereditary and nonhereditary. The same causal agent may be responsible for single or multiple defects, as observed in the sequelae to rubella in pregnancy. Similarly, it is possible for isolated or combined malformations to be transmitted to different members of the same family, as in cleft lip or palate.

REFERENCES

Bergstrom L: Congenital deafness, in Northern JL (ed): Hearing Disorders, Boston, Little, Brown, 1976

Feinmesser M, Tell L, Neonatal screening for detection of deafness. Archives of Otolaryngol 102:297–299, 1976

Fraser GR: Genetic approaches to the nosology of deafness, in Bergsma D (ed): The Clinical Delineation of Birth Defects: Part IX, Ear. Baltimore, Williams and Wilkins for the National Foundation/March of Dimes, 1971

Johannsson B, Wedenberg E, Westin B: Measurement of tone responses by the human foetus. Acta Otolaryngol (Stockh) 57:188–192, 1964

Konigsmark BW: Syndromal approaches to the nosology of hereditary deafness, in

Bergsma D (ed): The Clinical Delineation of Birth Defects: Part IX, Ear. Baltimore, Williams and Wilkins, for the National Foundation/March of Dimes, 1971

Kroger WS, Freed SC: Psychosomatic Gynecology. Glencoe, Ill., Free Pr, 1956

Nance WE, Sweeney A: Genetic factors in deafness of early life, in Glassock M (ed) Sensorineural hearing loss in children. Otolaryngol Clin North Am 8:19–48, 1975

Nance WE, Setleff R, McLeod A, et al.: X-linked mixed deafness with congenital fixation of the stapedial footplate and perilymphatic gusher, in Bergsma D (ed): The Clinical Delineation of Birth Defects; Part IX, Ear. Baltimore, Williams and Wilkins for the Natoinal Foundation/March of Dimes, 1971.

Ormerod FC: The pathology of congenital deafness. J Laryngol Otol 74:923–926, 1960

Proctor CA, Proctor B: Understanding hereditary nerve deafness. Arch Otolaryngol 85:23–40, 1967

Silverman SR: Rehabilitative audiology, in Paparella MM, Shumrick DA (eds): Otolaryngology. Philadelphia, Saunders, 1973

Stewart J: HRS screening. Paper presented to the Western Society for Pediatric Research, Carmel, 1974

Wright MJ: The Pathology of Deafness. Manchester, Univ Pr, 1971

Sanford E. Gerber

3
High-Risk Conditions

Deafness is caused. Knowledge of the causes of deafness should enable one to detect severe auditory deficit at birth and thereby to prevent or to ameliorate handicap. The issue, then, is to determine the causes of deafness, and to employ this determination diagnostically in an economic and beneficial manner. That is to say, a high-risk register should contain the smallest number of questions with which to identify the largest number of hearing-impaired infants. Several attempts at producing such registers have been made with varying degrees of success. Certainly one would expect that if a register were very long, such that it contained all known causes of congenital deafness, its success rate ought to be very high, as would its expense. One needs to be willing to accept a certain small number of both false positives and false negatives in order to make a register useful.

In 1973, the Joint Committee on Newborn Hearing recommended a five-item register. Over a period of the last few years the items on that register have been employed in various places, so that we now have fair knowledge of its utility. The substance of this chapter is a consideration of the several high-risk items individually. A proposed modification of the 1973 statement of the Joint Committee on Newborn Hearing says:

> In light of the urgent need to detect hearing impairment as early as possible, a 1970 statement of the Joint Committee urged further investigation of screening methods, but discouraged routine hearing screening unless it is specifically research oriented. In consonance with that statement, and in view of the information that application of high-risk data may increase the detectability of congenital hearing impairment, the committe considered it appropriate to make an additional 1973 state-

ment. Experience with the recommendations of that statement has led to the modifications below.

The Joint Committee on Newborn Hearing recommends that infants at risk for hearing impairment should be identified by history, tested, and followed-up. The criterion for identification of a newborn in the high risk category for hearing impairment is the presence of one or more of the following conditions:

I. Family history of hereditary childhood hearing impairment.
II. Maternal rubella or other transplacental infection (e.g., cytomegalovirus infections, Herpes infections, syphilis).
III. Congenital defects of the ear, nose, or throat. Malformed, low-set, or absent pinnae; cleft lip or palate (including submucous cleft); any residual abnormality of the otorhinolaryngeal system.
IV. Birth weight less than 1500 grams.
V. Any free or indirect serum bilirubin concentration which is judged to be potentially toxic.

Recommendations:

A. All infants falling in the high risk category should be referred for audiologic evaluation during their first two months of life.
B. Even if hearing appears to be normal among those with family histories or history of maternal rubella, they should receive regular audiologic evaluations thereafter. This additional measure is particularly important since hearing impairment in these groups is not necessarily present at birth but may develop at an uncertain time later.
C. All infants at risk for hearing impairment, whether or not they have passed an initial test, should be screened at office or well baby clinic visits using a questionnaire for the parents and an arousal test for the infant. Again, routine follow-up testing is necessary because hearing impairments may appear in this group at some time after birth.

These five items constitute the content of this chapter. Following the discussion of these items is a discussion of studies and clinics using various forms of this register.

HEREDITARY FAMILIAL DEAFNESS

The most common cause of congenital severe hearing impairment is familial. About one-half of the children who are born deaf are so for genetic reasons. Some familial discorders arise from a dominant pattern of inheritance, while others arise from recessive patterns. The single largest category of congenital deafness is dominant inherited severe sensory-neural hearing impairment without associated handicap. Inherited deafness takes many forms, including those which are not congenital; any practicing audiologist or otolaryngologist can report his experience with patients who seem to display presbycusis at an age earlier than that of most people. Clearly this is not a category to be considered here. Additionally, otosclerosis is not to be considered although it too is dominantly inherited (Konigsmark and McKusick, 1966). We are concerned only with those forms of genetic deafness that are present at birth or that appear in infancy or childhood. Therefore, we can speak of congenital genetic deafness and we can also speak of early onset severe sensory-neural impairment (Konigsmark, 1971a).

Some of the dominant forms of inherited congenital deafness are well known and can be identified with relative ease. These would include, for example, Waardenburg's syndrome, which probably is the example most often cited (1951). There are two reasons for it being cited so frequently: one is that it is rather common, and the other is that it exemplifies so many of the features of genetic disorders. The symptoms of Waardenburg's syndrome —alterations of hair pigmentation, heterochromia iridis, characteristic facies, and hearing impairment—appear with varying penetrance. As a consequence, many patients with Waardenburg's syndrome have no hearing loss, some have unilateral hearing losses, and some are severely impaired (Fraser, 1976). In this writer's experience, for example, was one family in which the signs of Waardenburg's syndrome appeared only in the females, although it is not due to a sex-linked gene. In this family the mother had a severe unilateral hearing impairment, while her daughter had a profound bilateral impairment. The mother's aunt similarly had a severe unilateral impairment and was the mother of a child with a profound bilateral impairment. As one familiar with Waardenburg's syndrome would have predicted, these four females looked very much alike. Another family in the writers' experience had had only one instance of hearing loss. All the family members displayed the alteration of hair pigmentation (i.e., a white forelock) and heterochromia iridis. The children examined looked very much like their father, all typical of Waardenburg's syndrome. Of the two little girls, one had normal hearing and the other was profoundly impaired. The father reported that they had known for many years the nature of the disorder in their family and were concerned about the incidence of severe hearing impairment; but, in fact, the hearing loss had appeared in only the one child. The father's hearing has been tested and found to be normal as is that of the younger child. The matter of variable penetrance tends to cloud the topic of dominant inheritance.

A genetic counselor would like to be able to say that since such a disorder is dominant, one can expect the handicap to appear in the descendants, but such is not the case in Waardenburg's syndrome. Such may be the case, however, with dominant hearing losses without associated handicaps or with other dominant impairments that do have associated handicaps. On the other hand, this problem does not arise with recessively inherited deafness. Fraser (1976) reports a case of one parent with Pendred's disease and the other with Usher's disease; their children are normal for hearing, vision, and thyroid function.

The subject of dominant early onset neural deafness is a very difficult one indeed. We are aware of hereditary degenerative hearing losses, but there are no clear data having to do with the time course of the degeneration. Frequently, these children are born with normal or nearly normal hearing. Without a high-risk register, such a child would be likely to pass a hearing screen in the newborn nursery. He then appears at a later age with a severe hearing loss. When did it occur? How long did it take for the hearing to degenerate? The answers to these questions are not known. In our center, a clear case of dominant hereditary degenerative early onset sensory impairment was a fourth child born to a deaf couple who already had three deaf children; a fact that causes the diagnostician to appear to be very wise indeed. Their fourth child was examined at the age of 1 week and appeared to be essentially a normally hearing child. At the age of 1 month her responses were poor, but there was as yet no evidence of severe hearing loss. By the age of 3 months she appeared to be quite severely impaired indeed. By the age of entrance into public school she was found to be the most severely impaired of the four children. While this is an example of the brilliance of hindsight, it is also an example of the point made in favor of using the high-risk register previously mentioned. The essential question is: Is there a history of severe hearing impairment which occurred in childhood in a near relative? This case is a striking instance of exactly such hearing impairment. This family has no associated handicaps, there has been no known history of prenatal disease, nor of any of the other deafness predicting conditions.

Recessive inheritance presents a much more difficult problem. An example from our center is a family where the parents are normally hearing, but they have three severely hearing-impaired children. In the absence of other information (e.g., metabolic disorder) one has to assume a recessive mode of inheritance in such a family. In the instance of autosomal recessive deafness occurring in a first-born child, where the parents have or claim to have no knowledge of a family history of hearing impairment, the high-risk register will fail. If the family denies knowledge of hearing loss, and if the answers to the other questions are all negative, such a child will pass a high-risk screen. This must be one category—probably the major one—which will account for the difference in detection between the use of the high-risk register alone and the use of a high-risk register supplemented by a behavioral screen. We return to this subject later. The fact is that this autosomal recessive inheritance is probably a very common mode. Konigsmark (1971b) predicted that perhaps at least as many as 35% of children who are born deaf would be classified in this category. That is a goodly number indeed, especially considering that many of them are not detectable by a high-risk register. On the other hand, if the family history is known and if deaf siblings already exist, then very careful consideration must be given to the probability of an autosomal recessive mode of inheritance. Certainly it ought to be clear that a normal hearing couple who has already produced two severely hearing-impaired children has an inordinately high probability of producing a third. The incidence of congenital deafness is not a random process.

Some forms of inheritance reflect severe hearing loss with associated handicaps. These are considered in a later section, the one on orofacial anomalies. Some of these are dominantly inherited while some others are recessively inherited.

In a recent report, Stewart (1974) found that about one-third of the hearing-impaired children in her program had a positive family history. This is a reasonably large program: during a period of 26 months, 220 hearing-impaired children were born to families with history of childhood hearing impairment. It must be seen, therefore, that determining family history becomes critical. It is perhaps the most essential of the several questions due to its significantly high incidence. It is important, however, that the person giving the information understands the question. When we ask about history of childhood hearing impairment we must also ask who had it. In the program we conduct at two hospitals[1] in Santa Barbara, this information is acquired by the obstetrics nurse as part of her history-taking procedure. We have found it to work effectively.

RUBELLA OR OTHER TRANSPLACENTAL INFECTIONS

Rubella, popularly called "German measles," is the most well known of the prenatal viral diseases leading to severe congenital hearing impairment and/or other neurosensory impairment. We are very sensitive to the issue of rubella, and tend to forget that our knowledge of the sequelae of prenatal rubella is fairly recent, dating from the 1939–41 epidemic in Australia. Until recently we had become unduly sanguine about prenatal rubella, as we have believed that the rubella vaccine will have solved our problems for us. That isn't true. At the same time, while we continue to want to concentrate on the incidence of prenatal rubella, we do not wish to overlook other prenatal viral

[1]Santa Barbara Cottage Hospital and Goleta Valley Hospital.

diseases. It is for this purpose that the Joint Committee, in its policy statement, cites examples of cytomegalovirus and Herpes infections, and suggests other infections as well.

The rubella virus is a nasty little creature that lives a long time. The last major rubella epidemic in this country was that of 1964–65. In an earlier paper (Gerber, 1969), we reported on nine deaf children who were products of that epidemic in our relatively small community. The major study of the auditory sequelae of that epidemic has been the ongoing program at Johns Hopkins University (Bordley et al., 1967). According to the Johns Hopkins' data, of women who were pregnant at the time of the epidemic and who contracted or were exposed to rubella, nearly half of those births had severe hearing impairment. The other commonly occurring sequelae of prenatal rubella are mental retardation, cataracts, and cardiac defects; some children have all. In addition, it needs to be noted that the long life of the rubella virus often makes it possible to diagnose this as a cause of deafness many months after birth.

At a recent meeting, Mencher (1977) reported a number of deaf infants consequent to prenatal rubella born during a rather short interval. This suggests again that we cannot be sanguine about the once proposed disappearance of prenatal rubella. At the same meeting, there were reports of histopathologic changes of the temporal bone following severe middle ear infection of viral origin in patients who had small pox, chicken pox, or measles (Kapur, 1977).

In the report of Bordley et al. on the first 79 of some projected 300 children, there were 47 who exhibited positive virus cultures. They, too, observed the long life of the rubella virus; in some instances positive cultures were obtained at postpartum ages of 4–6 months and in one child at the age of 15 months. Two of their patients were born to mothers who had contracted rubella prior to conception. Of 48 children who had hearing tests, 31 failed. The failure was defined as no consistent responses at or above 50 dB sound pressure level, using a Ewing method of testing. Of these 31 children, slightly more than half were among the group from whom live virus could be cultured. In addition, it is essential to note the finding that the ability to isolate the virus was not limited to those patients in whom rubella occurred during the first trimester. In fact Bordley et al. reported "that 23 percent of the children born following infection during the second trimester failed their hearing tests." The temporal bones were obtained from one child who died at the age of 31 days. While no assessment of his hearing had been made, they noted that he had failed to show responses to simple sounds. Both temporal bones showed Scheibe-type alterations, although his left ear seemed to be changed less markedly than the right. Two very important conclusions were derived by Bordley et al. One was the strong reminder that children can be severely damaged due to prenatal rubella, which may be present with no clinical symptoms in the mother. The other is to repeat that the effects of this prenatal infection are very severe.

However, rubella is not the only viral disease of concern. The viruses which have been suspected to cause deafness include mumps, measles, chicken pox, influenza, the common cold, and poliomyelitis (Hemenway and Bergstrom, 1967). The frequency of neurosensory sequelae of prenatal forms of these viral diseases is not well established, but probably accounts for substantially less than the incidences of neurosensory sequelae following prenatal rubella. This may be due to the relatively long life of the rubella virus. However, many years ago it was shown that the measles virus does cross the placental barrier, although it is likely to cause spontaneous abortion. On the other hand, development of severe sensory-neural deafness postnatally in infancy is likely to be caused by viral endolabyrinthitis.

Cytomegalovirus presents a confusing picture. While Hemenway and Bergstrom (1967) claimed that the cytomegalovirus has not yet been implicated as a source of cochlear pathology, they did refer to a case reported by Ward et al. (1965) of cytomegalic inclusion in an adult. More recently Dahle et al. (1974) have reported a few cases of apparently progressive cochlear impairment following prenatal cytomegalic inclusion disease. This viral disease constitutes a very difficult problem. For one thing, it is hard to diagnose. For another, its effects on audition are not well known and, if the observations of Dahle et al. are correct, its auditory effects may not be observable soon after birth. We need to be attentive to this problem in order to establish some sense of its significance for deafness or other neurosensory deficits in infancy.

Congenital syphilis frequently causes permanent and progressive sensory-neural hearing loss. With the recently increased incidence of venereal disease, we may find more cases of syphilis deafness. Congenital syphilis is transmitted from mother to child after the fourth or fifth month of fetal development. Its progress is similar to that of acquired syphilis. During the third stage, the spirochetes may attack many tissues of the body but have a propensity for blood vessels and nerve cells.

It is in the tertiary (or late secondary) stage that deafness can occur. Although congenital syphilis will affect the eyes more frequently than ears, when deafness does occur it appears to affect females primarily. Paparella and Capps (1973) report that usually one ear is affected first, then the other.

Since a fetus will not be infected until the fourth or fifth month, spontaneous abortions do not usually occur; but, in severe cases, stillbirth can be the result. In less severe cases, an apparently healthy infant may appear jaundiced and have no other symptoms at birth. Deafness can occur with sudden onset any time from late childhood to age 20, and will most often be permanent.

DEFECTS OF THE OTORHINOLARYNGEAL SYSTEM

Oral facial anomalies frequently incorporate hearing impairment among their stigmata. Sometimes the hearing impairment is limited to the conductive apparatus, as in Treacher–Collins syndrome (i.e., mandibulofacial dysostosis); cochlear, as in Waardenburg's syndrome; and sometimes they may be mixed, as in Hurler's disease. Of course many (even most) oral facial anomalies are sufficiently bizarre as to be immediately obvious at birth. A questionnaire is not required to determine if an infant is born with a bilateral cleft of the lip and palate. On the other hand, it is important to note, as did Stool (1975), that any child with an unusual facial appearance should be assumed to have a hearing impairment until it can be demonstrated otherwise. For this reason the Joint Committee on Newborn Hearing in its 1973 statement called attention to "residual anomalies of the otorhinolaryngeal system."

Congenital anomalies of the middle ear conductive mechanism are not always as gross or as apparent as those which accompany (e.g.) Treacher–Collins disease. In a recent paper, Jaffe (1976) called attention to variations in the appearance of the pinna occurring in children with confirmed middle ear anomalies. DiBartolomeo (1974) mentioned a case of a preauricular pit not discovered until adulthood. We have seen a deaf child of prenatal rubella who had a unilateral conductive overlay first noted by the fact that his pinnae did not match. Later studies revealed a middle ear anomaly on the side of the smaller pinna. Oral facial anomalies presenting with conductive hearing impairment (Figs. 3-1 through 3-6) include the following: Treacher–Collins disease, Pierre Robin syndrome, Otopalatodigital syndrome, Crouzon's disease, Apert's syndrome, and cryptophthalmos.

Most notable among the oral facial anomalies which include cochlear impairments is Waardenburg's syndrome (Fig. 3-7). First described by P. J. Waardenburg in 1951, the syndrome that bears his name incorporates anomalies of pigmentation reflected in hair and eye colors with alterations of the eye lid and nose root, and sometimes with cochlear deafness. There is considerable variation in the expression of these several traits. Waardenburg considered them to be genetically the same, and general opinion today describes Waardenburg's syndrome as dominantly inherited, although Fisch in 1959 raised some doubt. Other oral facial anomalies which incorporate cochlear impairment (Figures 3-8 through 3-11) include: Klippel–Feil syndrome, Wildervanck's syndrome, Usher's syndrome, and Cockayne's syndrome.

Other congenital defects are often seen accompanying deafness. In his study of the distribution of various causes of deafness, Fraser (1964) reported that 2½% of the deaf children he studied had a cranial–facial syndrome that affected hearing, but 7½% had goiters, 3% had retinitis pigmentosa, and

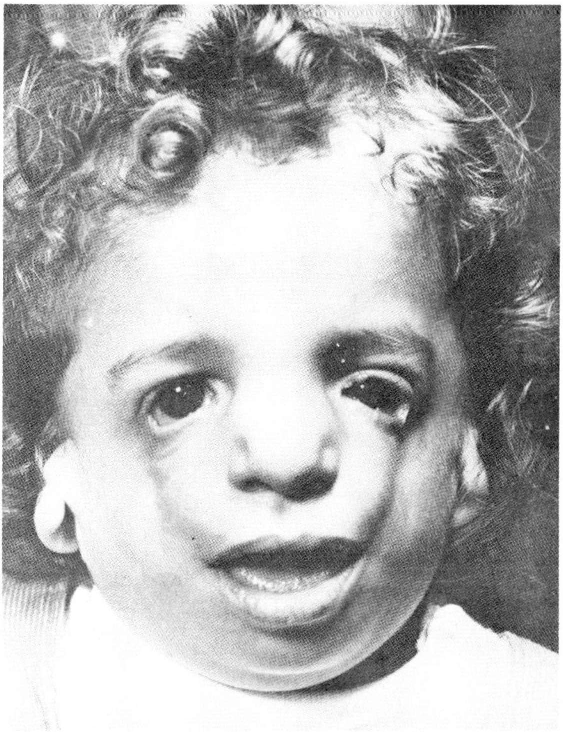

Fig. 3-1. Treacher–Collins syndrome. Manidibulofacial dysostosis or Berry –Treacher–Collins syndrome, characterized by antimongoloid slant of the eyes, underdevelopment of the zygomatic-maxillary complex, colobomata of the lower eyelids, and mircrotia. (From Rogers BO (ed): Facial Disfigurement. Washington, D.C., HEW, Vocational Rehabilitation Administration, 1964.)

another 2¼% had pigment abnormalities. Brown (1967) reported that the most common syndrome which includes deafness in children is the syndrome of Pendred, that is the one with congenital profound deafness and goiter developing during childhood (Fig. 3-12). He points out that other enzyme defects are associated with deafness as well. Usher's syndrome, also fairly common, is heritable as an autosomal recessive trait presenting with congenital severe deafness and the progressive blindness associated with retinitis pigmentosa. Brown reports Fraser's observations that this is the second most commonly occuring identifiable syndrome. Another category would be cardiac defects which, according to Fraser, constitute 1% of the syndromes of childhood deafness. Probably some examples of this are to be found in the Jervell and Lange–Nielson syndrome, which is fatal. Pigmentary abnor-

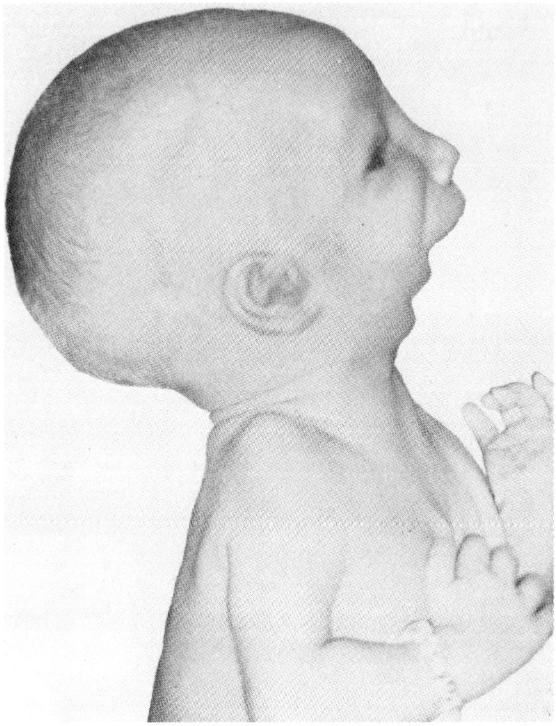

Fig. 3-2. Pierre Robin syndrome. Severe micrognathia leading to glossoptosis and respiratory embarrassment. [From Paparella MM and Shumrick D (eds): Otolaryngology. Philadelphia, Saunders, 1973]

malities other than Waardenburg's syndrome also occur with congenital deafness. These would include partial albinism as well as total albinism and Leopard's disease (Konigsmark, 1971b). Also reported is dominant piebaldness with deafness.

Other anomalies of the skeletal system have been associated with congenital deafness. These include especially such syndromes as Apert's, with marked abnormalities of the hands and feet (Fig. 3-13); the elongation of long bones plus temporal bone difficulties encountered in Englemannn's Disease (Fig. 3-14); and deafness associated with syndactyly or polydactyly. All told, congenital severe deafness with other associated handicaps of the integumentary and/or skeletal systems including the cranium account for nearly 20% of those who are born deaf. One sees, therefore, that examination of the head and neck with special reference to intraural examination and otoscopy is a

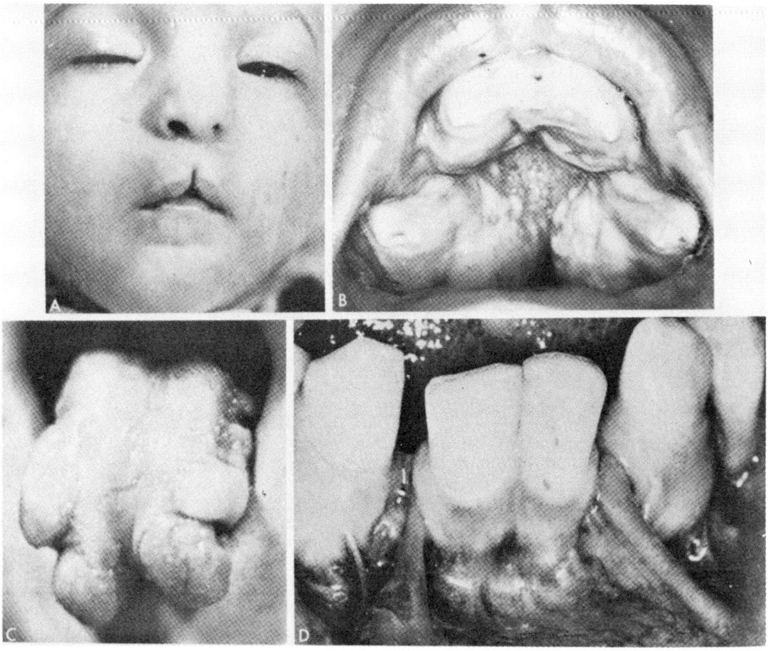

Fig. 3-3.. Oral-palatal-digital syndrome. Oral-facial-digital syndrome. A. Pseudocleft in middle of upper lip, one nostril smaller. B. Note lateral clefts in premolar area. Patient had asymmetric cleft of soft palate. C. Tetrafurcation of tongue. D. Hyperplastic frenula traverse mucobuccal fold in region of missing lower lateral incisors. (From Gorlin RJ, Psaume J: J Pediat 61:520-530, 1962.)

matter of some importance in the diagnosis of deafness in early infancy. Quite a thorough review of this topic is to be found in the small book by Black et al. (1971) in which the several syndromes are separately described, and in the nosology by Konigsmark (1971c).

LOW BIRTH WEIGHT

The small-for-gestational-age infant is at risk for a variety of respiratory and/or neurosensory deficits. In a report by Stewart (1974), of nine high-risk children with confirmed hearing losses, two were reported to be due to "prematurity." In Doctor Stewart's sample, low birth weight was defined as it had been by the Joint Committee on Newborn Hearing at 1500 g or less. In their paper before the Nova Scotia Conference on Early Identification of Hearing

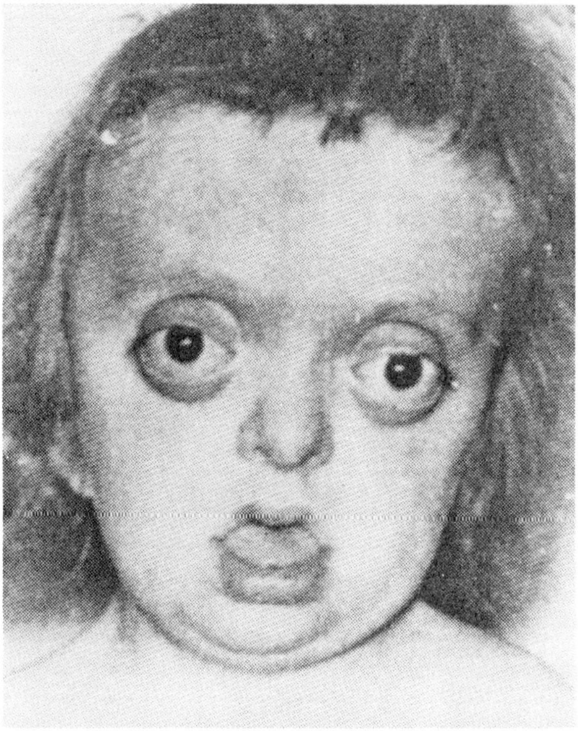

Fig. 3-4. Crouzon's disease. Note proptosis and bulging forehead. (From Baldwin J: Dysostosis craniofacialis of Crouzon. Laryngoscope 78:10, 1660–1675, 1968.)

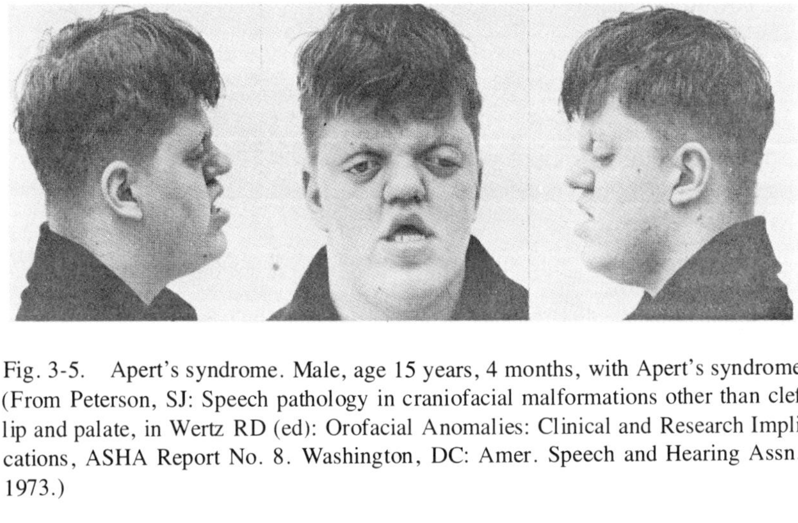

Fig. 3-5. Apert's syndrome. Male, age 15 years, 4 months, with Apert's syndrome. (From Peterson, SJ: Speech pathology in craniofacial malformations other than cleft lip and palate, in Wertz RD (ed): Orofacial Anomalies: Clinical and Research Implications, ASHA Report No. 8. Washington, DC: Amer. Speech and Hearing Assn., 1973.)

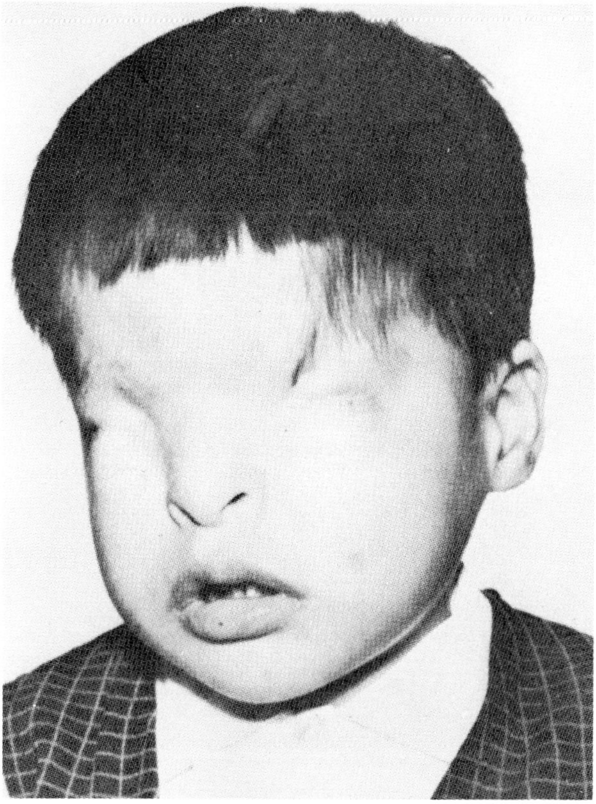

Fig. 3-6. Cryptophthalmos. Cryphthalmia syndrome and mixed deafness in a Greenlandic boy of normal intelligence. He had unilateral renal aplasia and hypospadias. (From Warburg M: Birth Defects 7(3):136, 1971.)

Loss, Feinmesser and Tell (1976) recommended an increase of the low birth weight criterion. In their extensive study, they had discovered 23 deaf infants; one of these infants would not have been on the recommended high-risk register had a 1500-g criterion been used, but would have been placed on the register were the criterion set at 2000 g. Many hospitals use as their definition of low birth weight a value of 4 lb, that is, about 1800 g. Many large scale samples of congenital deafness show that 8–10% of children who are born deaf would be classified in the low birth weight category, as previously redefined, and may or may not be found under any of the other categories of risk. Recent considerations by the Joint Committee on Newborn Hearing, however, have reaffirmed the 1500-g criterion. It is their opinion that an increase would lead to an unduly large number of hearing children being referred for further evaluation.

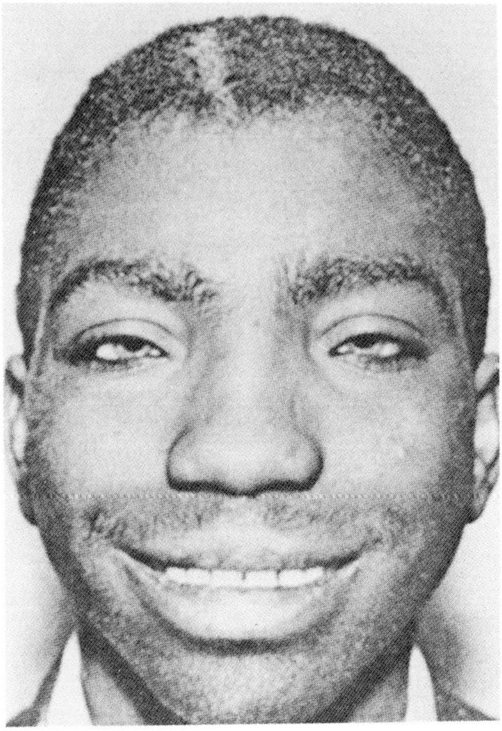

Fig. 3-7. Waardenburg's syndrome. Note white streak in center of hair, broad nasal root, and light-colored irises in this patient. (From DiGeorge A, Olmsted RW, Harley RD: Waardenburg's syndrome. J. Pediat 57:649–669, 1960.)

Low birth weight infants frequently are classified in other high risk categories not listed on the Joint Committee's register. In this context we consider especially perinatal hypoxia. In our center, for example, we have seen one child of a marginally low weight who took one breath at birth and then stopped. He was intubated for seven minutes before resuming respiration on his own. The hypoxic infant has long been known to be at risk for neurosensory deficits including hearing impairment, sensory-motor difficulties, and mental retardation.

Ototoxicity of the newborn seems to be an unduly mysterious subject. Drugs of well-established and well-known ototoxicity, such as kanamycin and gentamycin, are frequently given to small birth weight infants who do not fare well. Many neonatologists prefer these drugs to other broad spectrum antibiotics because they are highly effective, broadly useful, and said to be

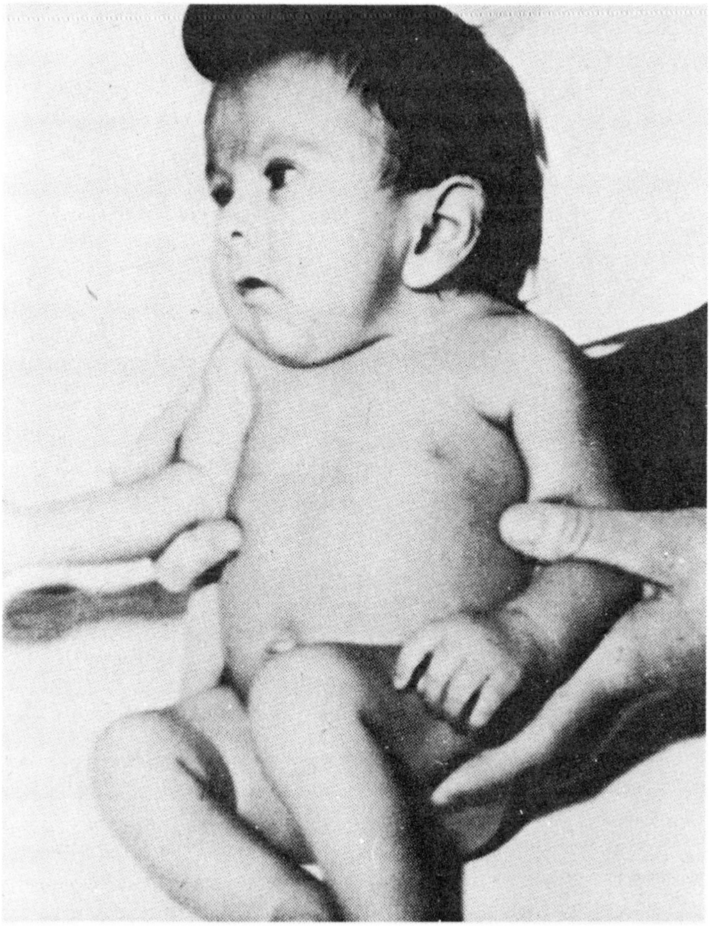

Fig. 3-8. Klippel-Feil syndrome. Note short neck giving impression that head is set directly on shoulders. (From Black FO et al., Congenital Deafness, Colorado Associated Univ Pr, 1971.)

not ototoxic in early infancy. It has been claimed that their potential ototoxicity is diminished due to the relatively high frequency of renal clearance in the newborn. On the other hand, inadequate renal function is a frequent hazard among premature infants, thereby increasing the susceptibility to ototoxicity; of course, impaired renal function is threatening to audition in its own right. Although it is uncommon for streptomycin to be used in infancy, as recently as 1965, one study reported a large number of infants who had received

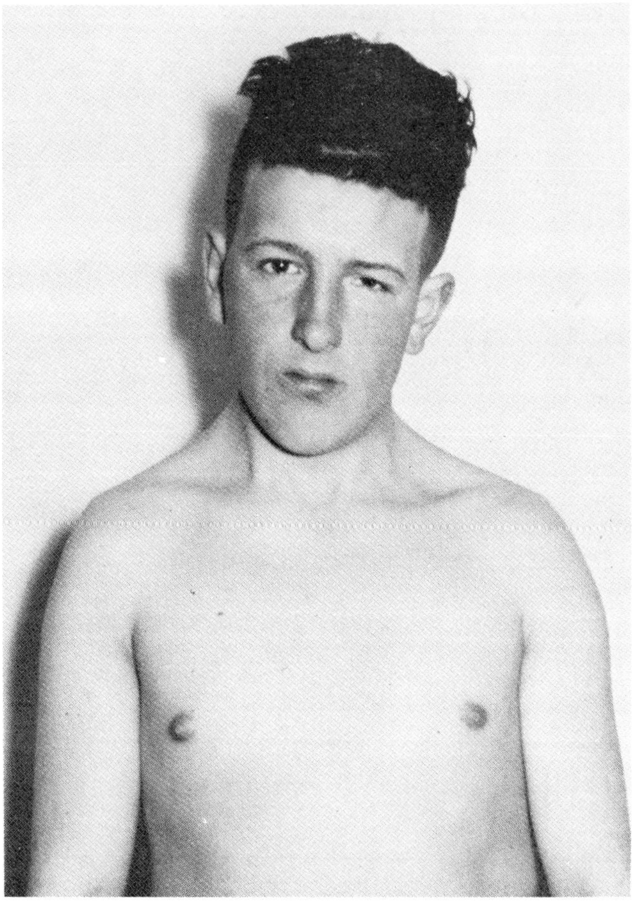

Fig. 3-9. Wildervanck syndrome. Klippel-Feil anomalad and abducens paralysis with retracted bulb and sensorineural or conductive deafness (Wildervanck syndrome; cervico-oculoacoustic dysplasia.) Twenty-two-year-old male with facial asymmetry and torticollis. Left eye exhibits strabismus, narrowed palpebral fissure, and retracted globe. Patient had unilateral sensorineural deafness and epibulbar dermoid. (From Franceschetti A, Klein D: J Genet Human 3:176, 1954.)

streptomycin, more than half of whom had hearing losses (Hawkins, 1967). Furthermore, although streptomycin is known to cross the placental barrier, it nevertheless has been used during pregnancy. Neomycin, perhaps the most threatening of the ototoxic drugs, is not commonly used in infancy. One can only hope that pediatricians are sufficiently sensitive to its side effects to

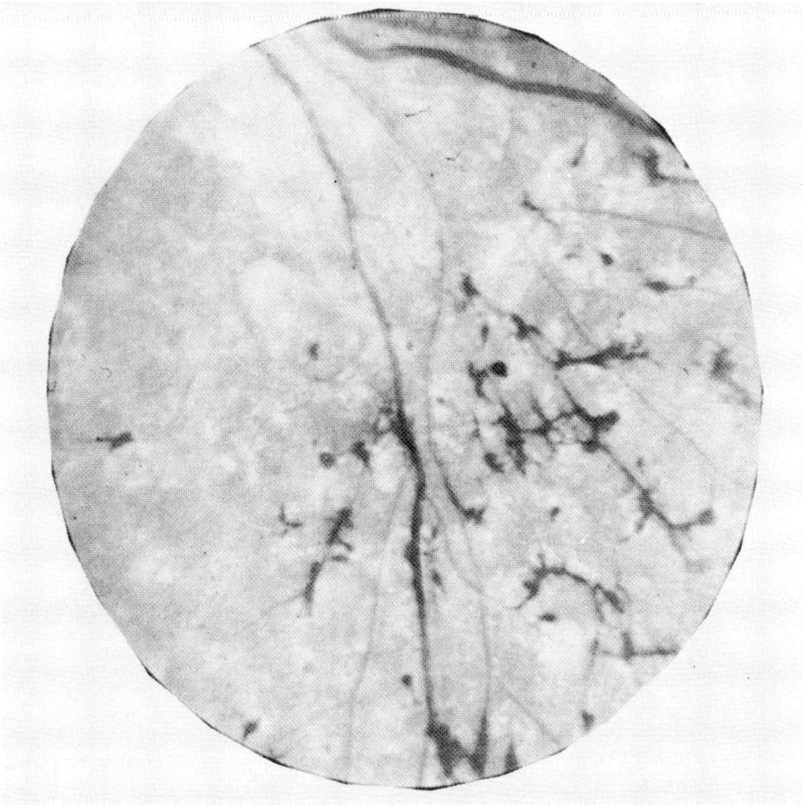

Fig. 3-10. Usher's syndrome. Retinitis pigmentosa and congenital sensorineural deafness (Usher syndrome). Equatorial view of fundus showing typical bone spicule pigmentary changes clustered around vessels. (From McLeod AC, et al.: Arch Otolaryngol 94:321, 1971.)

avoid its use. We have to agree with Hawkins, especially with reference to the very young child, that these antibiotic drugs "are a threat to hearing, and a serious one, unless they are employed with the greatest circumspection and only in cases where no other antimicrobial agent will serve." Sometimes it appears that other antimicrobial agents are not considered for use in the small birth weight infant. Only recently have perinatologists begun to consider the long-term effects of the use of such drugs as gentamycin in the high-risk nursery. We must await further reports.

HYPERBILIRUBINEMIA

The Joint Committee on Newborn Hearing recommends the use of a high-risk register that defines hyperbilirubinemia as "any free or indirect serum bilirubin concentration judged to be potentially toxic." An earlier version of this register item defined hyperbilirubinemia as 20 mg/100 ml; however, 20 mg/100 ml is far beyond the toxic level for some infants, while it is not toxic in others. In Stewart's 1974 report, about ⅛ of the births were children with bilirubin levels greater than 20 mg/100 ml and/or children who had had exchange transfusions. This amounted to 82 infants, 2 of whom had

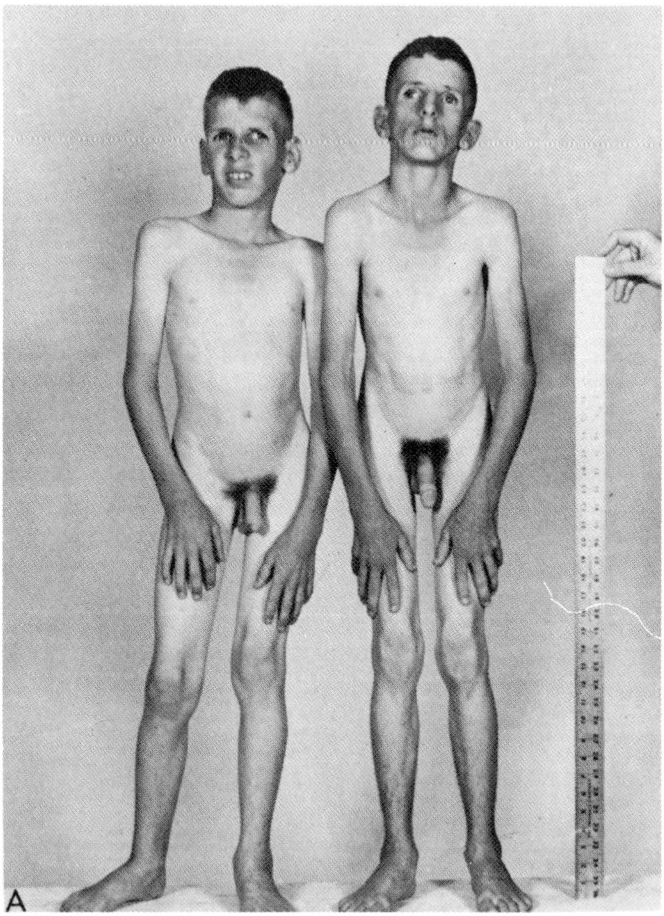

confirmed hearing losses and 1 other of whom had a suspected hearing loss. Putting it differently, Stewart found eight high-risk children in whom she could confirm the hearing loss, and two of the eight were products of hyperbilirubinemia, as she defined it. Hyperbilirubinemia accounts for about 7% of those who are congenitally deaf (Paparella and Capps, 1973). According to Altenau (1975), hyperbilirubinemic "deafness is thought to result from damage to the cochlear nuclei." This has been suggested by Dublin (1974) also.

Hyperbilirubinemia should not be confused with kernicterus. Bilirubin levels in the newborn that exceed 12 mg/100 ml for full-term infants or 15 mg/100 ml in premature infants frequently result in physiologic jaundice. Such hyperbilirubinemia is a contributory factor in kernicterus, but is not the sole culprit. Similarly, while our concern for kernicterus arises from Rh incompata-

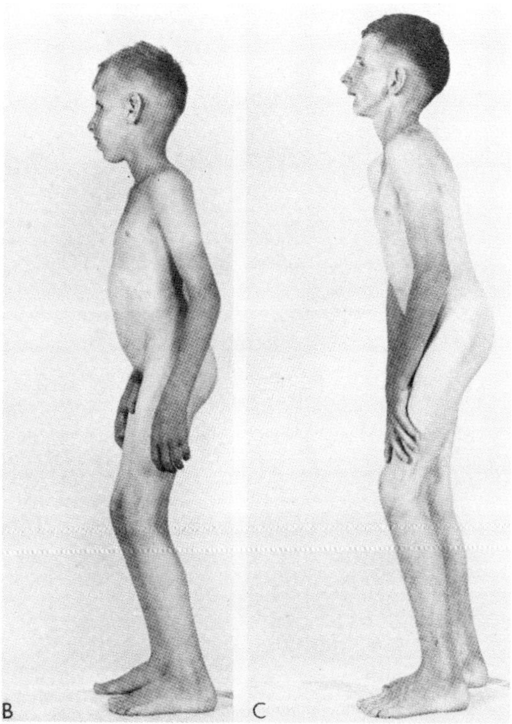

Fig. 3-11. Cockayne syndrome. A *(opposite)*, B, and C. Fourteen- and 16-year-old sibs with marked mental and somatic retardation, eye difficulties, and sensorineural deafness. Note wizened appearance, photodermatitis of sun exposed areas, horseriding stance, and large hands and feet. (From Paddison RM et al.: Derm Trop 2:196, 1963.)

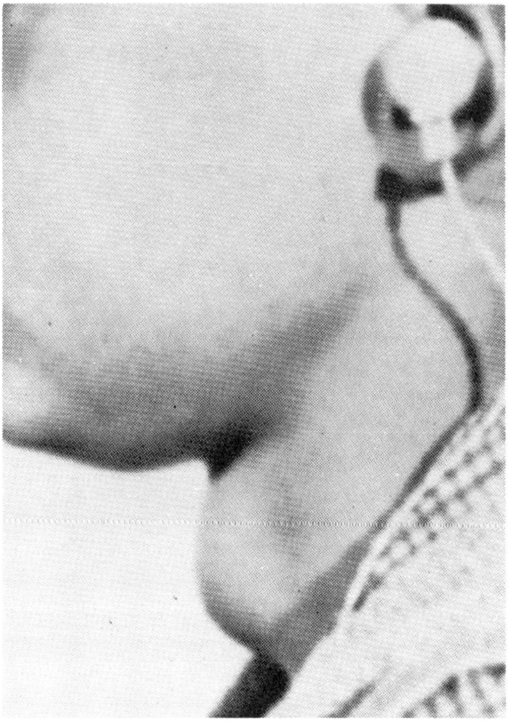

Fig. 3-12. Pendred's syndrome demonstrating the association of sensorineural deafness, goiter, and normal function. [From Fraser GR: The genetics of congenital deafness, in Hemenway WF, Bergstrom L (eds): Symposium on Congenital Deafness. Otolaryngolical Clinic North America. June, 1971.]

bility, other things lead to hyperbilirubinemia. Goodhill (1967) pointed out that indirect bilirubin can accumulate and result in jaundice due to any condition that causes hemolysis and these could be Rh incompatability, ABO incompatability, and other blood incompatabilities, as well as syphilis. So the Rh factor is not the only potential source of kernicterus. Furthermore, Goodhill continued, it is not only the icterus that produces lesions of the nervous system, including the auditory nervous system. It was his view that the deposits of icterus lead to cellular anoxia which, in turn, "destroys the integrity of the neural auditory pathway." Furthermore, he pointed out that kernicterus could be simulated by hypoxia with or without icterus.

The essential problem is to find a quantifiable way to live up to the directive of the Joint Committee's high-risk register. That register recom-

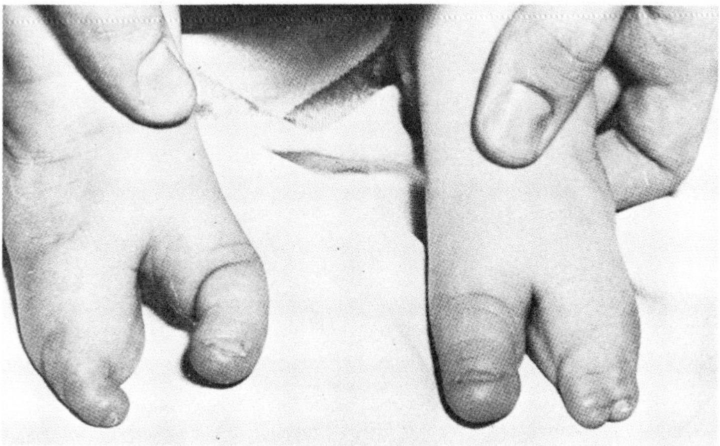

Fig. 3-13. Syndactyly (lobster claw hands) typical of Apert's syndrome. (From Nelson WE: Pediatrics, ed. 9. Philadelphia, Saunders.)

mends "any free or indirect serum bilirubin concentration which is judged to be potentially toxic." Judged by whom? What is the consequence of the judgment? What is the bilirubin level that leads to such a judgment? These quantitative questions remain unanswered. But, in our experience, pediatric examination of the child which suggests to the examiner that the infant is jaundiced occurs frequently at bilirubin levels substantially lower than 20 mg/100 ml. Perhaps we should return to Goodhill's criterion of 12 mg/100 ml in the full-term infant and 15 mg/100 ml in the low birth weight infant. Again, good pediatric judgment is required in every case.

RESULTS OF EXPERIENCE

In general, employment of the high-risk register described at the beginning of this chapter has been fairly successful. Reports of its success have been made by Mencher (1974), Stewart (1974), and Feinmesser and Tell (1976), while Meyer and Wolfe (1975) have had less success. Using the 1973 version of the high-risk register, Downs (1976) reported "the finding of one deaf child in 57 in the High Risk Register." Furthermore, she found that all of the deaf infants discovered also failed an arousal screening test, and there was a very small number of false positives. In the same proceedings, Rossi and Guidotti (1976) reported finding five deaf children, three of whom were

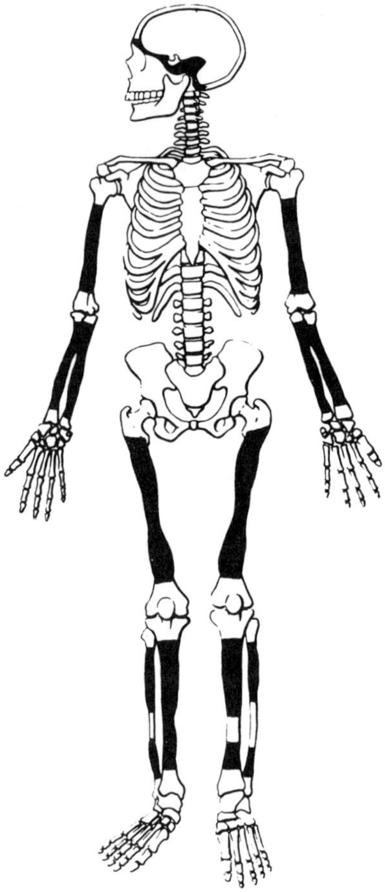

Fig. 3-14. Englemann's Disease. This schematic drawing of the skeleton shows the affected bones in a case at 18 years of age. Only short segments of the leg bones are uninvolved. (From Sparkes RS, Graham CB: Camurati-Englemann disease. Genetic and clinical manifestations with a review of the literature. J. Med Gen 9:73–85, 1972.)

in the high-risk group. Also Feinmesser and Tell reported that 17 of their 23 deaf children would have been placed on a six-item high-risk register.

Mencher (1974) has shown that the use of this high-risk register leads to better detection in the newborn nursery than does the use of behavioral screening. He applied the five-item register retrospectively to data from a number of sources. His principal finding was that it would have correctly detected about

60% of all the true positives. Specifically, he reported that five of nine children with confirmed hearing impairments would have been placed on this register. In general, it is observed that the five-item high-risk register includes about 6–8% of the newborn population; 2–4% of the high-risk population will prove to have a hearing loss, and of these perhaps half will be severely impaired.

The high-risk register succeeds when behavioral methods fail. Mencher (1974) showed that the use of the high-risk register leads to much higher correct detection in the newborn nursery than does the use of various screening methods. Remember that Feinmesser and Tell found 23 deaf infants, 17 of whom were at risk; but only 6 of the 23 failed the behavioral test. Conversely this means that 17 hearing-impaired infants passed the behavioral screen. As a result, they concluded that "the assumption that newborns with severe hearing loss will fail to arouse if tested, is open to conjecture."

There are some interesting side benefits as well. Gerber (1972) directed attention to the fact that children who are at risk and/or fail to respond to intense acoustic stimuli frequently have neurosensory deficits other than deafness. Mencher, in the 1974 paper previously cited, observed that 3.3% of infants who are not at risk fail to respond to any acoustic signal, while 5.4% of the high-risk children fail to respond. When we attempt to diagnosis deafness in infancy, we often discover other things. There will be a greater number of children who are at risk and who are not severely hearing-impaired. These children, also, merit intensive study and follow-up. We must always have in mind Hardy's (1965) admonition that if a child does not respond, we cannot conclude that he doesn't hear; we can only conclude that he doesn't respond.

It is to be hoped that intensive and extensive application of the high-risk register will diminish the necessary truthfulness of Dr. Hardy's comments. Furthermore, we must observe with Greenough (1975) that the early release of sensory deprivation should be expected to lead to increased neuronal growth. Extrapolating from that observation, one hopes that application of the high-risk register and action taken thereon will serve to minimize the handicap associated with congenital deafness.

REFERENCES

Altenau MM: Histopathology of sensorineural hearing loss in children, in Glasscock ME (ed): Symposium on sensorineural hearing loss in children: Early detection and intervention, Otolaryngol Clin North Am 8:49–58, 1975

Black, FO, Bergstrom L, Downs M, et al: Congenital Deafness. Boulder, Colorado Associated University Press, 1971.

Bordley JE, Brookhouser PE, Hardy J, et al: Observations on the effect of prenatal rubella in hearing, in McConnell F, Ward PH (eds): Deafness in Childhood. Nashville, Vanderbilt University Press, 1967.

Brown KS: The genetics of childhood deafness, in McConnell F, Ward PH (eds): Deafness in Childhood. Nashville, Vanderbilt University Press, 1967.

Dahle AJ, McCollister FP, Hamner BA, et al: Subclinical congenital cytomegalovirus infection and hearing impairment. J Speech Hear Dis 39:320–329, 1974

DiBartolomeo JR: The auditory system: Pre and post natal development, in Sensory and Perceptual Dysfunctioning in Infants: Identification, Diagnosis and Current Research. Los Angeles, University of Southern California, School of Medicine, Postgraduate Division, 1974

Downs MP: Early identification of hearing loss: Where are we? Where do we go from here? in Mencher GT (ed): Early Identification of Hearing Loss. Basel, Karger, 1976.

Dublin WJ: Cytoarchitecture of the cochlear nuclei. Arch Otolaryngol 100:355–359, 1974

Feinmesser M, Tell L: Evaluation of methods for detecting hearing impairment in infancy and early childhood, in Mencher GT (ed): Early Identification of Hearing Loss. Basel, Karger, 1976.

Fisch L: Deafness as part of an hereditary syndrome. J Laryngol 73:355–382, 1959

Fraser GR: Profound childhood deafness. J Med Genet 1:118–151, 1964

Fraser GR: Heredity, early identification of hearing loss, and the risk register, in Mencher GT (ed): Early Identification of Hearing Loss. Basel, Karger, 1976.

Gerber SE: Auditory behavioral responses of some hearing infants. Volta Rev 71:340–346, 1969

Gerber SE: Biomedical technology and the detection of birth defects. Rehabil Lit 33:322–325, 329, 1972

Goodhill V: Auditory pathway lesions resulting from Rh incompatability, in McConnell F, Ward PH (eds): Deafness in Childhood. Nashville, Vanderbilt University Press, 1967.

Greenough WT: Experiential modification of the developing brain. Am Sci 63:37–46, 1975

Hardy WG: Evaluation of hearing in infants and young children, in Glorig A (ed): Audiometry: Principles and Practices. Baltimore, Williams and Wilkins, 1965

Hawkins JE Jr: Iatrogenic toxic deafness in children, in McConnell F, Ward PH (eds): Deafness in Childhood. Nashville, Vanderbilt University Press, 1967.

Hemenway WG, Bergstrom L: The pathology of acquired viral endolabyrinthitis, in McConnell F, Ward PH (eds): Deafness in Childhood. Nashville, Vanderbilt University Press, 1967.

Jaffe BF: Pinna anomalies associated with congenital conductive hearing loss. Pediatrics 57:332–341, 1976

Kapur YP: Panel discussion in Jazbi B (ed): Pediatric otorhinolaryngology in Otolaryngol. Clin North Am 10:248–252, 1977

Konigsmark BW: Hereditary congenital severe deafness syndromes. Ann Oto Rhino Laryngol 80:269–289, 1971a

Konigsmark BW: Hereditary and congenital factors affecting newborn sensorineural hearing, in Cunningham GC (ed): Conference on Newborn Hearing Screening. Berkeley, Bureau of Maternal and Child Health, California State Department of Public Health, 1971b

Konigsmark BW, McKusick VA: Hereditary Deafness. Volta Rev 68:336–341, 380, 1966

Mencher GT: A program for neonatal hearing screening. Audiology 13:495–500, 1974

Mencher GT: Perinatal hearing assessment, in Jazbi B (ed): Pediatric Otorhinolaryngology. Otolaryngol Clin North Am 10:177–182, 1977

Meyer DH, Wolfe VI: Use of a high-risk register in newborn hearing screening. J Speech Hear Dis 40:493–498, 1975

Paparella MM, Capps MJ: Sensorineural deafness in children—nongenetic, in Paparella MM, Shumrick DA (eds): Otolaryngology. Philadelphia, Saunders, 1973

Rossi P, Guidotti E: Problems associated with the early diagnosis of deafness in newborn babies, in Mencher GT (ed): Early Identification of Hearing Loss. Basel, Karger, 1976.

Stewart J: High risk screening. Paper presented to Western Society for Pediatric Research, Carmel, 1974

Stool SE: The identification of hearing loss in children, a miniseminar presented to American Speech and Hearing Association, Washington, DC 1975

Waardenburg PJ: A new syndrome combining developmental anomalies of the eyelids, eyebrows and nose root with pigmentary defects of the iris and head hair and with congenital deafness. Am J Human Genet 3:195–253, 1951

Ward PH, Lindsay JR, Warner NE: Cytomegalic inclusion disease affecting the temporal bone. Laryngoscope 75:628–636, 1965

Sanford E. Gerber

4 Auditory Development

This brief chapter has two purposes. The first is to describe the neurologic development of the very young child, and the second is to describe auditory behavior in infancy. Additional details of auditory behavior are to be found in the next chapter, which deals with the matter of using such behavior for audiometric purposes.

An essential point with respect to early auditory development is that, anatomically and physiologically, the auditory system develops very early. As a consequence, it is possible to assess auditory function prenatally and perinatally, as well as neonatally. To be sure, such things as gestational age and birth weight are significant in this context, and they are discussed in the following. Moreover, of considerable significance is the normal infant's development of speech and language, which results from auditory input.

PRENATAL DEVELOPMENT

If a viable infant is born prematurely, it is possible to demonstrate that he "hears" in some sense of the word. This is an observation that is so apparent that many of us have failed to notice it; it was the work of Vasiliu (1968) that made this "obvious" fact well known. The significance of this observation—that a premature infant hears at birth—lies not only in its own right, but also in the necessary conclusion that that same infant would have been hearing at that time had he not been born. That is to say, if we can demonstrate that an infant of, say, 30-weeks gestational age hears after birth, then he must have been able to hear at that gestational age had he not yet been born.

Embryology

It is not our purpose to describe in detail the embryology of the human auditory system. An outstanding paper on this subject is the chapter by Anson (1973) to which the interested reader is referred. What follows is a brief summary.

The external, middle, and inner ears arise from separate primordial tissues. Embryologists describe three types of primordial tissues: ectoderm, mesoderm, and endoderm. All three of these tissues are involved in the development of the human ear. Ectoderm and endoderm appear as early as the eighth day of fetal life; shortly afterward, mesoderm appears between them. During the succeeding stages of embryonic and fetal development the ectoderm will give rise to the external ear, the outer layers of the tympanic membrane, the membraneous labyrinth, thc organ of Corti, and the vestibular organs (semicircular canals, utricle, and saccule). It is important to note that all of the cochlear structures arise from ectoderm; hence, failure of ectodermal development will be expected to lead to cochlear anomalies. Meanwhile, the endoderm forms the inner surface of the tympanic membrane and the Eustachian tube; while mesoderm differentiates into the ossicles, the middle layers of the tympanic membrane, and the mastoid and petrous portions of the temporal bones.

At the time of the division of embryonic cells, the neural groove begins to appear along with a number of other structures. By 3 weeks of gestational age there is marked growth of the neural groove leading to the formation of five pharyngeal pouches and their arches and grooves. The mandible develops from the first arch and the hyoid bone from the second arch. The pharyngeal pouches are separated from each other by a series of clefts; the external auditory meatus develops from the first of these clefts. As the first cleft grows and invaginates, it develops a layer of ectodermal cells, which eventually form the tympanic membrane. The tubotympanic recess thus created becomes the Eustachian tube. Above this first external groove, there appears the otic placode, which invaginates into a pit becoming closed over by ectoderm and surrounded by mesoderm. As the tubotympanic recess grows, it eventually establishes the gross divisions of the three major parts of the ear. The middle ear develops from the endoderm of the tubotympanic recess, while the ossicles form from the adjacent mesoderm. By the eighth gestational week, a cartilaginous incus and malleus may be identified. By this time, one also can identify sensory cells of the vestibular system. By the eleventh fetal week, the two-and-one-half turns of the cochlea are present and the cochlear duct is attached to the VIII nerve. In the following week, the membraneous labyrinth is complete, the otic capsule begins to ossify, and there are sensory cells in the cochlea. By the twentieth week of gestation, the fetal inner ear has achieved adult size, although development of the middle and external ear continues. Details of this development are listed in Table 4-1 (Northern and Downs, 1974) and are illustrated in Fig. 4-1 (Anson, 1973). Examination of the table reveals to the informed reader how and when various auditory anomalies might arise.

Fetal Responses

An extensive review of the responsivity of the human fetus to acoustic events was published by Tanaka and Arayama in 1969. They write that fetal movements in response to loud sounds have been reported since 1924. Beginning in 1947, observations of the change of fetal heart rate as a response to intense acoustic stimulation were investigated. The signal report of this phenomenon was the study of Johansson, Wedenberg, and Westin (1964) in which they identified reliable heart rate changes as responses to acoustic stimulation at an average gestational age of 26 weeks. Table 4-1 indicates that the anatomy is well established by this age. In fact, Wedenberg's reports have shown responses as early as 24 weeks and never later than 28 weeks. Johansson, Wedenberg, and Westin examined 12 fetuses, while Tanaka and Arayama examined 134; their technique—phonocardiograpy—was the same. A summary of the data of Tanaka and Arayama is shown in Table 4-2. Notice that 10 of the 134 fetuses did not respond, and unfortunately, their paper does not say why. Notice also that none of the 124 responsive fetuses responded in the sixth month, and only 5 in the seventh month. This is a bit later than the Swedish data but may reflect only differences of sample size. A very interesting difference, however, relates to the older age groups. The Swedish data report that all infants had responded by the twenty-eighth week of fetal life, but the Japanese data show that about half of them did not respond until the "tenth month of pregnancy." It is important to observe that the form of response reported virtually always is one of heart rate change (the cardiovascular response to sound is discussed at considerable length and constitutes the subject matter of Chap. 8). In this context it is important to note that alterations of fetal heart rate have been shown to be independent of maternal heart rate.

Responses other than changes of cardiovascular rate are observed prepartum. These observations, however, are limited to fetal movement. Such motor responses were reported by both the Japanese and the Swedish researchers, but these responses hold less validity than heart rate changes.

Table 4-1.
Summary of the Embryology of the Ear

Fetal Week	Inner Ear	Middle Ear	External Ear
3rd	Auditory placode; auditory pit	Tubo-tympanic recess begins to develop	
4th	Auditory vesicle (otocyst); vestibular-cochlear division		Tissue thickenings begin to form
5th			Primary auditory meatus begins
6th	Utricle and saccule present; semi-circular canals begin		6 hillocks evident; cartilage begins to form
7th	One cochlear coil present; sensory cells in utricle and saccule		Auricles move dorsolaterally
8th	Ductus reuniens present: sensory cells in semicircular canals	Incus and malleus present in cartilage; lower half of tympanic cavity formed	Outer cartilagenous third of external canal formed
9th		3 tissue layers at tympanic membrane are present	
11th	2½ cochlear coils present; VIII nerve attaches to cochlear duct		

12th	Sensory cells in cochlea; membranous labyrinth complete; otic capsule begins to ossify		
15th		Cartilagenous stapes formed	
16th		Ossification of malleus and incus begins	
18th		Stapes begins to ossify	
20th	Maturation of inner ear; inner ear adult size		Auricle is adult shape, but continues to grow until age 9
21st		Meatal plug disintegrates exposing tympanic membrane	
30th		Pneumatization of tympanum	External auditory canal continues to mature until age 7
32nd		Malleus and incus complete ossification	
34th		Mastoid air cells develop	
35th		Epitympanum is pneumatized	
37th		Stapes continues to develop until adulthood; tympanic membrane changes relative position during first 2 years of life	

From Northern and Downs: Hearing in Children. Baltimore, Williams and Wilkins, 1974.

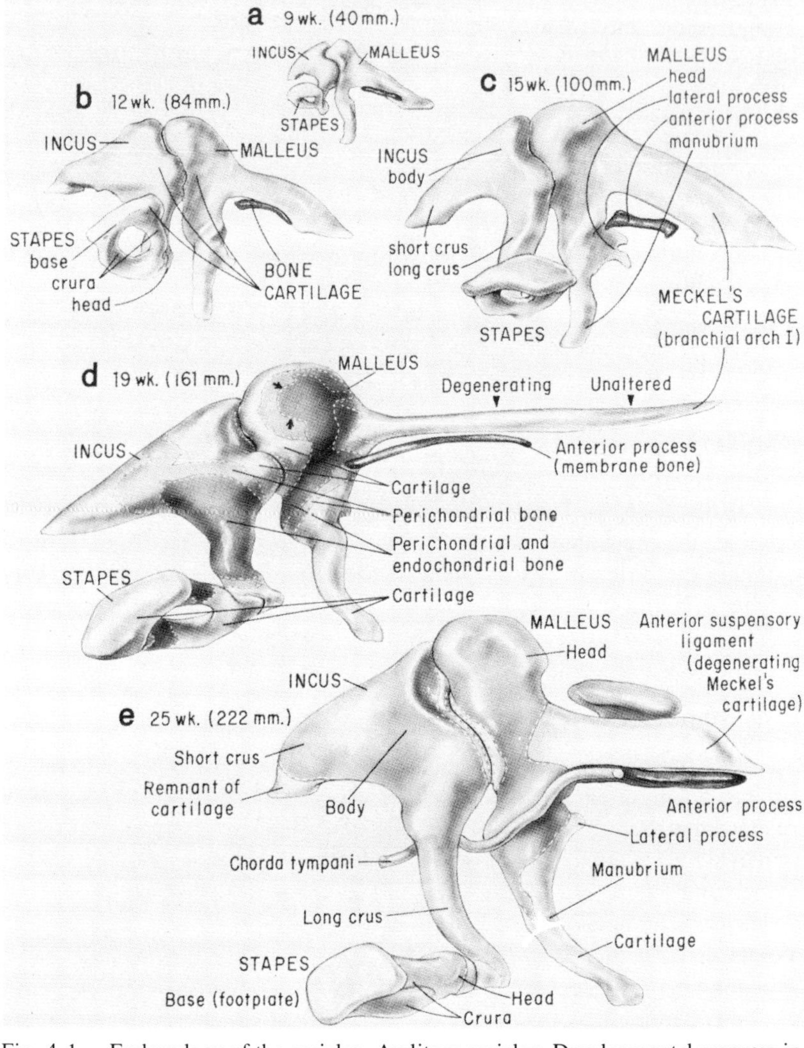

Fig. 4-1. Embryology of the ossicles. Auditory ossicles: Developmental progress in a 4-month period. A. Fetus of 9 weeks (40 mm CR length). B. Fetus of 12 weeks (84 mm). C. Fetus of 15 weeks (100 mm). Wisconsin Collection, series 168, 162, 22, 13, and 46, respectively. A–C. Cartilage models, in assuming characteristic form, reach their maximum dimensions in cartilage at the 4-month stage. D. Bone formation, well under way in the 5-month fetus, is both periosteal and endosteal (at darker areas at arrows). The anterior process of the malleus (formed in membrane bone) gains malleal attachment. E. At approximately 6 months the ossicles are full size. (From Anson: Embryology and anatomy, in Paparella and Shumrick (eds): *Otolaryngology*. Philadelphia, Saunders, 1973.)

Table 4-2.
Fetal Responses to Acoustic Stimuli

	Response		
Month of Pregnancy	*Positive*	*Negative*	Sum
6th	0	2	2
7th	5	4	9
8th	22	1	23
9th	29	0	29
10th	68	3	71
Sum	124	10	134

From Tanaka and Arayama: Pract ORL 31:269-273, 1969.

NEONATAL DEVELOPMENT

In discussing perinatal and early neonatal development, it is important to consider the premature as well as the full-term infant. In this section we examine the differences (or similarities) between premature and full-term infants as a function of postpartum gestational age and as a function of the behavior observed.

Premature and Mature Infants

One must again refer to the observation of Vasiliu (1968) that premature infants do make observable responses to sound. In fact, Wright (1971) claimed that premature children were hypersensitive to auditory stimuli. This apparent hyperresponsivity of premature infants may be an artifact, however. Bench and Parker (1971) also noted that premature infants appeared to be hypersensitive, but considered this "hyper-acoustic behavior" to result from the generally higher level of spontaneous activity of premature infants, and thought it may be due to the increased probability that some of their responses are false alarms. In fact, Bench and Parker claimed that full-term babies were "better sound detectors."

One of the problems in discussing "prematurity" is that this word has two meanings. Sometimes when we speak of premature infants we mean low gestational age infants, and sometimes we mean small-for-age infants. The distinction is neurologically important as these two categories of prematurity differ from each other. For example, neurologic maturation has been studied and reported by Graziani, Weitzman, and Velasco (1968), who found that auditory evoked encephalic responses were similar among low birth weight infants at the same postconception age regardless of birth weight or postnatal weight. In other words, the responsivity of the low birth weight infant is related to gestational age rather than to birth weight. Moreover, small-for-age infants appeared to have "more mature" evoked responses than younger infants who are not too small for age. Examination of the latencies of evoked potentials (Akiyama et al., 1969) does not reveal maturational changes such that conceptional age could be determined. One is concerned about the low birth weight infant, but not necessarily because of his lack of responsivity; low birth weight infants tend to exhibit neurologic and respiratory difficulties requiring medical intervention. Sometimes that intervention takes the form of the use of ototoxic drugs (note the discussion of this subject in the previous chapter). On the other hand, the small-for-date infant tends to be responsive in much the same way and to approximately the same extent as the full-sized full-term infant. Eisenberg (1969) has noted that neonates process sound in much the same way as adults.

Reflexes and Responses

Clearly the most obvious auditory reflex observed very early in life is the auropalpebral or cochleopalpebral reflex. This primitive reflex—usually called APR—is an example of those low-level neurologic behaviors that link two sensory modalities (Taft and Cohen, 1967). In this case, of course, it is the visual and auditory systems that are linked. Notice also that the APR is a reflex that is never completely lost: all normally hearing persons will exhibit an eye blink immediately following a sudden burst of noise. This is more often true in the early neonatal period. It was demonstrated in a large study by Wedenberg (1956) and in a most important investigation by Fröding (1960). Fröding examined 2000 children all within the first 30 minutes of life. All of the infants who repeatedly failed to demonstrate an APR turned out to be severely damaged. Wedenberg earlier had demonstrated the APR to be the most reliable auditory reflex among newborns. Grisanti, Restivo, and LaBarbera (1971) claimed that infants were most responsive on the fourth day of life. In the next chapter, which deals with behavioral responses, the reader will find a discussion of how to emply the APR audiometrically.

While the auropalpebral reflex has been shown to be highly reliable, much doubt has been cast on the Moro reflex. It was thought for quite a long time that the Moro reflex was a response to sound, but that mistaken notion was thoroughly put aside by Taft and Cohen in 1967. It is now clear that the Moro reflex is one elicited by activity of the muscles of the neck, and may often be as easily elicited from a deaf infant as from a hearing one if the test is done properly.

Some other responses to sound do appear among neonates. Crying, for example, is an apparent one, as well as changes in respiratory rate or pattern which are also seen (see Chap. 7). The cardiovascular responses seen prenatally may also be observed postnatally, but their form has recently been questioned (Gerber, Mulac, and Swain, 1976) and the reader will find a detailed discussion of this in Chapter 8. Similarly, if motor responses occur prenatally, they will also be observed postnatally. These limb movements become very useful in the arousal test (Chap. 5).

INFANT DEVELOPMENT

Development of reflexive and nonreflexive behavior is quite rapid during the first several months of life. Hardy (1965) described the infants' readiness to listen and readiness to speak. The latter phenomenon is evidenced, of course, by the fact that he does so. What may be more striking, however is the infant who doesn't. Friedlander (1971), for example, has again directed our attention to those "children who began to vocalize and babble in normal fashion," but in whom "expressive language patterns became dissipated toward the end of the first year in the absence of auditory experience and self-reinforcement." In other words, the readiness to speak never fully matures into the act of speaking in those children who don't hear; they stop vocalizing entirely.

Immobilization and Localization

The readiness to listen is easily observable in very young children. Downs (1967) has observed the cessation of activity, especially among crying infants. Gerber (1969) described immobilization in children as young as 2 months of age. This cessation of motor activity, or immobilization, is an overt display of listening behavior. In a sense, the baby stops to listen.

The term localization has been used to describe a variety of motor behaviors which arise in response to sound. For example, Frisina (1963) reported eye turning at ages as young as 2–4 months. More recently, Cohen and Peters (1974) reported that 4-month-old infants will seem to follow an apparently moving sound source with their eyes. Northern and Downs (1974) discussed turning the head toward or away from the source of sound, and considered both of these responses to be valid. Gerber (1969) described localization as a complete turning toward the source of sound located on one side only. This form of localization was not seen much before the seventh month. Northern and Downs claim that an infant will localize to speech by the age of 6 months and will begin to imitate some sounds by 8 months. Vertical localization, a rather difficult task, appears toward the end of the first year of life.

Speech

The development of speech—not to be confused with the development of language—is a phenomenon not at all understood in infancy. As is mentioned in Chapter 14, there has been virtually no research on phonological development during the first year of life. In general, it seems that very early phonological development consists largely of excluding from one's vocal repertoire those sounds which are not heard in the linguistic milieu. In other words, the notion of acquisition of phonology is, in a sense, an erroneous one. It appears that one does not acquire speech sounds, but rather one divests himself of speech sounds. Modern researchers such as Lenneberg (1967), Menyuk (1972), or Weir (1966) have all shown that young children babble in their native tongue. Clearly, this kind of speech readiness is not only language specific, but also reflects a high level of auditory accomplishment, and, as all parents know, this occurs quite early in life.

REFERENCES

Akiyama Y, Schulte FJ, Schultz MA, et al: Acoustically evoked responses in premature and full term newborn infants. Electroencephalog Clin Neurophysiol 26:371–380, 1969

Anson BJ: Developmental anatomy of the ear, in Paparella MM, Shumrick DA (eds): Otolaryngology. Philadelphia, Saunders, 1973

Bench J, Parker A: Hyper-responsivity to sounds in the short-gestation baby. Dev Med Child Neurol 13:15–19, 1971

Cohen L, Peters R: Response behaviors of infants to simulated moving sound stimuli. Paper presented to the Eighth International Congress on Acoustics, London, 1974

Downs MP: Testing hearing in infancy and early childhood, in McConnell F, Ward PH (eds): Deafness in Childhood. Nashville, Vanderbilt University Press, 1967

Eisenberg RB: Auditory behavior in the human neonate: Functional properties of sound and their ontogenetic implications. Int Audiol 8:34–45, 1969

Friedlander BA: Listening, language, and the auditory environment, in Hellmuth J (ed): Exceptional Infant, Vol 2 Studies in Abnormalities. New York, Brunner/Mazel, 1971

Frisina R: Measurement of hearing in children, in Jerger JF (ed): Modern Developments in Audiology. New York, Academic, 1963

Fröding CA: Acoustic investigation of newborn infants. Acta Otolaryngol (Stockh) 52:31–40, 1960

Gerber SE: Auditory behavioral responses of some hearing infants. Volta Rev 71:340–346, 1969

Gerber SE, Mulac A, Swain BJ: Cardiovascular responses to sound in human neonates. J Am Audiol Soc 1:185–191, 1976

Graziani LJ, Weitzman ED, Velasco MSA: Neurologic maturation and auditory evoked responses in low birth weight infants. Pediatrics 41:483–494, 1968

Grisanti G, Restivo S, LaBarbera L: Risultati dell'audiometria comportamentale nei neonati a termine. Il Valsalva 47:161–170, 1971

Hardy WG: Evaluation of hearing in infants and young children, in Glorig A (ed): Audiometry, Principles and Practice. Baltimore, Williams and Wilkins, 1965

Johansson B, Wedenberg E, Westin B: Measurement of tone response by the human foetus. Acta Otolaryngol (Stockh) 57:188–192, 1964

Lenneberg EH: Biological Foundations of Language. New York, Wiley, 1967

Menyuk P: The Development of Speech. Indianapolis, Bobbs-Merrill, 1972

Northern JL, Downs MP: Hearing in Children. Baltimore, Williams and Wilkins, 1974

Taft LT, Cohen HJ: Neonatal and infant reflexology, in Hellmuth J (ed): Exceptional Infant, Vol. 1, The Normal Infant. New York, Brunner/Mazel, 1967

Tanaka Y, Arayama T: Fetal responses to acoustic stimuli. Pract Otorhinolaryngol 31:269–273, 1969

Vasiliu DI: L'enfant est prêt a entendre même dans la vie intrauterine. Contributions sur l'embryogenese de l'orielle et la pneumatisation de la mastoïde et du rocher. Int. Audiol 7:181–185, 1968

Wedenberg, E: Auditory tests on new-born infants. Acta Otolaryngol (Stockh) 46:446–461, 1956

Weir RH: Some questions on the child's learning of phonology, in Smith F, Miller G (eds): The Genesis of Language. Cambridge, MIT Press, 1966

Wright L: The theoretical and research base for a program of early stimulation care and training of premature infants, in Hellmuth J (ed): Exceptional Infant, Vol. 2, Studies in Abnormalities. New York, Brunner/Mazel, 1971

II

The Methods

Sanford E. Gerber
Bronwyn L. Jones
and Janis M. Costello

5
Behavioral Measures

As we observed in Chapter 4, the normal newborn should be expected to hear at birth. In fact, he should be expected to hear before birth. We need to develop our expectations vis-a-vis the auditory behavior of an infant at any given age so that we can employ them clinically (Gerber, 1969). One can talk about auditory behavior, one may speak of unconditioned responses to various acoustic events, and one may consider conditioned responses to audible signals. However, in discussing these various kinds of responses, one needs to continue to be alert to the variables recommended by the 1970 statement of the Joint Committee on Newborn Hearing: stimuli, response patterns, environmental factors, status at the time of testing, and behavior of observers.

STIMULI

What constitutes an appropriate stimulus for the auditory testing of an infant? We raised this question in an earlier paper (Gerber, 1969) by asking "What stimuli will cause an infant to behave in a way that would permit observers to determine if he responds to sound?" Eisenberg (1965), in one of her many brilliant papers on the subject, observed that acoustic events probably have differential functional properties that are innate, unconditioned, and relevant to the ontogeny of communicative functions. She concluded (1969) that the discriminable property of sound for newborns is the organization of the stimulus envelope. On the other hand, Gerber, Mulac, and Swain (1976) reported that they were unable to find that the response to sound varied as a function of spectrum. This, however, was a narrow observation limited to the conclusion that "a narrow band of noise centered at 3150 Hz is neither more nor less effective than a pure tone of 3150 Hz." It was further reported by Turkewitz et al. (1972) that ineffective stimuli were not rendered effective by changes of duration nor were effective stimuli rendered ineffective. They —like Gerber, Mulac, and Swain—were concerned with cardiovascular responses; this subject is discussed at length in Chapter 8.

If one could make a generalization, it would be that there has been a historical preference for frequencies around 3000 Hz. Stubbs (1934) claimed that neonates' response activity would be proportional to pitch up to 4000 Hz, although earlier Marquis (1931) had demonstrated neonates' auditory responses using a buzzer presumably with low frequency emphasis. In fact, during the early 1930s, the subject of neonatal auditory behavior and maturation had attracted substantial attention. The nature of neonates' responses and the stimuli by which they could be elicited had been investigated by Pratt, Nelson, and Sun in 1930, by Marquis in 1931, by Haller in 1932, and by Stubbs in 1934. While a variety of signals has been employed, there does seem to have been a trend to higher frequencies. While early researchers used buzzers, clappers, and bells, more modern researchers have used complex signals such as one which descends continuously from 5000 to 200 Hz (Eisenberg et al. 1966). Roberts and Campbell (1967) preferred the sound of human heartbeats. It seems, however, that most researchers have preferred signals in the neighborhood of 3000 Hz. Downs and Sterritt (1964) used a narrow band of noise which peaked at 3000 Hz; Heron and Jacobs (1968), along with many others, preferred a tone frequency-modulated around 3000 Hz; Gerber, Mulac, and Swain used both tones and a narrow band of noise distributed around 3150 Hz. On the other hand, Ling et al. (1970) were unable to find stimuli of 3000 Hz any more effective than stimuli of 2000 Hz. Rudmose (1967) described an instrument using a frequency-modulated tone of 3000 ±150 Hz which varied at a 40 cycle rate. Feinmesser and Tell (1976), using a narrow-band signal that peaked at 3000 Hz, eventually concluded that this stimulus was not valid for screening. On the other hand, Bench et al. (1976 a, b, c) compared a wide-band signal extending from 200 to 5000 Hz at several levels to such other signals as narrow bands and speech. They concluded that a wide band was a more effective stimulus than the narrow bands at high sound pressures. Given the findings that high-frequency tones (or narrow-band noises distributed around a high frequency) seem to be relatively ineffective, the Nova Scotia Conference on Early Identification of Hearing Loss (Mencher, 1976) recommended a specific stimulus spectrum. For the test stimulus it recommended a random noise having a low-frequency attenuation of 30 dB/octave below 750 Hz, a maximum of 90 dB sound pressure level at the pinna, a rise-decay time of 5 milliseconds or more, a duration of 0.5–2.0 seconds, and an intertest interval minimum of 15 seconds.

Spectrum, of course, is not the only consideration and, undoubtedly, the primary consideration is the intensity of the signal. After all, what we want to know in audiometry is how quiet a signal can be heard. Neonates seem to be uninterested in quiet sounds. Consequently, using behavioral procedures only, we can hope to discriminate only those infants who are profoundly impaired from those who are not. That is, we should expect to identify only those neonates who fail to respond to intense signals. Neonates' behavioral responses to sound depend on a high level of stimulation. Responsivity seems to depend on Pavlov's rule of force: strong stimuli elicit strong responses with short latencies, while weak stimuli elicit only weak responses with longer latencies. As early as 1932, Haller observed that infants' motor activity increased with intensity, although Stubbs (1934) claimed that such increased activity was irregular. More contemporary researchers (e.g., Eisenberg, 1969) consider the responses of neonates to sound to be intensity bound; rather intense signals apparently produce more reliable responses. Rudmose (1967) predicted that reactions from newborns would not be repeatable unless signals were in the order of 80–90-dB sound pressure level. Repeatability refers to test–retest reliability.

As in all other audiometry, the duration of the stimulus is significant. Not only is the duration of a given signal event significant, but so, also, is the number of signals required to serve as stimuli. Stubbs (1934) found that response activity was proportional to duration up to 15 seconds; that is, the longer the duration, the greater the response activity. Clifton, Graham, and Hatton (1968) observed that heart rate responses did not habituate for signals whose duration extended up to 2 seconds, but they did observe habituation for longer signals. Neonates seem to react to those stimuli which have rapid rise times and are of relatively brief duration (Gerber, 1971). Repetition seems to lead to habituation or adaptation; although Pratt, in 1934, observed signal repetition every 10 seconds led to a clearer response than repetition of the same stimulus every 60 seconds. Herer (1967) cautioned us to ". . . observe the first stimulus administered because, frequently, repetition of the stimulus is not helpful and often confuses the picture." What may eventually prove to be more interesting and important than either stimulus duration or interstimulus interval will be stimulus pattern. Eisenberg (1969) attached a great deal of significance to pattern-bound behavior, and this is a topic that merits a great deal of investigation.

The customary audiometric parameters—frequency, intensity, and duration—apply to infants just as well as they do to older children or to adults. They contribute independently as well as interactively. Equal loudness functions in infancy have not been determined, but one should expect them to have the same shape as they do in adults. One may also expect that infants would have greater sensitivity than older persons for extremely high frequencies; von Békésy calculated that we normally lose 80 Hz from the high end every 6 months of life.

RESPONSE PATTERNS

How can we tell if an infant's response is to the noise we make? While that appears to be a simple question, a moment's reflection points out that it is, in fact, fairly complex. We have raised this question previously (Gerber, 1969) by asking "What does the responsive infant do that the unresponsive infant does not do?" What, then, should be accepted as a response?

The most common and reliably observed response in very early infancy is the auropalpebral reflex. This response has also been called the cochleopalpebral reflex and the auditory eye blink response. The auropalpebral reflex (APR) is an example of a startle reaction, the presentation of sound eliciting an eye blink by stimulation of the auditory system. It has been said to be "the only consistent auditory reflex found in infants" and it is thought to be "dependent upon a normal auditory conduction and neuronal system" (Taft and Cohen, 1967). The APR was thought to be the most common response 30 years ago (Froeschels and Beebe, 1946). The major large investigations of the APR were those of Wedenberg (1956) and of Fröding (1960). Both of these scientists investigated infants during the earliest time of life. Fröding's 2000 subjects were all under the age of 30 minutes, and he discovered the APR to be a reliable response. In fact, Fröding's infants who consistently failed to exhibit an APR were neurologically impaired.

How can we tell that a particular eye blink is in response to a sound and not a random behavior? After all, we all do blink our eyes fairly often. How does the audiometrist in the nursery or well-baby clinic tell that this particular baby's particular eye blink is any way related to what he (the tester) did? It seems, a priori, that he cannot tell since the vast majority of eye blinks will occur whether or not one makes a noise. Ling, Ling, and Doehring (1970) masked the observers' hearing so that they did not know when a stimulus was presented to the subject infants. In this study, then, 70% of the recorded "responses" occurred in the absence of external stimuli. In other words, observers don't know which eye blinks are responses to sound and which are random.

On the other hand, if we employ the APR as a test response, and prepare an experimental paradigm which accounts for its apparent randomness, then these errors seem not to occur. For example, Mencher (1972) reported that the probability of mistakenly recording a response during a fixed observation interval was only about 3%; and if two observers agree, the error is thereby cut by a factor of 2 to 1½%. Furthermore, the probability of making the kind of error described by Ling, Ling, and Doehring drops essentially to zero if one follows Mencher's paradigm. Mencher requires that two observers record two motor responses during a fixed observation interval following presentation of a real stimulus. If the baby opens his eyes and moves a limb and if two independent observers note both movements within a few seconds, then one must call that a response. Subsequently, Mencher (1976), in reporting the recommendations of the Nova Scotia Conference on Early Identification of Hearing Loss, stated that an infant's response is any generalized body movement which involves more than one limb and which is accompanied by some form of eye movement. Furthermore, scoring of such a response must be controlled either by two observers' independent score or the scoring of a single observer who does not know when the stimulus is present. Still furthermore, all of these things must occur twice in eight consecutive trials for the infant to be cleared, that is, thought to be normal. When we discuss the APR—or, more appropriately in light of the previous statement, the arousal test—we are talking about responses which occur in early infancy. It is apparent that our willingness to accept 25% (two of eight) responses as clear indicates that there are many unknowns.

For a number of years the literature on audiometry for newborns has reported the Moro reflex to be a valid and reliable response to sound. It seems, however, that there has been considerable confusion between the Moro reflex and some other whole body startle responses. This confusion was evident, for example, in a statement by Newby (1964) that "the response of a newborn infant . . . is a startle or Moro's reflex." Similarly, Frisina (1963) included the Moro reflex among those responses that he considered to be readily observable. The issue is not whether an infant responds with the whole body startle but whether the true Moro response has anything to do with audition. Taft and Cohen (1967) concluded that "the Moro reflex occurs as the result of any sudden movement of the head and neck causing retroflection." Therefore, must current thinking would not accept the Moro reflex to be a valid response of a newborn to sound.

Other behavioral responses have been observed. In general, these behaviors have taken the form of some alteration of ongoing motor activity. That is to say: if the infant is moving, he stops; if he is not moving, he starts; if he is crying, he stops; if he is not crying, he starts; etc. The alteration, cessation, or beginning of motor activity is no longer considered sufficiently valid for clinical purposes.

For children beyond the neonatal stage, behavioral criteria remain to be established. Frisina (1963) reported that hearing infants should turn their eyes in the direction of the sound source somewhere between the ages of two and four months. Northern and Downs (1974) expect lateral head turning in response to sound usually before the age of six months, although Gerber (1969) reported the average age of head turning to be nearer 7½ months. Similarly, localization in a vertical plane should occur by the age of 1 year. These differences in age at which certain responses are reported to appear are likely not real differences but instead are differences of observers' interpretations.

Beyond the age of about 18 months, an infant's ability to localize becomes useful in its own right as an audiometric procedure. This involves the use of the so-called conditioned orientating response (COR), which has given rise to a method known as COR audiometry. Suzuki and Ogiba (1960; 1961) and Suzuki, Ogiba, and Takei (1972) have described and reviewed the use of COR audiometry with children aged one to three years. Making use of the natural visual orienting response, a child is conditioned to look at a toy, internally illuminated, which lights up approximately one second after an acoustic simulus (usually a pure tone) is presented (Fig. 5-1). This procedure is repcated three or four times for the conditioning to take effect when the child should look for the toy to light up if he hears the stimulus tone. Suzuki, Ogiba, and Takei suggested beginning the conditioning "about 30 dB above the estimated threshold . . ." The stimulus intensity is then reduced and the procedure repeated until hearing threshold is reached. They have reported latencies from ½–two seconds for the orienting response, and a success rate of more than 80% with children aged one to two years. Children over the age of three years do not test successfully with this method presumably because the task is uninteresting and too easy for them. When using the COR method one expects that conditioning would occur in three or four trails, but that the conditioned response would extinguish in about three more trials. Of course, COR methodology assumes that a lighted toy is a reinforcer for all subjects and that sound would become a conditioned reinforcer by three or four pairings with the toy. Not only does sound itself become a conditioned reinforcer, it also becomes a discriminative stimulus intended to evoke a looking response. Unfortunately, the toy doesn't maintain its reinforcing function.

Barr and Junker (1969) have described a similar technique using a rattle or jingle bell and a music box as they thought that pure tones would not hold a child's interest. They wanted to discriminate between simple "organic" hearing and the more integrated process of "functional" hearing. Therefore, they used a "distracting technique." This required making sure that the child's visual attention was occupied, and then distracting him with noise makers to observe an orienting response. Barr and Junker held that this type of orienting response insures "the intact capacity of interpretation and selection." It seems doubtful to us, however, that such a conclusion is really possible; orientation need not suggest interpretation.

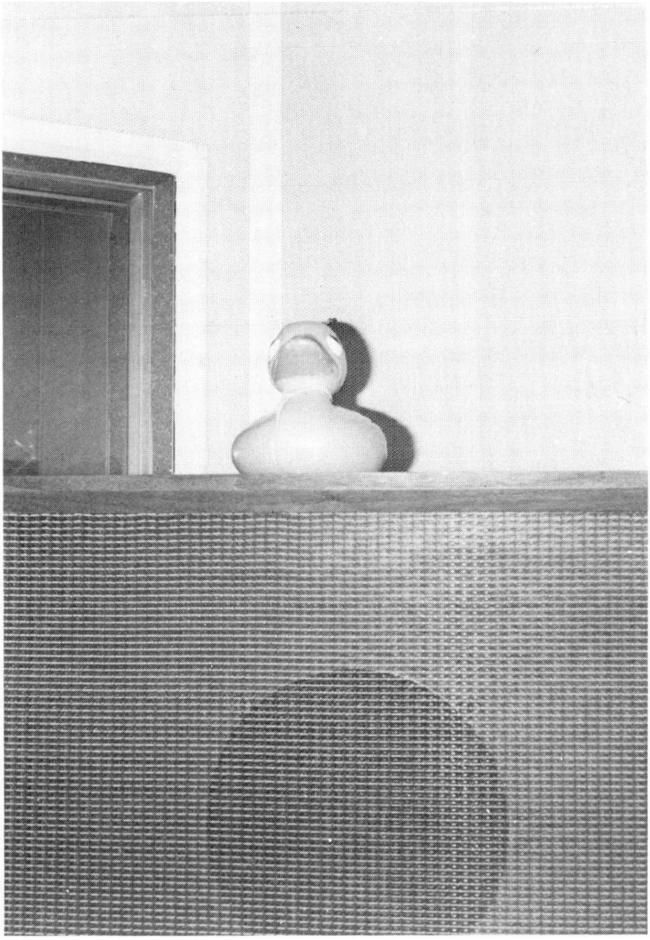

Fig. 5-1. Conditioned orienting response apparatus, the UCSB duck.

Miyazaki (1970) also developed a distraction procedure which he called the teddy bear test (Fig. 5-2). He built two toys with loud speakers, tone generators, and lights. They can be used for COR as well as play audiometry, and were employed with children from five months to two years of age and with older mentally retarded children. Miyazaki reports that the responses of female infants were more mature than males' responses; this was reported by Gerber (1969) also.

Tangible reinforcement operant conditioned audiometry (TROCA) is a more elaborate, and apparently more reliable, procedure for conditioned be-

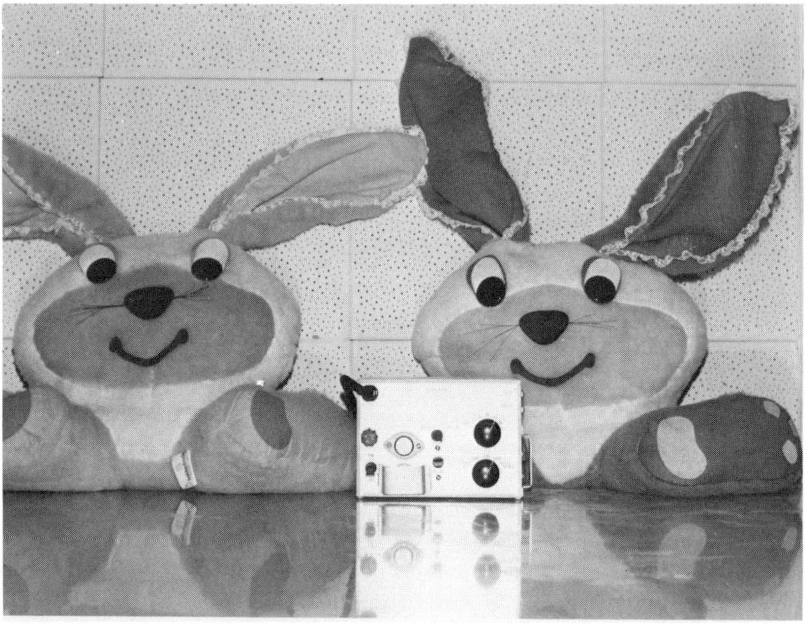

Fig. 5-2. A version of a teddy bear test, the UCSB rabbit-tone.

havioral testing of very young children or of persons with developmental delay. Described by Spradlin and Lloyd (1965), Lloyd (1966), Lloyd, Spradlin, and Reid (1968), and by Lloyd and Cox (1975), this technique has proved successful with the difficult-to-test patient and especially with the profoundly retarded (IQ<25). Essentially the same method has been employed with infants by (e.g.) Wilson, Moore, and Thompson (1976) who call it "Visual Reinforcement Audiometry" and who report 60% success at 5 months of age. The use of tangible reinforcers—whether candy, trinkets, or visible displays—has permitted behavioral testing of many patients who had not previously been considered testable. The first step in TROCA is to choose a reinforcer for the child to be tested. That may seem trivial, but what is reinforcing for one child may not be for another. Threshold testing proceeds using a reinforcement schedule best suited to the patient. Of course, rigidity has no place in this sort of testing as things may change quickly and a new reinforcement schedule or perhaps a new reinforcer may be needed. Sometimes shaping procedures are needed even to place the earphones.

For the child over two years of age, the peep show technique has been employed. Recommended by Dix and Hallpike in 1947, the peep show employs allowing the child to view a set of cartoon or puppet characters through a peephole as a reward for correct response. Illumination of the show is possible only when responses are made to actual stimuli. Green's (1958) version of this technique uses a moving toy, and is called a "pup show." Of course, there are many variations of this theme, and many clinicians have developed their own. One should be aware, though, that Hillis and Oyer (1960) could find no high correlations between chronologic age and test–retest reliability; maybe it works for some younger children.

ENVIRONMENTAL FACTORS

While the literature on infant audiometry, as on audiometry in general, concerns itself with the desirability of having an appropriate environment in which to conduct the tests, there seems to have been rather little concern for what makes an environment appropriate for infants. Even the recent Nova Scotia Conference (Mencher, 1976) dealt with the test environment only by saying that "the ambient noise level at the time of a typical test should be measured and reported." It has been recommended (e.g., by Feinmesser and Tell, 1976) that children who fail either behavioral tests or high risk screens in the newborn nursery should be followed at an audiology center. At the same time, many testers do perform their examinations not only in audiology centers, but in newborn nurseries, in well baby clinics, in pediatrician's offices, and wherever the child happens to be. Most of the standard textbooks on audiometry (e.g., O'Neill and Oyer, 1966) recommend that the sound field in which audiometry is performed should not exceed 50 dBA. We don't really know if 50 dBA is a proper level for the testing of the very young, as it is probable that their sensitivity is greater than that of an adult. Certainly this better sensitivity is well established by the data of the Pittsburgh Study (Jordan, 1971). Therefore, it may be that the environment in which we conduct our tests on infants should have lower maximally acceptable ambient levels than otherwise thought needed.

Other aspects of the environment have not been thoroughly investigated. Only Eisenberg (e.g., 1966) has considered variations of the environment as potential influences on responsivity on the newborn. Such things as temperature of the room, color of testers' clothing, number of persons in the room, etc. need to be considered. These kinds of considerations are less relevant, of course, for the older child except insofar as he may have a learning history with such variables. Nevertheless, one should hope that pediatricians' offices or well baby clinics or other environments in which infants would have their hearing tested would be reasonably controlled. One also hopes that experimental studies regarding the effects of variables commonly present during testing will be done.

INFANT STATUS

In general, by infant status we mean his state of arousal at the moment of the test. In fact, Bench (1969) has shown that responses of newborns may be elicited by modifying their state of arousal. Moreover, he observed that children under the age of six days will quiet more readily when stimulated by sound than when not stimulated. This same observation had been made by Birns et al. in 1965 and still earlier by Frisina in 1963. Bench (1970) has also cautioned that one must account for the law of initial values (Lacey, 1956) by noting the prestimulus state of the infant. Behavioral scales of activity have been attempted. Such descriptions vary widely from asleep versus awake (Lewis et al., 1967) to Brown's (1964) scale of (1) deep sleep, (2) regular sleep, (3) disturbed sleep, (4) drowsy, (5) alert activity, (6) alert and focussed, and (7) inflexibly focussed. No reliability has been reported across several observers using such scales.

In addition, the state of infant arousal can be described by monitoring various autonomic response systems. However, the terms "state" and "level of arousal" should not be used interchangeably as one refers to behavior and the other to autonomic status (Ashton, 1973; Prechtl, 1974).

BEHAVIOR OF OBSERVERS

It has been noted (particularly by Hamilton, Derbyshire, and Joseph, 1970) that the observer is part of the total test situation. In fact, Jazbi (1968) and Gerber (1971) have suggested that audiometric testing of newborns is best conducted with the observer located elsewhere.

Nevertheless, observers do seem to agree with each other fairly well. Earlier (Gerber, 1969) we have referred to "consensus audiometry" meaning that a response is recoded if the observers agree with each other that it has occurred. This was explicit in the Nova Scotia recommendations (Mencher, 1976) that two observers must independently agree on at least two occasions. Downs and Sterritt (1964) found very high interobserver reliability. That means that one observer seemed to be responding to the same thing as another observer. Remember, however, that reliability does not imply validity; it is possible that all the observers are making the same mistake. This was certainly underlined by the findings of Ling et al. (1970). Their observers also agreed with each other; but they were wrong more often than not. Hence, they concluded that "observers are likely to accept behavioral changes arising for other reasons as positive responses." Nevertheless, relevant controls, such as those in Mencher's (1972) paradigm, can be employed. It is for these reasons that the recommendations of the Nova Scotia Conference applied to the behavior of observers as well as other properties of the test and the test situation. It is curious, though, that no one has published a training program for observers since volunteers are used and there are studies on training observers for other things.

Clearly, beyond the neonatal period, the observer's behavior is explicitly part of the examination. It is not explicit enough in testing of neonates, although there is abundant literature on examining situations with young children. Most of us have found that children respond fairly well to normal conversation. One should be reminded in this context of the thoughtful admonition of Dale (1962) that one should smile at the child and one should also smile at his mother; she is frightened too.

REFERENCES

Ashton R: The state variable in neonatal research: A review. Merrill-Palmer Q Behav Dev 19:1–9, 1973

Barr B, Junker KS: Functional Contact Test for Babies as a Screening Method. Stockholm, Lekatekek Pa Blockhusudden, 1969

Bench RJ: Audio-frequency and audio-intensity discrimination in the human neonate. Int Audiol 8:615–625, 1969

Bench RJ: The law of initial value: A neglected source of variance in infant audiometry. Int Audiol 9:314–322, 1970

Bench J, Collyer Y, Mentz L, et al: Studies in infant behavioural audiometry: I. Neonate. Audiology 15:85–105, 1976

Bench J, Collyer Y, Mentz L, et al: Studies in infant behavioural audiometry: II. Six-week-old infants. Audiology 15:302–314, 1976

Bench J, Collyer Y, Mentz L, et al: Studies in infant behavioural audiometry: III. Six-month-old infants. Audiology 15:384–394, 1976

Birns B, Blank M, Bridger WH, et al: Behavioral inhibition in neonates produced by auditory stimuli. Child Dev 36:639–645, 1965

Brown JL: States in newborn infants. Merill-Palmer Q Behav Dev 10, 313–327, 1964

Clifton RK, Graham FK, and Hatton HM: Newborn heart-rate response and response habituation as a function of simulus duration. J Exp Child Psychol 6:265–278, 1968

Dale D: Applied Audiometry for Children. Springfield, IL, Thomas, 1962

Dix MR, Hallpike CS: The pup show: A new technique for pure tone audiometry in children. Br Med J 2:719–723, 1947

Downs MP, Sterritt GM: Identification audiometry in neonates: a preliminary report. J Aud Res 4:69–80, 1964

Eisenberg RB: Auditory behavior in the human neonate. A paper presented at the biennial meeting of the Society for Research in Child Development, Minneapolis, 1965

Eisenberg RB: Auditory behavior in the human neonate: Functional properties of sound and their ontogenetic implications. Int Audiol 8:34–45, 1969

Eisenberg RB, Coursin DB, and Rupp NR: Habituation to an acoustic pattern as an index of differences among human neonates. J Aud Res 6:239–248, 1966

Feinmesser M, Tell L: Neonatal screening for detection of deafness. Arch Otolaryngol 102:297–299, 1976

Frisina R: Measurement of hearing in children, in Jerger JF (ed.): Modern Developments in Audiology. New York, Academic, 1963

Fröding CA: Acoustic investigation of newborn infants. Acta Otolaryngol 52:31–40, 1960

Froeschels E, Beebe H: Testing the hearing of newborn infants. Arch Otolaryngol 44:710–714, 1946

Gerber SE: Auditory behavioral responses of some hearing infants. Volta Rev 71:340–346, 1969

Gerber SE: Neonatal auditory testing: A review, in Cunningham GC (ed): Conference on Newborn Hearing Screening, Berkeley, California Department of Health, 1971

Gerber SE, Mulac A, Swain BJ: Idiosyncratic cardiovascular response of human neonates to acoustic stimuli. J Am Audiol Soc 1:185–191, 1976

Green DS: The pup-show: A simple inexpensive modification of the peep-show. J Speech Hear Dis 23:118–120, 1958

Haller MW: The reactions of infants to changes in the intensity and pitch of pure tones. J Genet Psychol 40:162–180, 1932

Hamilton LR, Derbyshire AJ, Joseph ME: Testing variables in infant audiometry. Paper presented to the annual convention of the American Speech and Hearing Association, New York, 1970

Herer GR: Evaluation of hearing in infants and young children. Clin Proceed Children's Hospital of Washington 23:18–33, 1967

Heron TG, Jacobs R: A physiological response of the neonate to auditory stimulation. Int Audiol 7:41–47, 1968

Hillis JW, Oyer HJ: Success of play audiometry as a function of chronological age. Paper presented to the American Speech and Hearing Association, Los Angeles, 1960

Jazbi B: Audiometry for children. Film presented to the Ninth International Congress of Audiology, London, 1968

Jordan RE: Symposium: Conservation of hearing in children. Trans Am Acad Ophthalmol Otolaryngol 76:340–342, 1971

Lacey JI: The evaluation of autonomic responses: Toward a general solution. Ann NY Acad Sci 67:123–164, 1956

Lewis M, Bartels B, Goldberg S: State as a determinant of infants' heart rate response to stimulation. Science 155:486–488, 1967

Ling D, Ling AH, Doehring DG: Stimulus, response, and observer variables in the auditory screening of newborn infants. J Speech Hear Res 13:9–18, 1970

Lloyd LL: Behavioral audiometry viewed as an operant procedure. J Speech Hear Dis 31:128–135, 1966

Lloyd LL, and Cox BP: Behavioral audiometry with children, in Glasscock M (ed): Sensorineural hearing loss in children. Otolaryngol Clin North Am 8:89–107, 1975

Lloyd LL, Spradlin JE, Reid MJ: An operant audiometric procedure for difficult-to-test patients. J Speech Hear Dis 33:236–245, 1968

Marquis DP: Can conditioned responses be conditioned in the newborn infant? J Genet Psychol 39:479–492, 1931

Mencher GT: The University of Nebraska neonatal hearing project. Paper presented to the Eleventh International Congress of Audiology, Budapest, 1972

Mencher GT (ed): Early Identification of Hearing Loss. Basel, Karger, 1976.

Miyazaki K: Teddy-bear screening audiometry for infants and mentally retarded children. Paper presented to the Tenth International Congress of Audiology, Dallas, 1970

Newby HA: Audiology, 2nd ed. New York, Appleton, 1964

Northern JL, Downs MP: Hearing in Children. Baltimore, Williams and Wilkins, 1974

O'Neill JJ, Oyer HJ: Applied Audiometry. New York, Dodd, Mead, 1966

Pratt KC: The effects of repeated auditory stimulation upon the general activity of newborn infants. J Genet Psychol 44:96–116, 1934

Pratt KC, Nelson AK, Sun KH: The Behavior of the Newborn Infant. Columbus, Ohio State Univ Pr, 1930

Prechtl HFR: The behavioral states of the newborn infant (a review). Brain Res 76:185–212, 1974

Roberts B, Campbell D: Activity in newborns and the sound of a human heart. Psychonom Sci 9:339–340, 1967

Rudmose W: Audiometric screening of the newborn. J Acoust Soc Am 41:868, 1967

Spradlin JE, Lloyd LL: Operant conditioning audiometry with low level retardates: A preliminary report, in Lloyd LL, Frisina DR (eds): The Audiological Assessment of the Mentally Retarded: Proceedings of a National Conference. Parsons, KS, Parsons State Hospital and Training Center, 1965

Stubbs EM: The effect of the factors of duration, intensity, and pitch of sound stimuli on the response of newborn infants. University of Iowa Studies on Child Welfare, #9, 1934

Suzuki T, Ogiba Y: A technique of pure tone audiometry for children under three years of age. Conditioned orienting reflex (C.O.R.) audiometry. Rev Laryngol Otol Rhinol (Bord) 81:33–43, 1960

Suzuki T, Ogiba Y: Conditioned orientation reflex audiometry. Arch Otolaryngol 74:192–198, 1961

Suzuki T, Ogiba Y, Takei T: Basic properties of conditioned orientation reflex audiometry. Minerva Otolaringolog 22:181–186, 1972

Taft LT, Cohen HJ: Neonatal and infant reflexology, in Hellmuth J (ed): Exceptional Infant, Vol. I. The Normal Infant. New York, Brunner/Mazel, 1967

Turkewitz G, Birch HG, Cooper KK: Patterns of response to different auditory stimuli in the human newborn. Develop Med Child Neurol 14:487–491, 1972

Wedenberg E: Auditory tests on newborn infants. Acta Otolaryngol 46:446–461, 1956

Wilson WR, Moore JM, Thompson G: Sound-field auditory thresholds of infants utilizing visual reinforcement audiometry. Paper presented at the annual convention of the American Speech and Hearing Association, Houston, 1976

Barbara K. Cone
and Sanford E. Gerber

6
Impedance Measurements

Because it is interposed between the source of an acoustic signal and the cochlea, the middle ear is of importance when one attempts to define the actual input to the cochlea (Weiss et al., 1962). Some of the elements of the middle ear, the stapedius muscle and its ossicular attachments, are involved in a reflex which is elicited by acoustic stimulation. Because the neural pathway of this reflex involves the lower afferent portions of the auditory tract, an understanding of its dynamics can be used to further one's knowledge of normal and pathological auditory function. For example, measurement of the acoustic reflex has been used clinically to discern the existence of a conductive lesion, as an objective measure of adaptation and recruitment, as an index of an individual's susceptability to noise, as a test of neonates' hearing acuity, and as a diagnostic indicator of brain stem lesions (Lilly, 1972). In addition, it has been used to validate and explain auditory phenomena such as critical bandwidths (Flottorp et al., 1971) and temporal summation (Djupesland and Zwislocki, 1971).

The tympanic muscles, tensor tympani and stapedius, are the smallest muscles of the human body. They are pennate muscles that consist of short fibers running obliquely to impinge on a tendon midline. Because of this structure, the muscles have capacity for exerting great tension, with very little linear displacement. The tensor tympani traverses the lumen of the tympanic cavity in a lateral direction and attaches to the manubrium of the malleus, which in turn is imbedded in the tympanic membrane. Upon tensor tympani contraction, the tympanic membrane is pulled medially and anteriorly into the middle ear cavity. The origin of the stapedius is on the pyramidal eminence

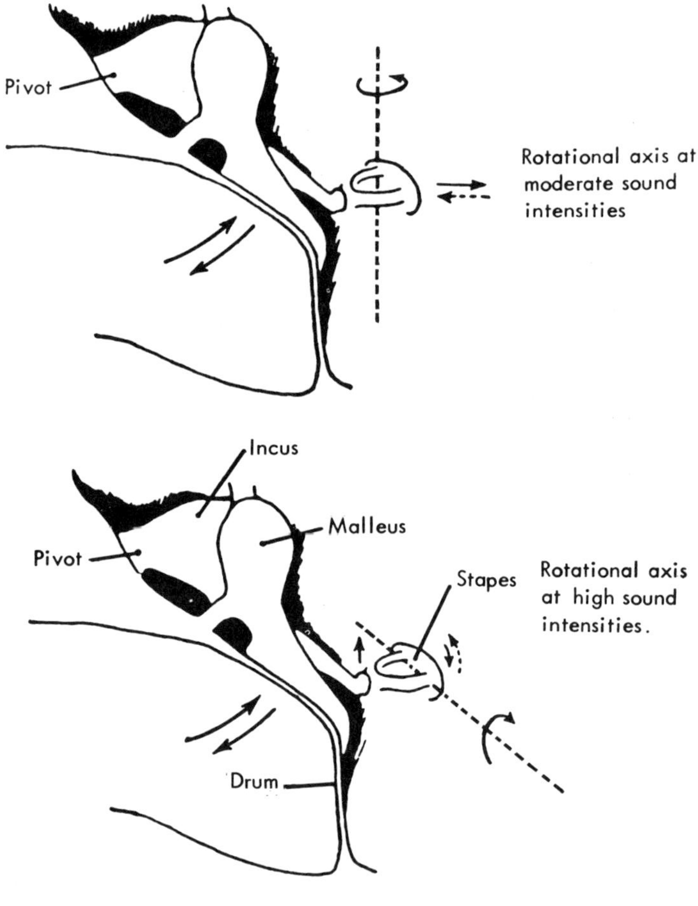

Fig. 6-1 Changes in mode of vibration of stapes as a function of sound intensities. (From: Zemlin W: Speech and Hearing Science. Prentice-Hall, 1971.)

on the posterior wall of the tympanic cavity. Its tendon emerges through an opening at its apex and inserts on the neck of the stapes. When the stapedius contracts, it pulls the head of the stapes sideways in the direction of greatest flexibility of the incudostapedial joint. When the muscles' contractions are simultaneous, they exert a force in opposite directions to one another and in a direction perpendicular to the primary rotational axis of the ossicular chain (Fig. 6-1). Dallos (1973) wrote that the innervation ratio of the stapedius—that is, the ratio of efferent nerve fibers to motor nerve fibers—was in the range of 1:5.6 to 1:3.5. This high innervation ratio makes possible fine gradations of contractions.

The ossicular chain functions to enhance the transmission of vibration from the tympanic membrane to the cochlear fluids. The ossicular chain is seen as a mechanical transducer of airborne acoustic energy to the fluid medium of energy transmission in the cochlea. The intratympanic muscles act simultaneously as a damping mechanism on the middle ear transmission system. Contraction of the muscles, elicited by acoustic or tactile stimulation, causes a reduced mobility of the ossicular chain. Though the contractions of the tensor tympani and the stapedius are anatomically antagonistic, they are seen as functional synergists for decreasing the sound transmission of the tympanic membrane and ossicular chain (Møller, 1972).

Goldstein (1974) has written about the function of the tympanic membrane and ossicles in terms of the mechanical linking which is provided between the tympanic membrane and the stapes to effect an impedance match between the airborne acoustic signal and the inner ear's fluid environment; without this mechanism there would be a 34-dB loss as sound traveled from the environment to the cochlea. He proposed three factors which provide for the impedance match: (1) the ratio of the area of the tympanic membrane to the area of the stapes footplate; (2) the lever system of the malleus and incus; and (3) the leverage that results from the curvature of the tympanic membrane and the manner in which it vibrates.

At rest this system has two natural resonance frequencies, 1200 Hz and 800 Hz. When the middle ear muscles contract, the principal resonance frequency (1200 Hz) is raised, resulting in a loss of transmission for lower frequencies which serves a protective function. The contraction of the middle ear muscles has been studied via electromyography (Simmons, 1964; 1965; Salomon, 1966; 1967) and extratympanic phonometry (Neergaard and Rasmussen, 1966), but most research used a change of the impedance of the middle ear as an indication of reflex activity.

When the force of acoustic events acts on the middle ear system, its components are set into motion. The amplitude of this motion is dependent upon the friction, mass, and stiffness of the system. The system's response to the force is twofold, consisting of a resistance part which dissipates energy, and a theoretical reactance part which stores energy. The vector sum of reactance and resistance is the impedance of the system. Since the driving force of the middle ear transmission system is a sound wave, the measurement of resistance and reactance to this force is called acoustic impedance. When input impedance and the cochlear microphonic are measured simultaneously in cats and rabbits, the magnitude of static impedance at the eardrum and the cochlear microphonic sensitivity curve are very similar over a significant portion of the frequency range. Thus, a measure of the impedance of the system, or a change of impedance caused by the contraction of middle ear muscles, is proportional to the sound transmission of the middle ear.

The exact change of impedance produced by contraction of the middle ear muscles is an increased reactive component, with increased stiffness. The resistive component may either increase or decrease. During contraction, the sound absorption by the middle ear is decreased and reflected sound energy from the drum membrane is increased. Dallos (1973) observed that the absolute magnitude of transmission change is not predicted with perfect accuracy from input impedance changes, but the alterations show a similar time course during muscle contraction. Thus, one is justified in using the recording of input impedance changes in order to measure the effects of middle ear muscle contraction.

Klockhoff (1961) used acoustic stimuli to attempt activation of the tensor tympani in subjects with some paralytic pathology of the stapedius muscle, and met with no success. Only an air jet directed at the orbital region of the eye was an appropriate stimulus for tensor tympani contraction. This middle ear reflex was habituated at a faster rate than a cutaneously elicited stapedius reflex, although cutaneous stimulation of the stapedius reflex caused faster habituation than that caused by acoustic stimulation. When using impedance measurement, or direct observation of the intra-aural muscles in human subjects, Djupesland (1963) found the cutaneously elicited stapedius reflex to be bilateral as it is when acoustically elicited. Except for reports which differentiate tensor tympani and stapedius responses to acoustic, cutaneous, and air jet stimulation, one can assume that unless very intense and/or unexpected acoustic stimuli are used, the acoustic reflex in humans is attributable only to the stapedius muscle. Thus, the term acoustic reflex has been used interchangeably with stapedius reflex.

The acoustic reflex in man has been studied in a population of normally hearing subjects in order to determine its exact functional nature. Its characteristic responses can be related to psychophysical data, as well as data from subjects with pathology of the peripheral auditory mechanism. Although some studies present normative data for threshold, dynamic range, and adaptation of the reflex, they are limited in their application because of the small number of subjects used. Differences in the sensitivity of the measuring equipment and stimuli used to elicit the reflex also make comparison difficult. Results must emphasize the frequency dependence and adaptation functions of the reflex threshold and the linear relationship of the magnitude of the response to the intensity of the stimulus over a designated range.

ACOUSTIC AND PSYCHOPHYSICAL CORRELATES

Psychophysical, as well as direct, measurements of the sound transmission of the middle ear have been made during contraction of the middle ear muscles in order to relate the physiology of the acoustic reflex to its functions.

By comparing results of studies which elucidate the attenuation properties with those which discuss the threshold growth and latency functions of the reflex, one can see that the reflex is most efficient at attenuating low frequencies, where it has the lowest thresholds, the most linear growth function, and the greatest resistance to decay. This evidence leads to a model in which the reflex works as a feedback regulator for acoustic stimuli in the lower part of the frequency range (Hung and Dallos, 1972).

Rather than ascribing a protective role to the action of the middle ear muscles in response to auditory stimuli, Simmons (1964) described the reflex as part of an orienting response. This is an observation especially relevant to infants. Low frequency attenuation was seen to be a masker of biological noise such that an organism could determine the source of a signal to be external or internal. Related to this was the observation that middle ear muscle contractions precede other somatic muscle activities, such as chewing or vocalization, and are maintained throughout the activity. Again seen as a signal-to-noise ratio improver, the contraction would be a valuable mechanism for animals that must graze and be alert to environmental noise, or in animals that must separate their own signals from those of the environment, such as the bat. For humans, the attenuation of both air- and bone-conducted low frequency sounds of the speech act via muscle contraction was also seen as a valuable signal-to-noise ratio improver. Because the environment does not usually provide the intense stimuli for which the acoustic reflex could protect the cochlea, and because the latency of the reflex does not contribute to a protective theory, Simmons' conclusions about the roles of the acoustic reflex provide an interesting view of its dynamics.

Clinical Application

Though the neuroanatomy, neurophysiology, and psychophysics of the acoustic reflex in man are incompletely understood, measurement of the phenomenon by impedance change is a valuable diagnostic tool in clinical audiology. Observation of the acoustic reflex in the clinical setting has added not only many normative data but also contributed new insights about processing in the peripheral auditory systems of normal and pathological subjects.

Anderson, Jepson, and Ratjen (1962) stated that an intact and mobile ossicular chain is prerequisite for acoustic or tactile elicitation of the stapedial muscle contraction. Thereafter, Feldman (1964), Djupesland (1969), Klockhoff (1971), and Lilly (1972) observed that the absence of an acoustic reflex is an indication of the presence or absence of middle ear pathology. Reflexes cannot be elicited when the middle ear mechanism is altered as with ossicular chain disruption or fixation, otosclerosis, or severe adhesive otitis media. They are absent even in subjects demonstrating moderately subnormal intratympanic pressures. Completing this comparison, stapedius paralysis, ossicular disruption, stapes ankylosis, or pathology that inhibits movement of the malleus are differentially diagnosed. McCandless (1972) noted, however, that reflexes could be measured in patients with middle ear pathology such as stapes fracture, monomeric tympanic membrane, and patent Eustachian tube; also that reflexes were present, absent, or reduced by diseases such as otosclerosis, otitis media, or other Eustachian tube dysfunction. He cautioned that reflex measures must be clarified by considering the results of the static impedance measure and tympanometry. Wilber (1972) also stressed the need to couple reflex measures with the static compliance and tympanometric tests for differential diagnosis.

Jerger (1970), Jerger et al. (1972) and Jerger et al. (1974a) collected acoustic reflex data on patients seen for audiological evaluations, and from them developed norms for a clinical population. When the population considered encompassed an age range of ten months to 81 years (sic) the modal hearing threshold level for elicitation of the reflex was 85 dB SL with a distribution around this mode of 40 dB. There was a tendency for the distribution of reflex thresholds to narrow and sharpen as the age of the subjects increased, and there was an increasing number of ears which showed a reflex with increasing age. Later studies defined 65–105 dB as the hearing threshold level needed to elicit a reflex in 99% of subjects with normal hearing or sensory-neural hearing losses. If the amount of sensory-neural loss was less than 60 dB, the percentage of absent reflexes was low; as the hearing loss increased, so did the number of missing reflexes. An air–bone gap as small as 10 dB indicates conductive pathology which could prohibit measure of a stapedius reflex.

In 1952, Metz found good agreement between results of binaural loudness balance tests and acoustic reflex threshold measures (Jepsen, 1963). Alberti (1972) measured the thresholds of the stapedius reflex in patients with Ménière's disease or another sensory type of hearing loss. Comparison of acoustic reflex thresholds and pure tone sensitivity thresholds showed that the gap between the pure tone audiometric threshold and the reflex threshold was much less in subjects with cochlear pathology than it was in normal hearing subjects; i.e., a patient with Ménière's disease or sensory hearing loss demonstrates an acoustic reflex at a lower sensation level. Alberti also found that reflex thresholds were not elevated beyond 30 dB of thresholds measured in the normally hearing subject, regardless of the amount of hearing loss of the pathologic ear. He concluded that, though loudness recruitment is believed to be demonstrated only by a loudness balance test, an acoustic reflex threshold measured at a lower sensation level than normal has clinical utility for the detection of recruitment.

Reasoning that the presence of an acoustic reflex was directly dependent on the physical integrity of the cochlear structures, Norris et al. (1974) looked for an alteration of the acoustic reflex response to be indicative of anomalies of the cochlear mechanism. They used pulsed stimuli at reflex threshold and at 10 and 35 dB above the reflex threshold, and calculated the amount of reflex relaxation that was produced by such stimuli. Reflex relaxation was defined as the amount of amplitude displacement of the pulsed component divided by the total reflex amplitude. Whereas normally hearing subjects showed different percentages of reflex relaxation according to the sensation level of the stimulus, subjects with hearing losses had a diminished and unchanging reflex relaxation ratio. There was no correlation between the slope of the audiogram and the reflex relaxation ratio. However, because of the smaller reflex relaxation ratios for the hearing-impaired group, the measure was thought to have efficacy for identifying those with hearing loss of a moderate or more severe degree (Letein and Bess, 1975).

Though both the reflex relaxation ratio and loudness summation tests at best suggest the possibility of hearing loss, it has been proposed that they be used for the testing of subjects who cannot respond to pure tone audiometric testing; the very young child is an obvious candidate. The literature on acoustic reflex testing of children and infants, however, reveals problems which preclude the use of these methods as predictive measures.

Impedance Measures in Children

Brooks (1971), in his study of children aged 4–11 years, wrote that subjects who exhibit a reflex threshold of 95 dB HTL or less were normal for middle ear function, but that only 70% of his subjects demonstrated normality in this way. Jerger (1970) reported a high incidence of middle ear disease detected by abnormal tympanograms and absent reflexes in a group of subjects aged two to five years. When reflexes were recorded, the children showed a higher mean threshold level than an adult group, with greater variability of threshold values. Later research (Jerger et al., 1974d), using a population aged three months to six years, indicated two systematic changes with age: the first was an increasing number of reflexes at lower hearing threshold levels as age increased; the second was a decreased number of missing reflexes at any level with increasing age. Habener and Snyder (1974) also recorded higher mean acoustic reflex threshold levels in the first two decades of life as compared to the last two decades in a population of subjects aged 3 years to 68 years.

Robertson, Peterson, and Lamb (1968) found reflexes in only three of ten subjects tested who were 12 months old. Other findings were that mean reflex threshold values were the same for age groups consisting of 12-, 18-, 24-, and 36-month old children. The greatest variability of reflex thresholds was seen in children aged 24–36 months. Absence of reflexes in the very young children was speculated to result from unknown maturational factors of the reflex arc, or even undetected middle ear pathology (Jerger et al., 1974d) though tympanometric and static compliance measures were made on these subjects and found to be normal.

The data on measurement of acoustic reflexes in children less than one year of age have been even more elusive. Keith (1973, 1976) attempted to measure reflexes in neonates of 36 to 151 hours and found that, in 160 trials, only 30% of these trials resulted in a clear reflex. Forty-four percent of the trials were inconclusive because of gross behavioral response that masked the measurement; but, in 26% of the trials, no reflex was elicited. Garrabrint, Robertson, and Biggers (undated) also attempted to elicit the acoustic reflex in neonates, and from a sample of 68 ears, only four exhibited a reflex. In the Margolis and Popelka (1975) study, acoustic reflexes for at least two activating stimuli were obtained from only 16 ears of a population of 14 infants aged 55–132 days. It should be remembered that most of these infants had normal tympanograms, though with high maximum compliances, but this was not seen as a factor which would prohibit measurement of a reflex. Instead, the lack of maturation of central nervous system development needed for an acoustic reflex was invoked to explain its absence.

In view of the data which indicate an inability to elicit or measure an acoustic reflex in infants and neonates, there is reason to doubt a statement concerning prediction of hearing losses from measures of the acoustic reflex:

> The technique is especially useful to us in confirming the presence of normal hearing in babies who, because of high risk or some other factor, have raised considerable apprehension in the mother . . . the fact that this can be done with a child of virtually any age, with or without sedation, in five to ten minutes with a minimum of difficulty, recommends the technique highly to those clinicians who are concerned with the accurate assessment of babies and small children (Jerger et al., 1974b).

Literature concerning the measure of acoustic reflexes in infants is ambiguous. Since the reflex measure is an indication of the afferent flow of information from the cochlea, with the potential of being predictive of hearing loss, the necessity for more data to be collected from infants is obvious.

Acoustic reflex threshold testing provides differential diagnosis of conductive and cochlear lesions, and is useful for the testing of subjects not considered testable by other audiometric techniques. One final area of utility may be the differential diagnosis of retrocochlear and other brain stem lesions, while anomalous reflex patterns have been used in the identification of normal hearing carriers of genes for deafness (Anderson and Wedenberg, 1968).

Developmental aspects of the acoustic reflex have yet to be clearly defined. It is ironic that a measurement which has been so highly praised as the solution to the problems of diagnosis presented by the infant (Jerger et al.,

1974b; 1974d) has not been studied with much success in this population because of the technical problems involved. Even when reflex measurement was successfully completed, the number of missing reflexes in the pediatric population, as well as the elevated reflex thresholds, raises questions as to what the normal acoustic reflex is in infants and young children. Not only must thresholds be studied, but other areas of the reflex behavior—latency, on-time, threshold duration, amplitude and decay of the reflex—have implication for the development of predictive tests.

It has been said that

> Measurement of the acoustic reflex adds an extremely valuable weapon to the clinician's armamentarium (Jerger et al., 1974c).

IMPEDANCE AUDIOMETRY IN INFANTS

A review of the literature on this subject reveals that, in very young children, norms for the static compliance of the middle ear are influenced in two ways. First, newborns have high static compliances which are probably due to tympanic membrane hypermobility and/or the relatively soft walls of the external auditory meatus. Secondly, norms which have been developed for children beyond the newborn period are probably influenced by a rather high incidence of middle ear disease which occurs in that age group and which decreases compliance. Further study of the body of published literature also reveals that most of the investigations have been concerned with rather broad age groups. As far as we know, only our own study (Gerber and Cone, 1975) investigated the range of compliance changes of infants' middle ears during the first year of life. The impetus for the study was this very lack of developmental data. In addition, rarely have acoustic reflexes been measured in subjects who are under the age of one year. Since the measure of the middle ear muscle reflex indicates the afferent flow of information from the cochlea, this measure is potentially indicative of hearing loss. Hence the necessity for more reflex data to be collected from infants was still another impetus for our 1975 study.

In that study, we attempted the measurement of static compliances, acoustic reflexes, and tympanograms on 31 infants, all of whom were younger than 14 months of age. The subjects were chosen from the caseloads of local pediatricians. The infants in the study were considered to be well babies on the basis of physical examinations by their pediatricians on the day of the impedance testing. A few infants in the study were not tested on the day of the physician's examination. They were examined otoscopically by one of us and a concommitant interview with the mothers cleared the infants for any recent illness. The children ranged in age from 5 days to 13 months. The data were

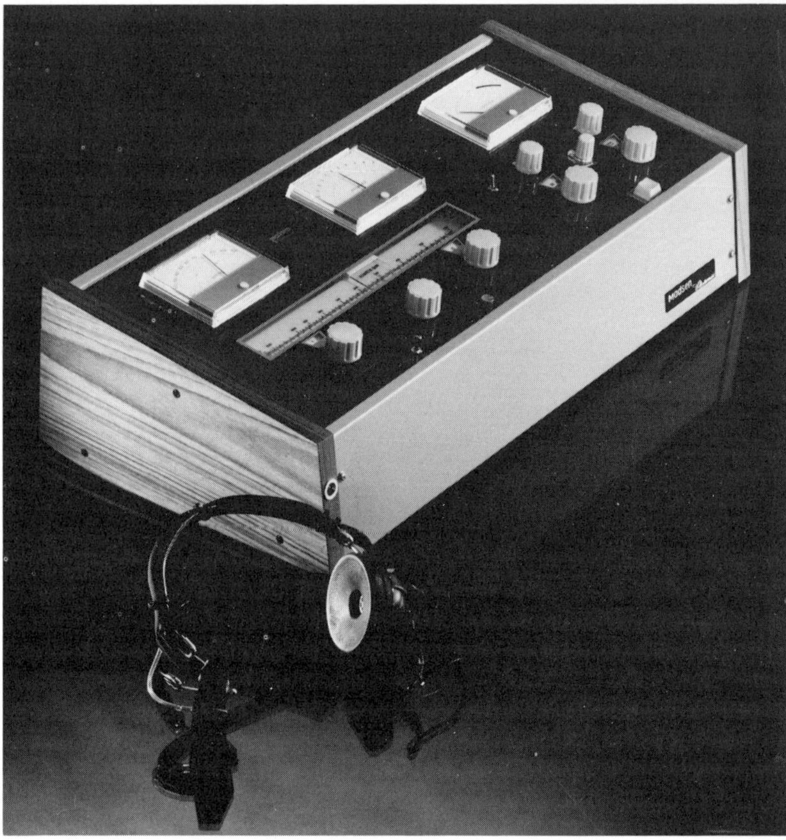

Fig. 6-2. Impedance audiometer. (Courtesy of Madsen Electronics.)

grouped accordingly: the three age groups studied were 0–3 months, 5–8 months, and 10–13 months.

For this study we used a Madsen Z072 impedance audiometer (Fig. 6-2). We modified this equipment somewhat by detaching the transducer housing with its tubes and probe tip from the headband. We also detached the earphone from the headband. The transducer housing was mounted on a ring stand so that it could be raised and lowered relative to the subject's head; hence, the only part of the bridge which touched the subject was the probe tip itself. The earphone was hand held on the ear contralateral to the impedance probe tip and acoustic signals were introduced through it. The stimuli were presented using an ascending approach to threshold. The lowest hearing threshold at which a positive needle deflection was observed after three approaches was recorded as the reflex threshold. The frequencies tested were 250, 500, 1000, 2000, and 4000 Hz.

Static compliance data were analyzed to determine the range and distribution of static compliance changes with age. Tympanometry data were tabulated to indicate the type of tympanometric functions recorded in each age group. The reflexes were analyzed in order to determine the mean reflex thresholds for each group, as well as to determine the existance of an acoustic reflex at all. The data collected in this manner are exhibited in Fig. 6-3. Overall, the range of static compliances was from 0.15 cc to 2.29 cc; the median compliance was 0.59 cc. In general it is observed that the median static compliance decreases as a function of age. For the youngest group the median compliance was 0.79 cc, in the 5–8 month age group the median was 0.35 cc, and in the oldest group the median was 0.39 cc. Furthermore, a median test revealed no significant differences between the median values for the two older groups, but these in turn were significantly less than the median compliance value for the youngest group. In other words, there is a significant decrease in the median and in the range of static compliances occuring between the ages of three months and five months but not thereafter.

Similarly, the number of each type of tympanogram which occurred in each age group was counted in order to discern the respective incidences and how they changed with age. These data are presented in Fig. 6-4. The type A tympanogram was the most common type of pressure-compliance function measured in our population, constituting 53% of all tympanograms. A contour which displayed an open-ended function in the vicinity of maximum compliance, which we called type A deep, occurred in 22% of the infants. A tympanogram with the pressure compliance function broader than usual and at least 1 unit wider than the normal type A, which we call type A wide, was found in 20% of the ears tested. Pathologic forms of the tympanogram were found in 6% of the ears tested: there was one occurrence of type B (indicative of serous otitis media) and two occurrences of type C (suggesting drumhead retraction) where the maximum compliance was measured at -200 mm H_2O. The largest number of tympanograms indicating highly compliant middle ear systems was found, as expected, in the age group from 0 to 3 months. About 30% of their tympanograms were of the A deep type and another 30% were of the A wide type. Nevertheless, the normal type A tympanogram occurred more often than either of the others. No A deep tympanograms occurred in the ten ears representing the group from 5 to 8 months of age. Nine of those ten ears displayed normal type A tympanograms and the other one was a type A wide. The B and C tympanograms occurred only in the oldest (10–13 month) age group, and that in only eight ears. The other tympanograms in this oldest group were all normal type A.

The predominance of the type A tympanogram, which indicates a normal pressure-compliance function according to adult norms, predominated in all the age groups. Nevertheless, there was a number of tympanograms indicative of very highly compliant middle ear systems. The largest number of

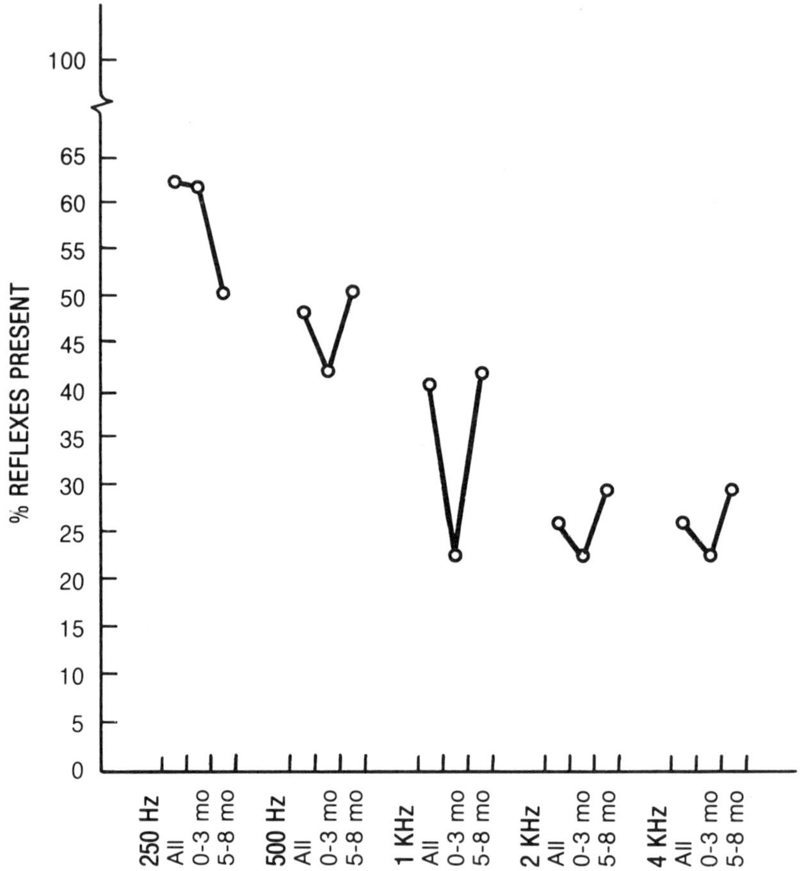

Fig. 6-3. Percent reflexes present.

these A deep and A wide tympanograms occurred in the youngest age group and accounted for 50% of all of their tympanograms.

The number of acoustic reflexes which we were able to measure at five different frequencies decreased as the frequency itself increased. Also the proportion of reflexes measured at any given frequency increased with age. More importantly, the mean hearing threshold needed to elicit an acoustic reflex at any frequency decreased with age. The mean threshold for all frequencies tested was 106 dB SPL (re 2 x $10^{-5} N/m^2$) in the youngest group; 97 dB in the middle group; and 98 dB in the oldest group. Again the two older

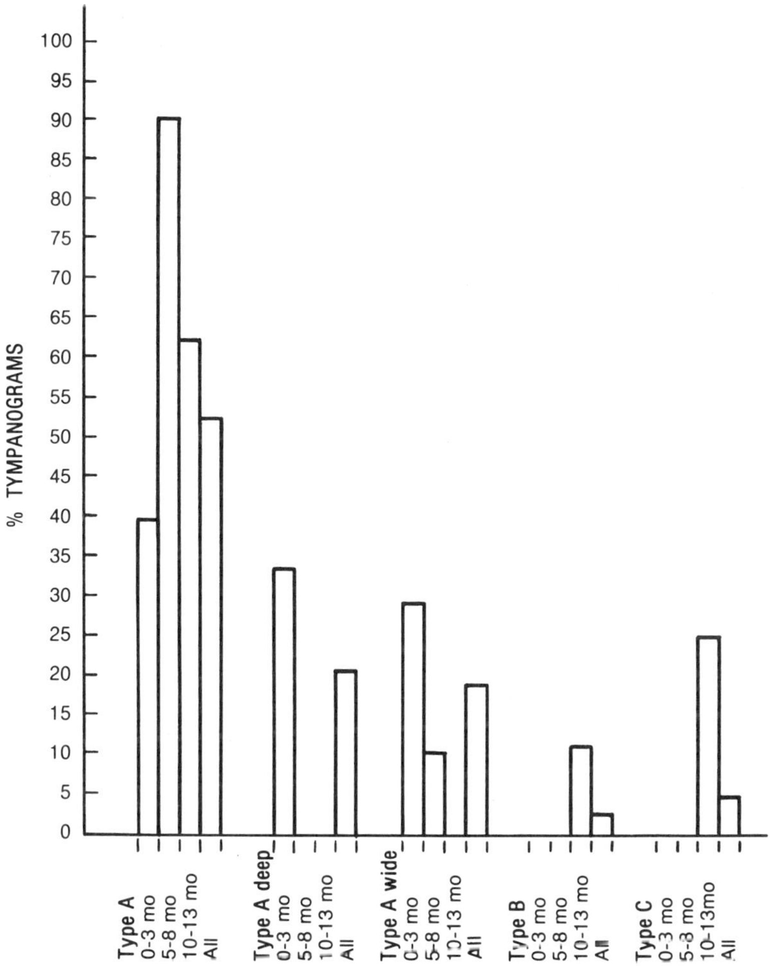

Fig. 6-4. Percent of tympanograms by type.

groups did not differ significantly from each other but they both differed from the youngest group.

Our conclusions about static compliance and about tympanometry are consistent with Keith's (1973, 1976) studies of the impedance in neonates in which he reported highly mobile middle ear systems in early infancy. Similarly our conclusions that the acoustic reflex threshold decreases as a function of age, and that the number of reflexes evoked increases with age, agree with data reported by Jerger et al. (1974b) even though their range of ages extended all the way up to 6 years. In general, we observed that the two older groups showed a rather restricted range of compliances and relatively low medians as compared to reports extant in the literature.

Perhaps most interesting was the fact that the pressure-compliance function recorded most frequently in the ears of these infants (type A) is the one defined as normal for adults. On the other hand, in the 0–3 month age group there was a very high incidence of tympanograms which indicated tympanic membrane hypermobility, and this occurred only in the ears of the youngest babies. This fact, coupled with the higher median static compliances of the youngest age group, confirms the notion that the hypermobility found in neonates' ears also is apparent in a population of babies up to 3 months of age. This is indicated additionally by the relatively high number of type A wide tympanograms in the same age group, although it did occur also in the 5–8 month old group.

CONCLUSIONS

The contribution of impedance data needs to be assessed. It has been observed that the static compliance measure does not rule out the pesence of middle ear pathology since values for pathologic ears overlap with values for some ears which have no evidence of pathology. Similarly the presence or absence of a reflex is not a clear indicator of pathology, as many infants with normal tympanograms have no measurable reflexes. Hence, developmental norms for the reflex need to be established in the infant population before the fact of its absence or presence can be employed as a diagnostic tool. Tympanometry, on the other hand, was clearly useful for the recognition of pathological conditions, at least in those cases where a type B or type C tympanogram was revealed. It seems also, at least according to our own data, that the type A deep tympanogram could be considered normal for infants under 3 months of age. However, it is important to observe that the incidence of this type of tympanometric curve diminished considerably as the children get older. As a consequence of that observation, the type A deep tympanogram may be considered suggestive of middle ear pathology in infants older than three months.

While there is still not sufficient data to establish developmental norms for any of the three impedance measures, one thing does seem to be clear:

there is an evident change that occurs after the age of three months. For this reason the user of the impedance audiometer should be forewarned that high compliances and moderately abnormal tympanograms ought to be expected in the very youngest population. However, using the same information, one should expect that children aged five months or older would adhere to the norms well established for adults. The impedance audiometer, then, is as useful a diagnostic tool in infancy as it is in adulthood.

REFERENCES

Alberti P: Stapedial reflex estimation and the loudness recruitment phenomenon, in Rose D, Keating L (comps): Impedance Symposium. Chicago, Zenith Hearing Instrument Corporation, 1972

Anderson H, Jepsen O, Ratjen E: Ossicular chain defects—diagnosis and treatment. Acta Otolaryngol (Stockh) 54:393–402, 1962

Anderson H, Wedenberg E: Audiometric identification of normal hearing carriers of genes for deafness. Acta Otolaryngol (Stockh) 65:535–554, 1968

Brooks D: Electro-acoustic impedance bridge studies on normal ears of children. J Speech Hear Res 14:247–253, 1971

Dallos P: The Auditory Periphery. New York, Academic, 1973

Djupesland G: Middle ear muscle reflexes elicited by acoustic and non-acoustic stimuli. Acta Otolaryngol (Suppl) (Stockh) 188:287–292, 1963

Djupesland G: Use of impedance indicator in diagnosis of middle ear pathology. Int Audiol 8:570–578, 1969

Djupesland G, Zwislocki J: The effect of temporal summation on the human stapedius reflex. Acta Otolaryngol (Stockh) 71:262–265, 1971

Feldman A: Acoustic impedance measurement as a clinical procedure. Int Audiol 3:156–165, 1964

Flottorp G, Djupesland G, Winther F: The acoustic reflex in relation to critical bandwidth. J. Acoust Soc Am 49:457–461, 1971

Garrabrint E, Robertson E, Biggers W: Tympanometry and acoustic impedance changes in newborns. (Unpublished paper)

Gerber SE, Cone BK: A study of impedance audiometry in infants. Paper presented to the Third Annual Convention of the Society for Ear, Nose, and Throat Advances in Children, Mexico City, 1975

Goldstein M: The auditory periphery, in Mountcastle V (ed): Medical Physiology Vol. 1. St. Louis, Mosby, 1974

Habener S, Snyder J: Stapedius reflex amplitude and decay in normal hearing ears. Arch Otolaryngol 100:294–297, 1974

Hung I, Dallos P: Study of the acoustic reflex in human beings. I: dynamic characteristics. J Acoust Soc Am 52:1168–1180, 1972
Jepsen O: Middle ear muscle reflexes in man, in Jerger J (ed): Modern Developments in Audiology. New York, Academic, 1963
Jerger J: Clinical experience with impedance audiometry. Arch Otolaryngol 92:311–324, 1970
Jerger J, Armstrong L, Jerger S, et al: Studies in impedance audiometry. III. middle ear disorders. Arch Otolaryngol 99:165–191, 1974a
Jerger J, Burney P, Mauldin L, et al: Predicting hearing loss from the acoustic reflex. J Speech Hear Dis 39:11–22, 1974b
Jerger J, Harford E, Clemis J, et al: The acoustic reflex in eighth nerve disorders. Arch Otolaryngol 99:409–413, 1974c
Jerger J, Jerger S, Mauldin L: Studies in impedance audiometry. I: normal and sensorineural ears. Arch Otolaryngol 96:513–523, 1972
Jerger S, Jerger J, Segal P, et al: Studies in impedance audiometry. II. children less than six years old. Arch Otolaryngol 99:1–9, 1974d
Keith R: Impedance audiometry with neonates. Arch Otolaryngol 97:465–467, 1973
Keith R: The use of impedance measurements in infant hearing programs, in Mencher GT (ed): Early Identification of Hearing Loss. Basel, Karger, 1976
Klockhoff I: Middle ear muscle reflexes in man. Acta Otolaryngol (Suppl) (Stockh) 164:1–92, 1961
Klockhoff I: Clinical use of ear impedance measurements. J Laryngol Otol 85:243–254, 1971
Letein W, Bess F: Acoustic reflex relaxation in sensorineural hearing loss. Arch Otolaryngol 101:617–621, 1975
Lilly D: Acoustic impedance at the tympanic membrane: An overview of clinical applications, in Rose D, Keating L (comps): Impedance Symposium. Chicago, Zenith Hearing Instrument Corporation, 1972
Margolis R, Popelka R: Static and dynamic acoustic impedance measurements in infant ears. J Speech Hear Res 18:435–443, 1975
McCandless G: Reflex measurement related to diagnosis, in Rose D, Keating L (comps): Impedance Symposium. Chicago, Zenith Hearing Instrument Corporation, 1972
Metz, O: Threshold of reflex contractions of muscles of middle ear and recruitment of loudness. Arch Otolaryngol 55:536–543, 1952
Møller A: The middle ear, in Tobias J (ed): Foundations of Modern Auditory Theory, Vol. 2. New York, Academic, 1972
Neergaard E, Rasmussen P: Latency of the stapedius muscle reflex in man. Arch Otolaryngol 84:173–180, 1966
Norris T, Stelmachowicz P, Taylor D: Acoustic reflex relaxation to identify sensorineural hearing impairment. Arch Otolaryngol 99:194–197, 1974
Robertson E, Peterson J, Lamb L: Relative impedance measurements in young children. Arch Otolaryngol 88:162–168, 1968
Salomon G: Middle ear muscle activity. Proc R Soc Med 54:966–971, 1966
Salomon G: On the continuous control of the middle ear muscle activity in cat. Acta Otolaryngol (Suppl) (Stockh) 224:218–219, 1967

Simmons FB: Binaural summation of the acoustic reflex. J Acoust Soc Am 37:834–836, 1965

Simmons FB: Perceptual theories of middle ear muscle function. Ann Otol Rhinol Laryngol 73:724–740, 1964

Weiss H, Mundie J, Cashin J, et al: The normal human intra-aural muscle reflex in response to sound. Acta Otolaryngol 55:505–515, 1962

Wilber L: Use of absolute and relative impedance in defining the nature of middle ear lesions in children, in Rose D, Keating L (comps): Impedance Symposium. Chicago, Zenith Hearing Instrument Corporation, 1972

Diane B. Gilchrist

7 Respiratory Measures

It has long been known that newborn infants respond to loud, sudden, and brief acoustic stimuli with changes of respiration. In 1882, Preyer isolated the auropalpebral reflex (APR), and noted the reactions of pupil dilation, nystagmus, facial and skeletal movement, and changes in respiration and pulse (Fröding, 1960). Canestrini in 1913 was the first to record infant physiologic responses to sound by recording changes in respiration and fontanelle pressures on a kymograph (Stubbs, 1934). In 1934, Stubbs determined that the rate of neonates' respiratory responses varied with changes in duration and intensity of pure tone stimuli. Suzuki et al. (1964) and Heron and Jacobs (1968, 1969) further demonstrated that changes in rate and pattern of respiration were observable responses to acoustic stimuli in newborn infants. Gerber and Gilchrist (unpublished) noted changes in rate of respiration associated with increases of intensity of filtered speech stimuli. Pilot research with two infants over a one year period at the Menninger Clinic (Bradford, 1975) indicated excellent test-retest reliability with pure-tone respiration audiometry at 1000 and 3000 Hz. Bradford suggested that respiration audiometry may be employed for determining neonatal and infant hearing sensitivity. In short, newborns and infants demonstrate measurable changes in respiratory pattern and rate when exposed to acoustic stimuli.

Most neonatal auditory screening programs—e.g., Downs and Sterritt (1967), Fröding (1960), Wedenberg (1956), and others—have been based on trained observation of infants' facial and skeletal movement or other behavioral responses to auditory stimuli. Hardy (1965) cited the failure of the behavioral observation method to differentiate the deaf or hard of hearing infant from others who are normal or abnormal. One viable alternative would be utilization of indirect measurements or observation of measurable physiologic responses to sound. Bradford et al. (1968) pointed out that respiratory changes accompanying auditory stimuli are useful for the indirect assessment of hearing sensitivity. Heron and Jacobs (1969) cited the increased sensitivity of neonates' respiratory responses to low intensity auditory stimuli and stated that a child may not exhibit a Moro or auropalpebral reflex. Therefore, a neonate may not appear to be responding.

The advantages of using recorded changes in respiration associated with an auditory stimulus as compared with other indirect methods used in the nursery, were summarized by Bradford, Rousey, and Bradford (1968):

> The advantages are that recording respiratory changes to acoustic stimuli does not require elaborate machinery, does not require extensive conditioning procedures or electrical shock, and it measures rib cage action which is difficult to suppress.

This might suggest that recording respiratory changes to measure neonatal response to acoustic stimuli might be a practical indirect method to use in the newborn nursery.

RESPIRATION IN INFANTS

Examination of neonates' respiratory cycles during the first few hours after birth has led researchers to conclude that rapid changes in breathing patterns occur as the infant adjusts to the new phenomenon of breathing. Normalization of respiratory function cannot be demonstrated until several hours after birth.

Reid (1967) has noted that the bronchial tree is developed by the sixteenth week of intrauterine life. However, the alveoli, as commonly understood, develop after this and increase in number until the age of eight years. According to Weibel (1967), at birth the organism has to shift from gas exchange from the placenta to the lung. The lung is structurally ready at birth, but the gas exchange apparatus has to grow concurrently with body growth. However, according to Purves (1967), "The peripheral chemoreceptors are, at birth or shortly after, mature . . ." so that, as Cotes (1968) has stated, the baby's respiratory apparatus normally adapts rapidly and totally to the stresses of extra-uterine life.

Investigators have noted changes in both rate and type of respiratory patterns in neonates. Desmond et al. (1963) stated that respiratory rate rose in an irregular fashion after the infant's first breath at birth to reach levels well above the norms of later ages. From birth to 15 minutes of age, a neonate's breathing is rapid and shallow. By 1 hour of age, there is a clear barreling of the chest, or an increase in the anteroposterior diameter of the chest. From two to six hours, respiratory rate is variable and related to activity. Data on respiratory rate from birth to six hours of age indicate that peak rates of respiration occur in infants from 15 to 30 minutes of age with a median of 82 breaths/minute and ranging from 50 to 108 breaths/minute. Individual low rates occur from 75 to 135 minutes of age with a median of 36 breaths/minute and a range of 20–56 breaths/minute. These rates are considerably higher than those reported by Deming and Washburn (1935, cited by Bradford, 1975) who found neonatal respiratory rates ranging from 24 to 76 cycles/minute, with a mean of 36 for females and 43 cycles/minute for males. Cross et al. (cited by Cotes, 1968) used a body plethysmograph and found that the frequency of oxygen exchange in normal neonates stabilized between five and forty breaths per minute. It may be concluded that neonatal respiratory rate is more variable and rapid than adult breathing rate, particularly during the first few hours of life.

Infants up to the age of six months seem to display predominantly abdominal and diaphragmatic respiration as contrasted with thoracic breathing, which is characteristic of adults. Even within the abdominal-diaphragmatic pattern, much variation has been observed in newborns as some thoracic breathing is also observed. Furthermore, vegetative breathing in infants may not display the regularity of respiratory cycles observed in adults who are at rest. Deming and Washburn also observed distinct normal breathing patterns in infants, in which inspiration–expiration cycles do not display the rhythmic characteristics of adult breathing.

It may be concluded that the respiratory apparatus adapts to extra-uterine life shortly after birth; but there is much variability in rate, type, and shape of pattern. Therefore, the individual breathing pattern of each infant subject should be carefully assessed before measuring changes in respiration as responses to acoustic stimuli.

PROCEDURES

State of the Infant

Because of the effect of bodily movement on respiration measurement devices, an infant should be at rest during audiometric assessment. This usually means that the infant is asleep. Does the depth of sleep—that is, light shallow sleep versus deep profound sleep—effect the regularity of infant breathing patterns?

Eisenberg (1965, 1966) postulated that auditory behavior of newborns is dependent, among other things, on the physiologic state of the subject. This is the infant's point on the activity state continuum or level of arousal. It was Canestrini who, in 1913, suggested that infants' respiratory patterns are more regular during light sleep. Heron and Jacobs (1968) found respiration patterns most regular during sleep that occurred 1½ hours after feeding. Bradford (1975) also preferred to test infants during the relaxed sleep that follows feeding. Gerber and Gilchrist (in press) tested sleeping infants ½ hour to 2½ hours after feeding. No observable difference was noted due to the amount of time post feeding as long as the infant was not awakened during the placement of the testing apparatus or during the testing procedure. Not all researchers, however, have limited infant respiration measures to the sleeping period. Suzuki et al. (1964) recorded infant respiration changes to acoustic stimuli while the infants were awake. However, if an examiner wishes to use a recording device measuring changes of thorax diameter, it is recommended that assessment be done during the period of least activity, as extraneous muscular movements can markedly interfere with recording procedures. Although the depth of sleep or amount of time post feeding may not have been established, this should not prevent an examiner from measuring respiration cycles that appear to be even and consistent for basal respiratory rate for an individual subject.

The Stimulus

The stimulus is probably the least defined variable in respiration audiometry. Although we know that infants do respond to acoustic stimuli by respiratory changes, the optimal stimulus for maximum change in respiratory rate or pattern has yet to be isolated. For this reason a review of a variety of stimuli used in various studies might be useful to the audiometrist.

Studies that are relevant to respiratory rate and pattern changes as measures of neonatal hearing acuity are: (1) those related to infant hearing testing in general; (2) those performed on adults' respiration changes as response; and (3) those few studies that have directly assessed hearing of infants by looking at changes in respiration rate or pattern. As studies using responses other than changes in respiration are discussed elsewhere in this book, only the highlights of the various types of stimuli used are discussed here.

Hearing testing of neonates, as reported by Fröding (1960), dates back to Pruger, who, in 1882, observed the auropalpebral reflex when exposing infants as young as six hours of age to "sudden short sounds," using various stimuli such as toys, hand claps, whistles, and tuning forks. Froeschels and Beebe (1946) studied the effects of pitch on neonatal response to sound using Urbantschitsch's whistles as stimuli. They concluded that newborns respond better to complex acoustic stimuli than to pure tone tuning forks. In recent years, newborn hearing screening programs have increased our knowledge of infants' responses to various stimuli. Fröding (1960) collected data on 2000 neonates within a half-hour of birth. Using a white noise stimulus ranging between 126 and 133 dB SPL, he observed the auropalpebral reflex (APR). Wedenberg (1956) used pure tone frequencies of 500, 1000, 1500, 2000, 3000, and 4000 Hz and intensities ranging from 50 to 115 dB in 5 dB steps to determine the optimum stimulus for evoking an APR in neonates. Downs and Sterritt (1967) used a frequency modulated tone of 3000 ± 150 Hz at 80, 90, and 100 dB SPL. Using paraprofessional or volunteer testers, various responses, such as APR and Moro's reflex, were observed on 10,000 infants.

Some researchers have examined responses to various stimuli to determine whether neonates can discriminate among acoustic signals. The results would, in theory, allow us to determine which stimuli would give us the most reliable results when performing infant audiometry. Most, but not all, research of this design has measured responses by the infants' APR or other observable changes in motor behavior. Such studies have left us with much contradictory information when selecting stimuli for neonatal audiometry. While Stubbs (1934) found changes in respiration as responses to variations in the duration and intensity of the stimulus tone, but no significant changes in neonatal response to various changes of pitch, other researchers disagreed. Wedenberg (1956) noted changes in the frequency of APR's in neonates due to changes of pitch. Downs and Sterritt (1967) found the greatest incidence of neonatal behavioral responses to a 3000 Hz tone warbled at ± 150 Hz, and at a 30–40 cycle rate; but Ling, Ling, and Doehring (1970) found no difference between a 2000- and 3000-Hz tone. Bench (1969) found significant audio–frequency discrimination in infants using an 85-dB pure tone stimulus at 200 and 5000 Hz. Neonatal audio-intensity discrimination using stimulus changes from 85 dB to 100 dB and back to 85 dB was not significant; yet Eimas et al. (1971), using habituation of a sucking response, noted that infants as young as 1 month of age can discriminate among speech sounds. Eisenberg (1965, 1966) concluded that, in addition to the effect of activity state, neonates can discriminate sound on the basis of bandwidth, duration, frequency, and pattern. Although researchers have come to varying conclusions about which acoustic parameters will evoke response, it appears that neonates do respond to differences in acoustic stimuli under certain conditions.

The wide variety of acoustic stimuli that has been used for testing neonates' hearing leaves the audiometrist in a dilemma. What is the optimal stimulus for infant respiration audiometry? Since so little research has been done using respiratory responses, the answer may well be in the preceding outline of various stimuli that have been used when measuring infant audition while examining non-respiratory responses. This leads to a very important question: can we conclude that stimuli which evoke maximal responses when observing other response classes will also evoke maximal responses when measuring changes in respiration? Presently there are insufficient data to make a conclusion regarding this issue. Although it may be logical to assume that infant responses will continue regardless of the stimulus, this is still conjecture. In the meantime, a description of stimuli and responses used in respiration hearing studies for all ages, and specifically those performed with infants, might be used as a guide when selecting stimuli for testing procedures as well as future research.

Respiratory Response Studies

Recent studies using respiratory responses have been described in some detail so that the audiometrist can model these procedures. Further details needed for replication can be found in the literature.

Poole, Goetzinger, and Rousey (1966) studied the effects of auditory stimuli on the respiration of 36 adults. They were particularly interested to see whether (1) respiration would be altered by changes in the intensity of the stimuli, (2) if the technique was valid when compared to voluntary threshold audiometry, and (3) if test-retest reliability could be obtained. Using the McNemar test of significance they found:

1. A significant slowing of the respiratory cycle of adults in the absence of tonal stimulation;
2. Greater slowing of the respiratory cycle for lower intensity sounds;
3. Respiration response thresholds which agree with conventional or voluntary thresholds;
4. Good test-retest agreement.

It appears that the use of respiratory responses is an effective measure of hearing thresholds in adults.

Teel et al. (1967) used respiration audiometry with 94 students between the ages of 7 and 21 years, all of whom had bilateral hearing losses. Assessing the degree of agreement between conventional hearing thresholds and those yielded by respiration audiometry, they selected a response criterion method as comparable measures. They concluded that the respiratory test made it possible to predict threshold within their selected criterion in 94% of the individuals tested.

Rousey et al. (1964) noted that respiratory rates seem to slow as the threshold of hearing is approached. Hence, responses to pure tone stimuli in respiration and conventional methods fail to show perfect agreement. This suggests a differential respiratory response (slowing of breathing) near thresholds, according to these authors.

A study using 381 subjects of all ages led Bradford et al. (1968) to conclude that "respiration changes in the presence of auditory stimuli can be a useful method for indirect assessment of hearing sensitivity." They also conducted a study comparing pure tone threshold levels obtained by respiration changes with those obtained by standard behavioral procedures with 29 preschool aged children. Using a mercury tube strain gauge pressure transducer to measure respiratory responses of expiratory phase, inspiratory phase, amplitude, and respiratory rate, they measured subjects' hearing thresholds at 500, 1000, and 4000 Hz. At 1000 Hz, in 85% of the cases it was possible to estimate thresholds within 10 dB of those thresholds given voluntarily, 81% of the subjects gave thresholds within 10 dB of those obtained voluntarily at 500 Hz, and 91% at 4000 Hz. In short, measurement of respiratory changes has been demonstrated as an adequate assessment of auditory threshold when compared to voluntary thresholds obtained from subjects of preschool age and older, including subjects with severe hearing losses.

NEONATAL RESPIRATORY RESPONSE STUDIES

Stubbs (1934) conducted three separate experiments on 75 infants from 1 to 10 days of age, assessing the effects of duration, intensity, and pitch on respiratory responses. She used a pneumograph consisting of a rubber air sack attached to a tambour, and was the first to use an audiometer in a study of neonates. She concluded that variables of stimulus duration and intensity yielded reliable differences in respiration rate and amplitude, but found no reliable differences in neonatal respiratory responses to pitch differences.

Suzuki et al. (1964) were the first in recent years to evaluate neonates' responses to pure tones and social sounds (a cow mooing) at 30, 40, 50, 60, 70, and 80 dB. They also observed auropalpebral responses and total body movement. Three changes in respiration were investigated: (1) changes in rate or depth of respiration; (2) decreases in regularity of respiratory movement; and (3) appearance of sudden deep inspiration. Their results indicated no significant difference between pure tone and social stimuli. Also, deep inspiration as a response increased in significance with stimulus sounds of 70–80 dB. The authors concluded that the most serviceable aural responses in newborns were a sudden deep inspiration, the auropalpebral response, and jerking of the body. Without exception, one of these three responses was displayed by each infant tested.

Heron and Jacobs (1968) have investigated neonates' responses to various acoustic stimuli in an attempt to discover viable alternatives to conventional infant auditory testing methods. Follow-up testing of 500 neonates at Bargwanth Hospital, South Africa, indicated 58% failure of correlation when conventional auditory testing was performed on infants at birth and again at one year of age. They tested 150 neonates within 7 days of normal birth and again at two and three weeks of age. Stimuli were five-second pure tones of 500, 1000, 2000, and 4000 Hz from 60 to 90 dB. Respiratory responses were recorded from a thermistor placed ½ cm from the nostril. They obtained the most consistent responses when two frequencies were exhibited alternately, for example, 200 and 500 Hz. In addition to recording respiratory response, body movement was observed. Heron and Jacobs isolated two important parameters for maximal neonatal respiratory response: (1) timing, one to 1½ hours after feeding; and (2) the optimal age for response, 7–14 days. The types of respiratory changes observed were increases or decreases in respiratory rate which bore no relation to the frequency or intensity of the stimulus; and breathholding or prolongation of inspiration, probably a gasp one to three respiratory cycles after cessation of the stimulus. Also, a respiratory response was elicited when no noticeable movement of the infant was observed.

Heron and Jacobs (1969) studied an additional two hundred infants using a four-second warbled tone at 40, 60, and 100 dB. Again, a thermistor acquired respiratory data. The investigators noted that respiratory changes were apparent, varied for each test tone in each infant, and from one infant to another. Respiratory responses most frequently associated with the stimuli were either a change in rate or a change in depth, the gasp reflex.

Gerber and Gilchrist (unpublished) studied respiratory rate changes in 15 neonates from eight to 72 hours of age. These babies were exposed to low-pass and high-pass filtered speech at 40, 60, and 90 dB. They concluded that the amount of respiratory rate change increased proportionately with the intensity of the stimulus. The direction of rate change (increase or decrease) was related to the intensity of the stimulus; the number of subjects who demonstrated an increment in rate increased as the intensity increased. Furthermore, the infants did not appear to discriminate between high-pass and low-pass filtered speech.

Bradford (1975) studied 25 newborns from 2 to 24 days after birth using pure tone stimuli at 1000 and 3000 Hz and respiratory measurement procedures similar to previous studies at the Menninger Foundation. Respiration thresholds at 1000 and 3000 Hz were 0 dB for all but one infant. When retested at four months of age the 23 subjects available for repeat testing displayed thresholds of 0 dB at 1000 and 3000 Hz. With a similar testing procedure for the fourteen subjects available at the age of 12 months, 13 of the 14 infants again demonstrated thresholds of 0 dB. Bradford stated:

> . . . normal infants during the first year of life demonstrated that pure tones alter newborn and infant's respiration patterns in a manner similar to that which has been observed with older children and adults. . . . This study suggested that respiration audiometry may be employed for determining neonatal and infant hearing sensitivity . . .

Up to this point, it has been presumed that the audiologist will measure changes in a subjects' respiratory rate or pattern to determine a response to acoustic stimuli. Such procedures require administering a stimulus, and then measuring a response by air pressure or thoracic changes which are graphically displayed. However, Kumpf and his associates (1966, 1968, 1970), working in Germany, have outlined an alternative procedure for assessing the respiratory mechanism's responses to sound by varying the stimulus, but more importantly, varying from the conventional procedure for measuring a respiratory response. He has tape recorded a subject's breathing sound as a response to both white noise and pure tone acoustic stimuli in both adults and neonates. This breathing sound is then used as stimuli for further testing of the subject. They describe a weakening of the breathing sound as a response when nearing a subject's threshold. Stimuli that are over threshold evoke responses of increased breathing sound. Kumpf has devised integrated level diagrams to aid in result interpretation. The audiometrist is advised to study Kumpf's works directly before utilizing this procedure due to the use of a recording procedure not in common use.

In summary, when selecting a stimulus, an audiometrist has a multitude of alternatives. One may wish to select a stimulus that has been utilized successfully in neonatal testing where nonrespiratory responses have yielded valid results. This would be based on the assumption that it is the stimulus, rather than the response recording technique, that is responsible for accurate measurement of neonatal acuity. Or, one may choose to use stimuli that have been used previously in respiratory studies with adults or infants and which have provided significant results for others. Hopefully, some audiometrists will choose to investigate the relationship between stimulus selection and respiration audiometry for standardized clinical application.

Apparatus and Procedures

After a stimulus has been selected, its presentation to the subject proves to be a simple procedure. If a pure tone stimulus is used, any portable pure tone audiometer may be introduced into the testing environment. If the acoustic stimulus is something other than pure tone, it may be recorded on any high fidelity, portable tape recorder. After the stimulus tape is prepared, the examiner can calibrate the intensity level from the tape recorder by use of an intensity measuring device. If the examiner wishes to use a stimulus tape recording, it is advisable to place interstimulus pauses directly on the tape. Interstimulus duration should be at least thirty seconds, but preferably closer to one minute. The inter-stimulus duration should be long enough to (1) allow respiratory responses to occur up to 30 seconds poststimulus (Suzuki et al., 1964), and (2) to prevent habituation or adaptation. It is possible, however, to present stimuli from either an audiometer or a tape recording by timing the interstimulus duration with a stop watch, as long as the stop watch is placed so that its click does not become another stimulus. Regardless of method, a standardized inter-stimulus duration will aid when examining results.

Infant respiration audiometry usually relies on stimulus presentation to one ear rather than two ears as with older subjects. There are two reasons for this. First, when an infant is asleep or at rest, usually only one ear is exposed. Second, it is not advisable or convenient to use the head band that attaches conventional headphones on the delicate neonatal skull. It is important, then, that a single earphone be handheld firmly in place over the subject's exposed ear. Some examiners prefer using a standard ear, such as always testing the right ear, while others will use whichever ear the infant has exposed. It is also a necessary procedure to place a sterile gauze between the infant's ear and the earphone. Free field testing is also acceptable, but calibration may not be practical if using portable equipment in the space available in a newborn nursery.

Recording respiratory responses to acoustic stimuli is again a simple procedure. Two major methods have proven to be popular. One is to measure changes in amount and direction of air pressure by changes in temperature or cooling of electrically heated wire directly from the babies' nostrils. This method (Heron and Jacobs, 1968, 1969) requires taping a thermistor within ½ cm of the infant's nostril. Heron and Jacobs cite the difficulty of air currents interfering with response recordings, and suggest that the thermistor may need to be placed within the nose.

The method that has become most popular in the United States is to measure respiratory responses by changes in the dimensions of a subject's thorax. A typical device used is a bellows type pneumograph. This pneumograph consists of a photoelectric cell, negative pressure transducer with a neoprene bellows, and an adjustable leather strap. The device is contained within an expandable rubber tube that can be comfortably placed around a baby's thorax. Girth measurements, or changes in the diameter of the rib cage, are monitored during inspiration and expiration. Data that may be obtained include changes in rate, time sequence, and respiratory patterns. This technique for measuring respiratory response was described by Ackner (1956), although he used an electrode connected to a mercury syringe rather than a photoelectric cell as a transducer. Ackner cited the disadvantages of other techniques of measuring respiration that would make them particularly undesirable for use with neonates. The spirometer requires a mouthpiece with a nose clamp. The conventional pneumograph is cumbersome and restrictive during inspiration. The principle of breath cooling electronically heated fine wires requires a support wire near the nose. Ackner cites the advantages of a thorax measurement device as:

> Because of its elastic properties, rubber tubing does not restrict the respiratory movements and is hardly noticeable to the subject. The sensitivity of the gauge is such that the slightest respiratory movement is immediately registered.

When using the bellows type pneumograph, Gerber and Gilchrist (unpublished) found it helpful to amplify the signal, using an E and M Physiograph transducer-monitor-coupler.

To record respiratory responses, any oscillograph may be used. Some require use of a manual event marker at the onset or the cessation of the stimulus, where other recording devices will mark this automatically. Hand examination of oscillograph recordings will permit study of both rate and pattern of respiration. If, however, one wishes to examine only rate, a computerized scanning device may be employed.

Placement of the pneumograph is a simple procedure. The infant is lifted by a nurse or an assistant while the examiner tightens the pneumograph around the infant's thorax. The placement of the pneumograph can be determined by observing the region of the thorax that shows maximal displacement as measured by amplitude on the oscillograph. After the infant appears to be asleep, the examiner may dust the neonate's eyelid with a sterile cotton ball to see if this will arouse him. If the infant is not awakened, the oscillograph and pneumograph may be started to collect normative respiratory data. When respiration cycles appear to be even and consistent, a basal respiratory rate may be recorded. Collection of an adequate and consistent basal response rate or pattern is most important as changes in poststimulus data will be compared to this prestimulus or basal period throughout testing. Once the basal respiratory data have been collected, presentation of the acoustic stimuli may commence. If the infant is awakened or displays bodily movement during testing, it may be necessary to cease testing, until he is again asleep or quiet. It is advisable to readminister baseline procedures at this time.

Interpretation of respiratory data may be accomplished in several ways, and the choice is determined by whether one wishes to observe changes in rate or pattern as responses to acoustic stimuli. Determination of respiratory rate change is calculated by comparing the number of respiratory cycles per time period exhibited by the subject before and after presentation of a stimulus. Respiratory rate is the frequency of inspiratory-expiratory cycles. One cycle equals one inspiration and one expiration. This may be done by calculating the number of cycles poststimulus and comparing this value to the initial basal respiratory rate, or by comparing the poststimulus rate and the respiratory cycle rate immediately preceding the stimulus. Most examiners have compared all poststimulus rates to the basal or pretesting respiratory data for ease of calculation.

The number of cylces needed or the amount of time to be recorded to calculate respiratory rate is a matter of question. According to Lipton, Steinschneider, and Richmond (1960) the minimum number of respiratory cycles needed to determine rate is a five second period before and after stimulation. In no case have we used less than a twenty second period to determine respiratory rate. After a certain poststimulus time, which varies from subject to subject, the examiner frequently notices a change in respiratory rate that tends to resemble the basal rate. This might be the point where changes in respiratory rate cease to be responses for a particular stimulus. Presently, however, there is no standard procedure for determining the number of cylces or amount of time to be used when calculating response or basal respiratory rate.

One advantage of using respiratory rate, rather than pattern, as a response is that it can easily be converted to a ratio or whole number integer to make intra or intersubject data comparable. These normalized or scaled data may be derived by the ratio, observation rate/basal rate, where observation rate equals the poststimulus respiratory rate in cycles/second, and basal rate equals average respiratory rate during basal measurement period in cycles/second. These positive integers allow comparison of data and ease statistical calculation of significance or correlation.

It should be noted that one is looking for a change of poststimulus respiratory rate, rather than an increase or a decrease. Most of the researchers in the field have found both increases and decreases depending upon the subject and/or the stimulus.

Calculating respiratory rate by hand counting pulses from oscillograph tracings is a long and tedious process. When one examines the respiratory cycle it appears as peaks and troughs representing inhalations and exhalations on a graphic representation. To determine one cycle, one may measure from peak to peak or trough to trough. To determine the rate, one counts per unit time the number of cycles by the rate of paper speed on the oscillograph. The use of a computer scanning method greatly simplifies this procedure. Using either method, however, does not eliminate a crucial question of data interpretation. How much does the poststimulus respiratory rate have to change (whether an increase or decrease) to be considered a response? Especially if the data are not statistically significant, it is up to the audiometrist to make this determination. Gerber and Gilchrist considered a 10% variation to be too strict a criterion.

A second area of data interpretation is the determination of change in respiratory pattern. Various researchers have presented characteristic shapes or graphic representations from oscillographs. Suzuki et al. (1964) observed decreases in regularity of respiratory movement and appearances of sudden deep inspiration when examining respiratory pattern changes. Heron and Jacobs also determined that breathholding or a prolonged inspiration one to three respiratory cycles after cessation of the stimulus is also a respiratory response. Bradford, in his book *Physiological Measures of the Audio-Vestibular System* (1975), has outlined a number of characteristic wave patterns that occur as respiratory responses to acoustic stimuli that have been

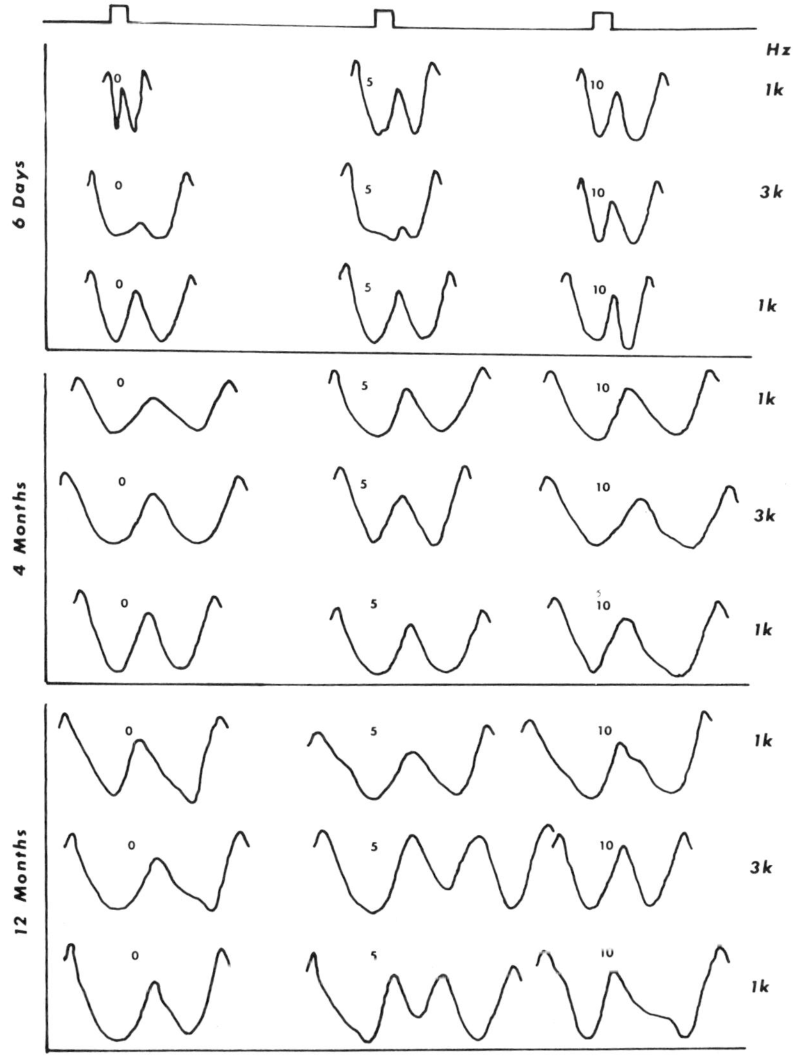

Fig. 7-1. Respiratory responses. Test–retest respiration alterations from 1- and 3-kHz pure tones presented through an earphone to the right ear of an infant at 6 days, at 4 months, and at 12 months of age, while sleeping naturally. The decibel levels of the stimuli are shown by the numbers in the response cycle. (From Bradford LJ: Physiological Measures of the Audio-Vestibular System, Academic, 1975.)

useful to the examiners at the Menninger Foundation (Fig. 7-1). He suggests examining the resting, response, and recovery cycles for the characteristic wave shapes he and his colleagues have observed. They determine auditory threshold by wave shapes representing a decrease in amplitude, a jammed or M-shaped pattern, or a flattening that must occur within a specific time period and over consecutive trials. Presently, this can be determined only by examining oscillographic traces visually rather than by summarizing results automatically. Some investigators have found it useful to examine both rate and pattern when analyzing changes in respiration as responses to acoustic stimuli.

SUMMARY

Respiration audiometry has yet to become a popular method for assessing infants' hearing acuity. However, it has some useful applications. It has certain advantages over other indirect methods of hearing assessment that might be performed in the newborn nursery. The equipment is portable; the method does not require the use of noxious stimuli; testing does not unduly disrupt hospital routine or disengage the nursing staff from their usual duties; and the test can be administered by paraprofessional personnel. Data interpretation, however, at this point still requires sophistication and considerable time. With the use of automatic scanners, more research in characteristic wave formation, and standardization of procedures, infant respiration audiometry could become a very useful audiometric tool.

REFERENCES

Ackner B: A simple method for recording respiration. J Psychosom Res 1:144–146, 1956

Bench J: Audio-frequency and audio-intensity discrimination in the human neonate. Int Audiol 8:615–625, 1969

Bradford LJ: Respiration audiometry, in Bradford LJ (ed): Physiological Measures of the Audio-Vestibular System. New York, Grune and Stratton, 1975

Bradford LJ, Rousey CL, Bradford MA: Respiration Audiometry with the Preschool Child. The Menninger Foundation, Topeka, 1968

Cotes JE: Lung Function: Assessment and Application in Medicine, 2nd ed. Oxford, Blackwell Scientific, 1968

Desmond MM, Franklin RR, Vallbona C, et al: The clinical behavior of the newlyborn. J Pediat 62:307–325, 1963

Downs MP, Sterritt GM: A guide to newborn and infant hearing screening programs. Arch Otolaryngol 85:15–22, 1967

Eimas P, Siqueland E, Jusczyk P, et al: Speech perception in infants. Science 171:303–306, 1971

Eisenberg RB: Auditory behavior in the human neonate. Paper presented at biennial meeting of the Society for Research in Child Development, Minneapolis, 1965

Eisenberg RB: Auditory behavior in the human neonate: functional properties of sound and their ontogenetic implications. Paper presented at the American Speech and Hearing Association annual convention, Washington, D.C., 1966

Fröding C: Acoustic investigation of newborn infants. Acta Otolaryngol 52:31–40, 1960

Froeschels E, Beebe H: Testing hearing in newborn infants. Arch Otolaryngol 44:710–714, 1946

Gerber SE, Gilchrist DB: Respiratory rate changes of neonates as responses to speech stimuli (unpublished)

Hardy JW: Studies in hearing in neonates. Acta Otolaryngol (Suppl) (Stockh) 206:34–36, 1965

Heron TG, Jacobs R: A physiological response of the neonate to auditory stimulation. Int Audiol 7:41–47, 1968

Heron TG, Jacobs R: Respiratory curve responses of the neonate to auditory stimulation. Int Audiol 8:71–84, 1969

Kumpf W: Objective hearing test by delayed acoustic stimuli-coupling with breathing sounds. Arch Klin Exp Ohren-Nasen Kehlkopf 186:80–97, 1966

Kumpf W, Landwehr FJ: Integrated level diagrams of breathing sounds. A useful supplement to breath sound audiometry. Monatsschrift Ohrenheil Laryngo Rhinol 12:535–539, 1970

Kumpf W, Munster W: Determination of the hearing threshold beginning with the age of infancy by stimulus synchronous level diagrams of the breathing sound. Arch Klin Exp Ohren-Nasen Kehlkopf 191:593–597, 1968

Ling D, Ling A, Doehring DG: Stimulus and observer variables in the auditory screening of newborn infants. J Speech Hear Res 13:9–13, 1970

Lipton EL, Steinschneider A, Richmond JB: Autonomic function in the neonate. Psychosom Med 22:57–65, 1960

Poole R, Goetzinger CP, Rousey CA: A study of the effects of auditory stimuli on respiration. Acta Otolaryngol (Stockh) 61:143–152, 1966

Purves MJ: Initiation of respiration, in De Reuch AVS, Porter R (eds): Ciba Foundation Symposium: Development of the Lungs. Boston, Little, Brown, 1965

Reid L: The embryology of the lung, in De Reuch AVS, Porter R (eds): Ciba Foundation Symposium: Development of the Lungs. Boston, Little, Brown, 1965

Rousey CL, Snyder C, Rousey CA: Changes in respiration as a function of auditory stimuli. J Aud Res 4:107–114, 1964

Stubbs EM: The effect of factors of duration, intensity and pitch of sound stimuli on the responses of newborn infants. Univ Iowa Stud Child Welf 9:77–134, 1934

Suzuki T, Kamijo Y, Kuichi W: Auditory test of newborn infants. Ann Otol 73:914–923, 1964

Teel J, Winston MA, Aspinall K, et al: Thresholds of hearing by respiration using a polygraph. Arch Otolaryngol 86:172–174, 1967

Wedenberg E: Auditory tests in newborn infants. Acta Otolaryngol (Stockh) 46:446–461, 1956

Weibel ER: Postnatal growth of the lung and pulmonary gas exchange capacity, in De Reuch AVS, Porter R (eds): Ciba Foundation Symposium: Development of the Lungs. Boston, Little Brown, 1965

Anthony Mulac
and Sanford E. Gerber

8
Cardiovascular Measures

As in the case of other methods discussed in this section, cardiovascular response measures have been suggested as having potential utility for audiometric measurement of the infant. As with other autonomic procedures, cardiac response measurement does not require subjects to make operant responses. Cardiovascular measures traditionally have taken the form of heart rate, that is, number of heart beats per minute. As the review of literature later in this chapter indicates, this commonality of units for cardiovascular response measurement is one of the few which has been consistent across the broad series of studies dealing with this phenomenon. One potential advantage of heart rate response is that it may not require an intact nervous system; another is that it does not employ noxious stimuli.

Questions addressed by this chapter include: (1) To what extent is the cardiovascular response a valid index of an infant's hearing? (2) What are some of the variables which may affect this response? (3) What results of experiments are relevant to these questions? (4) What research and clinical implications can be drawn from investigations of the cardiovascular response phenomenon with regard to acoustic stimulation?

VARIABLES

An analysis of research on the cardiac response to acoustic stimulation indicates that researchers have failed to agree on a wide variety of aspects relevant to this issue. Among these are: (1) variables affecting the cardiac response, (2) statistical procedures appropriate to cardiac response data analysis, and therefore (3) the form and direction of the cardiac response. Experience in our laboratory, along with an extensive review of pertinent literature, indicates the importance of these variables with relation to the potential validity and clinical applicability of the cardiovascular response as an indicator of infants' hearing. In fact, many of the apparently conflicting findings would appear to be potentially attributable to differences in stimulus variables, response variables, analysis variables, and statistical procedures applied to the resulting data. The following summary of relevant research suggests the importance of these variables.

Stimulus Variables

Since the presence or absence of a cardiac response raises the issue of reaction to acoustic stimulation, at least three properties of acoustic signals need to be considered: spectrum, sound pressure, and duration. It is not unusual for investigations to fail to indicate the nature of the sound spectrum utilized in cardiac response studies (e.g., Shock and Schlatter, 1942; Graham and Clifton, 1966). On the other hand, signal spectrum may not differentially affect the cardiovascular response (Schulman and Kreiter, 1971; Turkewitz et al., 1972).

A second stimulus variable which may or may not affect the cardiovascular response, but which requires consistent calibration across investigations in order for those investigations to be comparable, is sound pressure level. Failure to specify this variable is common and include: Lewis (1971) who used a "C chord at 65 dB," Moreau et al. (1970) who used white noise at "90 dB," and Graham and Clifton (1966) who employed "a 75 dB sound." Since none of these investigations specified the dB scale used, that is, the reference level, apparently conflicting results may or may not have resulted from this potential inconsistency in sound pressure level of the signals employed as stimuli.

A third stimulus variable which has failed to receive sufficient investigation in terms of cardiovascular response is stimulus duration. While we know that signal energy varies as a function of duration, we do not know whether the cardiovascular response varies as a function of energy. Researchers have applied a wide variety of stimulus durations with no clear-cut conclusions being derived as to their effect. At one extreme, Schachter et al. (1971) used clicks lasting 0.3 ms; while, at the other extreme, Clifton and Meyers (1969) used stimuli varying randomly from 40 to 60 seconds. In a series of studies, Schulman has used 3-second stimuli (Schulman, 1970; Schulman et al., 1970; Schulman and Kreiter, 1971). In an earlier investigation of the effect of stimulus duration, Clifton, Graham, and Hatton (1968) concluded that a

10-second signal was preferable, in terms of cardiovascular response, to stimuli lasting 2, 6, 18, and 30 seconds. On the other hand, Turkewitz et al. (1972) failed to find differential responses to stimuli lasting 1, 2, 4, or 8 seconds. While the psychoacoustic phenomenon of loudness has been shown to initially increase with duration, then decrease (Gerber, 1974), the effect of this stimulus variable on the cardiac response has not been clearly shown.

Response Variables

Much of the published research on cardiac response (notably by Bartoshuk, 1962a, 1962b; Graham and Clifton, 1966; and Schulman et al., 1970) has claimed that the heart rate of a human newborn increases during a period from 2 to 6 seconds following the onset of an acoustic stimulus. Furthermore, the literature not only leads one to expect this accelerative response in early infancy, but also to expect a decelerative response at a later age in infancy (Clifton and Meyers, 1969). Such a consistent variation in response direction may well be a function of age, and an experiment conducted in our laboratory (discussed later in this chapter) has dealt with this question. It also appears possible that the cardiac response to sound is better revealed, especially during the first month of life, by measuring the absolute amount of change, without regard to direction of change (Gerber, Mulac, and Swain, 1976).

Nor has the relationship between stimulus level and response magnitude been clearly established. Some researchers have claimed that the size of the heart change varies as a function of signal level, at least at some point above threshold (Bartoshuk, 1964; Graham and Clifton, 1966; Steinscheider and Richmond, 1966). On the other hand, several investigators have been unable to find a significant correlation between the response magnitude and signal level (Barnet and Goodwin, 1967; Davis, Buchwald, and Frankmann, 1955; Gerber et al., 1977; Schulman et al., 1970; Schulman, 1974). Results of this latter group of studies have suggested that the cardiac response is an all-or-none type of response.

Analysis Variables

The literature has demonstrated a surprising lack of consistency of post-stimulus duration during which the cardiac response was investigated. For example, Lewis (1971) began averaging three heartbeats *prior to* stimulus onset; Schachter et al. (1971) began three seconds *before* onset; Schulman and Kreiter (1971) began 16.6 seconds *after* onset; and Schulman (1974) began *at* stimulus onset.

Not only is it important to view the effect of how close to stimulus onset cardiac response measurement is begun, it is equally important to consider the effect of poststimulus analysis procedures. Even in the absence of stimuli, heart rate sometimes increases and sometimes decreases (Välimäki, 1970). Therefore, if one were to look at a sufficiently long period of time, both an accelerative and decelerative pseudobiphasic response (i.e., returning to and crossing the prestimulus heart rate value) would be likely to appear. Conversely, if one examined data for a sufficiently short period of time, only a monophasic response would be observed (i.e., accelerating or decelerating, but not crossing the prestimulus heart rate level). The importance of analysis duration is emphasized by the results of studies conducted by Graham, Clifton, and Hatton (1968) which indicated that "acceleration began within the first second and reached a peak by the fourth second after which there was a decrease to approximately the post-stimulus level." On the other hand, Schulman and Kreiter (1971) refrained from analyzing data until 16.6 seconds after stimulus onset and still claimed to find heart rate changes. Clifton and her associates (1968, 1969) have employed the analysis period extending from 1 second before stimulus onset to 30 seconds after onset. Schulman (1970) began analyzing 2 seconds prior to stimulus onset and continued for 20 seconds. It is only reasonable to suspect that such variations in analysis times would lead to differences in reported cardiovascular response.

Varying Procedures of Statistical Analysis

The law of initial values (Wilder, 1950) states that the relative level of autonomonic function previous to stimulation of a perceptual system affects any response that an autonomic mechanism may demonstrate following such stimulation. The applicability of this law to cardiovascular responses has been demonstrated by Bridger and Reiser (1959) among others. In order to control statistically for this effect, Lacey (1956) employed a form of multiple regression analysis and Benjamin (1963) recommended analysis of covariance. The utility of covariance analysis (Winer, 1962), which employs regression analysis, is suggested by the following facts: (1) it is reasonable to presume that the response of any physiological mechanism to stimulation should be affected by its initial state of excitation or relaxation; (2) data on cardiovascular responses have shown the relevance of the law of initial values to this autonomic response; (3) if there is no correlation between prestimulation rate and ensuing cardiac response, that is, if the law of initial values does not apply to this response, then analysis of covariance has no statistical effect which differentiates it from analysis of variance of these data. Hence, it seems only prudent to use the covariance approach to control statistically for any influence of the heart rate previous to stimulus onset upon the poststimulus heart rate.

SERIES OF EXPERIMENTS

In order to assess the validity and potential clinical utility of the cardiac response for infants, a series of experimental studies is being conducted by the audiology laboratory of the Speech and Hearing Center, University of California at Santa Barbara. While this ongoing investigation has not been concluded at this writing, results bearing on a number of questions raised by earlier studies are available. In these studies, we have generally sought to investigate the effects of stimulus variables, while holding response variables, analysis variables, and statistical analytical procedures constant. Several of these variables held constant in the completed studies (discussed below) are currently under investigation for their potential effect on the cardiac response.

Several aspects of research design employed in the majority of studies conducted in our laboratory tend to differentiate this series from the majority of investigations published recently. (1) The subjects themselves have been studied as a source of variation by inclusion as one of the independent variables in the factorial design. This has permitted the assessment of possible idiosyncracies in responses of the various subjects. (2) Nonsignal or blank events have often been randomly inserted among the stimulus events in order to test directly the validity of the cardiac response. (3) Finally, analysis of covariance has been employed with prestimulus heart rate the covariate in order to control statistically for the law of initial values.

Experiment 1

To establish directly the validity of the cardiovascular response as an audiometric measure Gerber, Mulac, and Lamb (1977) utilized stimulus and nonstimulus events. Subjects were 14 females between the ages of 21 and 23 years, with a mean age of 22.4. All had passed a 15 dB HTL (ANSI, 1969) screening test and had reported negative audiologic histories. Stimulus signals were bursts of narrow-band noise centered at 1000 Hz, dropping 22 dB/octave, and were presented diotically through earphones with each burst having a stimulus rise-time of 0.5 milliseconds and a duration of one second. This stimulus was presented at four signal levels: 20, 40, 60, and 80 dB above 20 $\mu N/m^2$. A fifth test condition was a 1-second interval in which no signal was presented. Hence, the stimulus conditions were four bursts of noise and blanks, arranged in five different presentation schedules in which the blank condition occurred as frequently as the four signal conditions combined. The nonsignal events were distributed randomly among the signal stimuli, which occurred in a prescribed order; each condition was presented five consecutive times in order of increasing intensity. Heart rate was measured as the output

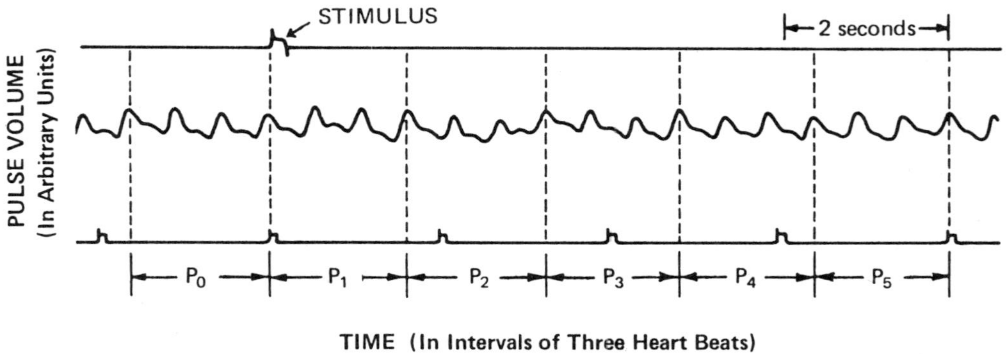

Fig. 8-1. Sample ECG oscillogram showing six measurement intervals. (From Gerber, Mulac, and Swain. J Am Audiol Soc, 1976.)

from a pulse volume transducer and recorded on a polygraph (Gilson M5) at a writing speed of 25 mm/s. An event marker recorded signal and non-signal presentations on the polygraph paper (Fig. 8-1).

Heart rate measurement was done in the manner suggested by Lewis (1971): the onset of each stimulus event marked the point from which the pre-stimulus and five poststimulus heart rate measures were taken. A Hewlett-Packard heart rate finder was employed to measure the heart rate averaged over three pulse cycles. (It should be noted that this method of analysis could conceivably obscure any biphasic response occurring during the first poststimulus interval, although such a rapid biphasic response seems unlikely because of the inertia of the heart muscles.) As Fig. 8-1 demonstrates, the prestimulus rate was determined by measuring backward from the pulse peak nearest the stimulus onset. This defines the interval called P_0. The five poststimulus heart rates were determined in the same way, measuring in beats/minute forward from signal onset, and were called P_1 through P_5. These measures were made for each signal and nonsignal event, with 30 seconds separating events. Heart rates were then converted into change scores from prestimulus rate to each poststimulus rate. In other words, the heart rate change between P_0 and P_1, P_0 and P_2, . . . P_0 and P_5 were computed for analysis. This procedure has been used with apparent success in other studies of our laboratory, some of which are discussed later in this chapter.

To determine whether stimulus magnitude differentially affected heart rate following onset of stimulus, a three-way analysis of covariance with repeated measures was employed (Winer, 1962) in which the covariate was the prestimulus heart rate (P_0) before each signal event. Independent variables for this analysis were: subjects, stimulus intensity level, and time interval. While both subjects and time interval were found to be sources of statistical significance ($p < 0.001$), signal intensity was not. Since signal intensity appeared to make no difference in apparent cardiovascular response (at least within the four intensities employed here), data for the subjects' heart rates under the four stimulus levels were combined and compared to the nonstimulus events in a second three-way analysis of covariance. These again showed significant difference among subjects and among changes in heart rate at various time intervals. More important, this analysis demonstrated a significant difference ($p < 0.001$) resulting from whether the signal was or was not presented preceding measurement. Figure 8-2 shows mean heart rates for subjects under stimulus and nonstimulus conditions. The pattern of the response is clearly monophasic decelerative.

Thus this study demonstrates that, for adults, a valid cardiac response to acoustic stimulation does exist. Using a somewhat different analysis procedure, Eisenberg, Marmarou, and Giovachino (1974) demonstrated the valid-

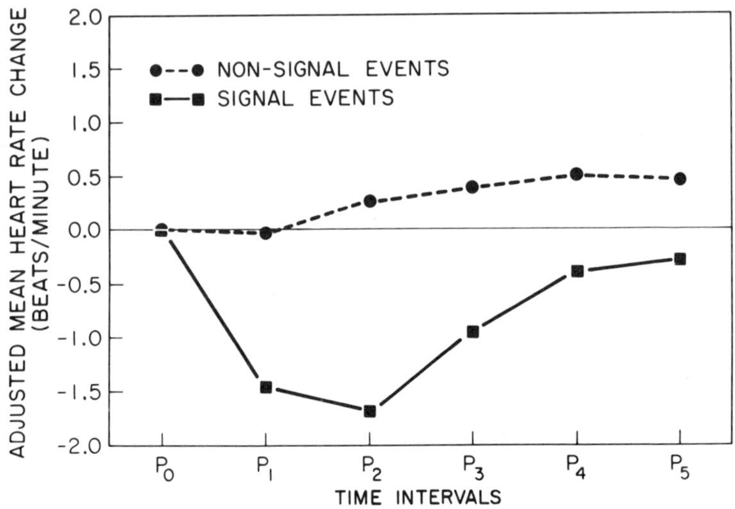

Fig. 8-2. Adjusted mean heart rate changes under signal and non-signal conditions. (From: Gerber, Mulac, and Lamb. Audiology 1977.)

ity of the cardiac response for infants. Further, it appears to be of an all-or-none variety; that is, response magnitude and latency were unaffected by stimulus magnitude.

Experiment 2

This study by Goldstein (1972) dealt with development of the cardiovascular response in infants at ages one month, 2 months, and 3 months through a longitudinal approach. Many of the procedures employed in experiment 1 were followed here. The infants in all cases were held in the arms of their mothers during testing, subjects generally were asleep during testing, but groupings of five heart beats rather than three were analyzed to determine heart rate per minute for a given time interval after onset of stimulus.

While statistical analyses were not employed for these data, trends indicated that the infants in general displayed accelerative responses to acoustic stimulation when they were one month old, showed a wide variety of directional responses at age two months, and by three months of age generally displayed a decelerative monophasic response. These general findings regarding the direction and latency of cardiac response were consistent with findings previously reported in the literature and gave further impetus to the investigation of the cardiac response as a potential measurement approach for hearing of the very young. Further, they suggest that by the age of three months, infants display an adult-like monophasic decelerative response to acoustic stimulation which is consistent with the findings of Clifton and Meyers (1969).

Experiment 3

Subjects for this study (Gerber, Mulac, and Swain, 1976) were 15 newborns, nine males and six females, between the ages of 24 and 48 hours. All were full-term, healthy infants of normal birthweight (i.e., $\geq$ 1500 grams) delivered at Cottage Hospital, Santa Barbara. Each was taken from the newborn nursery to an examining room for purposes of data collection.

All subjects received in randomized order 20 tape-recorded, calibrated, acoustic stimuli of two different spectra and two different durations via a single earphone. The signals were a one-third octave band of noise centered at 3150 Hz and a 3150 Hz sine wave; each had durations of 300 and 1500 milliseconds. All presented had a measured output sound pressure level of 50 dB above 20 $\mu N/m^2$. Calibration was accomplished through use of an artificial ear input to a B&K Model 2112 spectrometer. Acoustic signals were omitted at five randomly selected points on the tape and these events, along with the four signal events, were separated by intervals of 60 seconds.

Unlike the earlier studies, heart rate was transduced by thorax electrodes; this was monitored continuously on an electrocardiograph, with stimulus events marked on the oscillogram. Heart rate was measured in beats/min. over sets of three R-to-R (i.e., pulse peak-to-peak) intervals on the cardiac oscillogram. Six such measurements were made for each stimulus event; one preceding stimulus onset, and five succeeding measurements beginning with stimulus onset.

Analyses were conducted on raw heart rates and the following four transformations of raw heart rates: (1) rate changes from prestimulus to each of the five poststimulus rates indicating direction of change, (2) rate changes from prestimulus to each of the five poststimulus rates without regard to direction of change, (3) rate changes from each poststimulus measurement interval to the succeeding one with regard to direction of change, (4) rate changes from each poststimulus measurement interval to the succeeding one without regard to direction of change.

Raw and transformed heart-rate data were subjected to analyses of covariance with repeated measures with prestimulus heart rate used as the covariate to control for effects of the law of initial values.

Analysis of raw data indicated wide differences among subjects in terms of overall heart rate, with prestimulus rates ranging from a low of 105 beats per minute to a high of 165 beats/minute. Also wide variability of prestimulus rates was noted within individual subjects.

Table 8-1.
Summary of Results of Four-Way Analyses of Covariance on Heart-Rate Data (Raw and Transformed)

		Raw Data	(1) Pre-to-Post with Sign	(2) Pre-to-Post without Sign	(3) Post-to-Post with Sign	(4) Post-to-Post without Sign
Subject	*F*	2.92*	2.92*	2.31	3.16*	2.61*
	p	0.003	0.003	0.014	0.001	0.006
Time interval	*F*	5.45*	5.45*	70.12*	0.71	0.56
	p	0.001	0.001	0.001	0.50	0.50
Subject X time interval	*F*	1.12	1.12	2.06*	0.86	0.92
	p	0.280	0.280	0.001	0.50	0.50

*These achieved the predetermined criterion level ($p < 0.01$) for rejection of the null hypothesis.

Results of the analyses of covariance on raw and transformed heart-rate data, summarized in Table 8-1, show that the subjects themselves were a significant source of variance in all but one case ($p < 0.01$). When the law of initial values was controlled through analysis of covariance, an especially clear picture of subject response idiosyncrasy was noted (Fig. 8-3). Thus, the notion that newborns may be expected as a group to display acceleration of cardiovascular rate cannot be sustained by these data. For example, while subject 12 accelerated dramatically, subjects 4 and 11 decelerated; subject 6 did both, and subject 10 did neither. Thus, it is clear that the direction, as well as the size, of cardiac rate change is idiosyncratic across individual infants. This finding is consistent with the observations of Porges (1974). Further, the high intrasubject variability demonstrated in these data clearly indicates that infants of this age must be repeatedly measured under a given stimulus condition in order to get a true picture of that individual's response.

Another significant source of variance was poststimulus time interval;

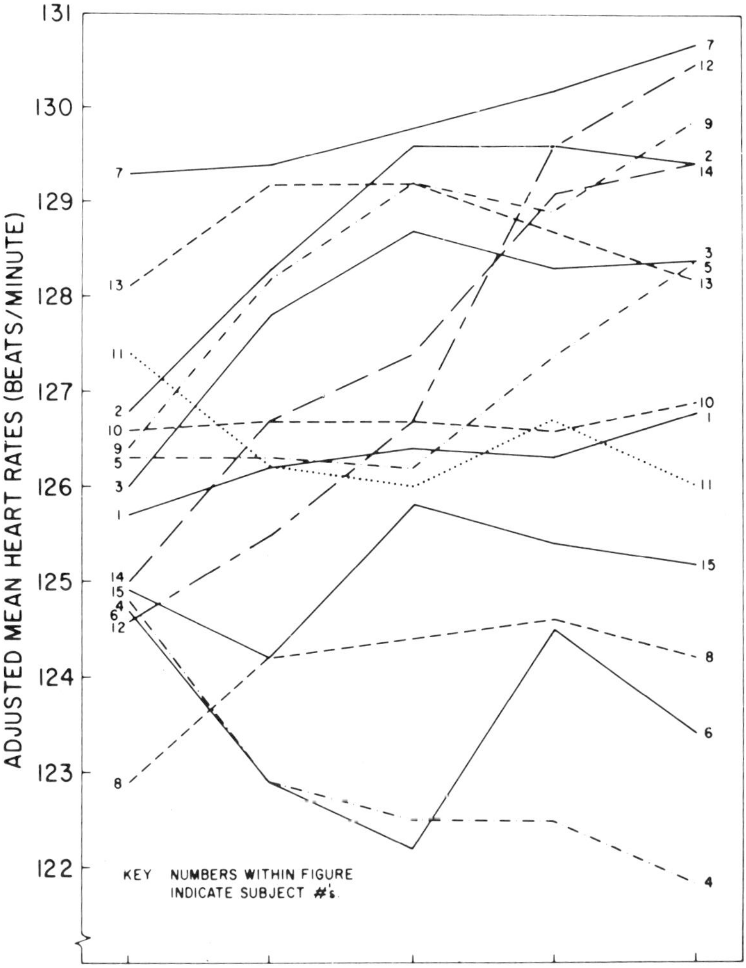

Fig. 8-3. Mean heart rate (adjusted for prestimulus rate) for each subject at five poststimulus time intervals. (From: Gerber, Mulac, and Swain, J Am Audiol Soc 1976.)

that is, the latency of response was significant across subjects ($p < 0.01$) for all data transformations except those comparing successive post-stimulus change scores. Specifically, poststimulus interval P_3 (seventh through ninth beats) was the one during which the group as a whole indicated the greatest cardiac rate differentiation from their prestimulus rates. This finding provides further evidence that acoustic stimuli induce changes of heart rate in the neonate. However, the fact that the examination of successive intervals revealed no significant changes from interval to interval demonstrates that each poststimulus rate should be compared to the prestimulus rate in order to get the clearest picture of the infant's response.

Another indication of the idiosyncrasy of subject response was found in the significant interaction between subject and poststimulus time interval on absolute pre-to-post-stimulus heart-rate changes. That is, the latency of a response differed from subject to subject. This significant interaction was found only when absolute changes were viewed. When signed changes (accelerations and decelerations) were combined, no such idiosyncrasy of subject latency was demonstrated. Thus it seems advisable to view absolute changes in the neonate rather than signed changes. Only when changes in both directions are taken together (i.e., absolute changes) were subjects seen to demonstrate different response patterns with respect to latency of maximal changes.

Finally, stimulus spectrum and duration were not found to be significant sources of variation for either raw scores or change scores. The failure of the four stimulus events to produce different heart rate changes from the blank events seems explainable on the basis of two statistical effects: the small number of blank conditions (five) as compared to the number of stimulus events, and the within-subject variability of heart rate.

Experiment 4

The fourth study was conducted to determine the potential effects of subject respiration cycle upon the cardiac response to acoustic stimulation (Gerber et al., in preparation). Porges (1974), among others, has suggested the potential importance of the variable upon the cardiac response. While this investigation was conducted using adult subjects, its findings may well have relevance to the infant cardiac response.

Subjects were 15 females between the ages of 21 and 27 years, with a mean age of 23.2. All subjects passed an audiometric screening examination with a narrow band noise centered at 1000 Hz at 15 dB SPL re 20 $\mu N/m^2$, and all indicated negative otological histories. As in experiment 1, subjects were seated in a darkened, sound-treated room during the test sessions.

Test stimuli were 1-second, 50 dB bursts of narrow-band noise centered at 1000 Hz with a 50 dB/octave roll-off. These were presented at approximately 30 second intervals under three respiration conditions: (1) at the peak of inhalation, (2) at the peak of exhalation, and (3) randomly with respect to the respiratory cycle. These three stimulus conditions were scheduled in three random orders in which each condition appeared ten times for each subject, and randomly assigned to subjects.

Subjects' respiration was monitored by an E&M bellows pneumograph and physiograph and recorded on a Gilson M5 polygraph. Subjects' heart rates were measured using a Gilson photoelectric transducer attached to the fingertip. These heart-rate data were recorded on another channel of the polygraph. The three remaining channels of the polygraph were used to record onset of acoustic stimulus, time in two-second intervals, and cardiotachometer output.

Heart rate was again measured in three-pulse units and converted to mean heart rate (beats/minute) for each three-pulse interval. Again, one prestimulus interval and five poststimulus intervals were used, each containing 3 beats.

Heart-rate data were subjected to a three-way analysis of covariance with prestimulus heart-rate as the covariate. Independent variables consisted of the subjects themselves, the three respiration conditions, and the five time intervals following onset of an acoustic stimulus. While both subjects and time interval were shown to be significant sources of variation ($p < 0.001$), the most important finding was the significant interaction between the three respiration conditions and time intervals ($p < 0.001$). The latter finding clearly

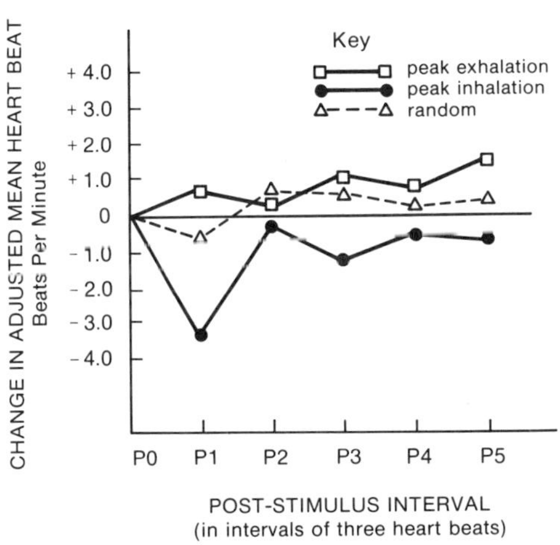

Fig. 8-4. Mean heart rate change at five post-stimulus intervals for three conditions of respiration.

indicates that the magnitude of the heart rate change due to acoustic stimuli varies as a function of the respiratory cycle. The differential effects of respiratory condition (peak inhalation, peak exhalation, or random) can be seen clearly upon the heart rate response pattern as shown in Fig. 8-4 for the combined group of subjects. When the stimulus was presented at peak inhalation, the response pattern appeared to be monophasic and markedly decelerative. When the stimulus was presented at peak exhalation, a monophasic and slightly accelerative response pattern occurred. Finally, when the stimulus was presented randomly in terms of the respiratory cycle, the pattern was biphasic with slight deceleration during the first poststimulus interval followed by an acceleration returning to a point above the pre-stimulus rate. Thus, it is clear that, at least in the case of adults, the magnitude, direction, and pattern of cardiac response are affected by the respiration cycle. Further, the significant interaction between subjects and time interval (without regard to respiratory cycle) suggested the possible idiosyncracy in adult cardiac response. The failure to find a significant three-way interaction among subjects, time interval, and respiratory cycle provides evidence suggesting that the infant idiosyncratic cardiac response found in experiment 3 was unlikely the result of respiratory cycle. Also, subjects in that study were measured in a condition comparable to the random condition of experiment 4.

CONCLUSIONS

It appears clear from the review of relevant literature and related studies by our laboratory that the cardiovascular response is a valid index of infants' hearing. However, the practical implication of this general finding is not so easily established. Not only have studies disagreed in their findings regarding the shape, direction, and magnitude of the cardiac response, our research clearly indicates that with very young infants the response to acoustic stimuli is idiosyncratic. While this research has indicated that neonates' heart rates do respond to acoustic stimuli, they do so with different magnitude, direction, and latency. Thus, generalizations about the general trend of infants of a given age would appear to be of little practical importance in testing an individual infant.

Further, a variety of stimulus variables has been identified which may well influence the cardiac response. Those which need to be considered include acoustic spectrum, sound pressure, duration, respiratory cycle, statistical data analysis, and the individual subjects. For cardiac response research to be meaningful, these variables, among others, either must be controlled or their effects assessed. A long-range goal of ours has been to assess the effects of these variables, while individual studies have generally held the majority of them constant so as to determine the effects of one or more others.

With regard to response variables, it is clear that until researchers come to greater agreement as to the interstimulus periods to be assessed and whether directional or absolute changes should be analyzed, wide discrepancies in infants' cardiac responses will continue to be reported.

Analysis variables, including the period relative to the stimulus to be analyzed, also need to be carefully considered. Also relevant to this issue is the question of the number of beats to be included in each temporal interval of analysis.

With regards to procedures for statistically analyzing cardiac response data, it appears clear that analysis of covariance is the most useful procedure available to date. To the extent that the law of initial values affects the cardiac response (and our data would suggest that in fact it does have such an effect) the covariance statistical procedure controls for it. Clearly no other procedure, such as waiting for the subject to return to baseline heart rate, would appropriately control for possible law of initial values effects, since such an approach would introduce in itself intervening variables such as differing inter-stimulus presentation time. Results of experiment 4 indicating the effect of respiration cycle upon the cardiac response suggest that analysis of covariance might properly employ two covariates: prestimulus heart rate and respiration cycle. Through multiple regression analysis, this procedure would control statistically for these two intervening variables (Winer, 1962).

Results of the third experiment described above clearly indicate that the cardiac responses of neonates are unique to each infant, or "idiosyncratic," except insofar as they may be influenced by respiration. Thus, it seems wise to investigate individual subjects' differences when conducting research in this area, especially as it is possible through the use of a repeated measures factorial design. Further, such a realization of neonate individuality should prompt both the researcher and clinician to search out the individual pattern of response for each individual subject, rather than assuming that one pattern holds for all. It would appear, based upon our studies, that if a consistent pattern exists, it does not stabilize until after the third month following birth. While it is possible that the majority of infants, by the age of three months, has established a nearly adult response which is monophasic and decelerative in nature, this hypothesis clearly needs further investigation. One further practical implication of these findings is that the researcher may well be required to take a larger number of stimulus and nonstimulus response readings in order to determine whether an individual infant in fact does hear the test stimulus.

On the basis of findings from our laboratory and some others, it would appear that stimulus duration and magnitude do not affect the cardiac response, at least in areas markedly above the normal threshold of hearing. This, along with other relevant literature, clearly supports the theory that the cardiac response is an all-or-none response. However, such an hypothesis requires further investigation.

Because of the obvious advantages of using the cardiac response for audiometric purposes, along with its demonstrated validity, its practical implementation would appear reasonable. However, the effects of a wide range of variables, many discussed in this chapter, require further investigation. Clearly a larger body of research, employing greater and more consistent controls, must be implemented before the potential value of the cardiac response as an expressly audiometric method is realized in the form of a standard clinical procedure.

REFERENCES

Barnet AB, Goodwin RS: Averaged evoked electroencephalographic responses to clicks in the human newborn, in Brackbill Y (ed): Behavior in Infancy and Early Childhood; A Book of Readings. New York, Free Press, 1967

Bartoshuk AK: Response decrement with repeated elicitation of human neonatal cardiac acceleration to sound. J Comp Physiol Psychol 55:9–13, 1962a

Bartoshuk AK: Human neonatal cardiac acceleration to sound; Habituation and dishabituation. Percept Mot Skills 15:15–27, 1962b

Bartoshuk AK: Human neonatal cardiac response to sound; A power function. Psychon Sci 1:151–152, 1964

Benjamin L: Statistical treatment of the law of initial values in automonic research: A review and recommendation. Psychosom Med 25:556–566, 1963

Bridger WH, Reiser MF: Psychophysiologic studies of the neonate: An approach toward the methodological and theoretical problems involved. Psychosom Med 21:265–276, 1959

Clifton RK, Graham FK, Hatton HM: Newborn heart-rate response and response habituation as a function of stimulus duration. J Exper Child Psychol 6:265–278, 1968

Clifton RK, Meyers WJ: The heart-rate response of four-month-old infants to auditory stimuli. J Exper Child Psychol 7:122–135, 1969

Davis RC, Buchwald AM, Frankmann RW: Autonomic and muscular responses and their relation to simple stimuli. Psychol Monographs No. 405, 1955

Eisenberg RB, Marmarou A, Giovachino P: Infant heart rate changes to a synthetic speech sound. J Audit Res 14:21–28, 1974

Gerber SE, Mulac A, Lamb ME: The cardiovascular response to acoustic stimuli. Audiology 16:1–10, 1977

Gerber SE, Mulac A, Kizziah KT: Effects of respiratory phase on the cardiovascular response to sound. (in preparation)

Gerber SE, Mulac A, Swain BJ: Idiosyncratic cardiovascular response of human neonates to acoustic stimuli. J Am Audiol Soc 1:185–191, 1976

Gerber SE: Introductory Hearing Science. Philadelphia, Saunders, 1974

Godlstein M: Cardiac rate response to acoustic stimuli in one-, two-, and three-month-old infants. Unpublished M.A. thesis, University of California, Santa Barbara, 1972

Graham FK, Clifton RK: Heart rate change as a component of the orienting response. Psychol Bull 65:305–320, 1966

Graham FK, Clifton RK, Hatton HM: Habituation of heart rate response to repeated auditory stimulation during the first five days of life. Child Dev 39:35–52, 1968

Lacey JI: The evaluation of autonomic responses: Toward a general solution. Ann NY Acad Sci 67:123–164, 1956

Lewis M: A developmental study of the cardiac response to stimulus onset and offset during the first year of life. Psychophysiology 8:689–698, 1971

Moreau T, Birch HG, Turkewitz G: Ease of habituation to repeated auditory and somesthetic stimulation in the human newborn. J Exp Child Psych 9:193–207, 1970

Porges SW: Heart rate indices of newborn attentional responsivity. Merrill Palmer Quart 20:231–234, 1974

Schachter J, Williams TA, Khachaturian Z, et al: Heart rate responses to auditory clicks in neonates. Psychophysiology 8:163–179, 1971

Schulman CA: Heart rate response habituation in high-risk premature infants. Psychophysiology 6:690–694, 1970

Schulman CA: Heart rate audiometry. Part II: The relationship between heart rate change threshold and audiometric threshold in hearing-impaired children. Neuropädiatrie 5:19–27, 1974

Schulman CA, Kreiter R: The contribution of heart-rate audiometry in the early identification of hearing impairment. Paper presented to the annual meeting of the California Speech and Hearing Association, Los Angeles, 1971

Schulman CA, Smith CR, Weisinger M, et al: The use of heart rate in the audiological evaluation of nonverbal children. Part I: Evaluation of children at risk for hearing impairment. Neuropädiatrie 2:187–196, 1970

Shock NW, Schlatter MJ: Pulse rate response of adolescents to auditory stimuli. J Exp Psych 30:414–425, 1942

Steinscheider A, Lipton, EL, Richmond JB: Auditory sensitivity in infant: Effect of intensity on cardiac and motor responsitivity. Child Dev 37:233–251, 1966

Turkewitz G, Birch HG, Cooper KK: Patterns of response to different auditory stimuli in the human newborn. Dev Med Child Neurol 14:487–491, 1972

Välimäki I: Postnatal alterations of cardiac rhythm. Clin Pediatr 9:652–655, 1970

Wilder J: The law of initial values. Psychosom Med 12:393, 1950

Winer BJ: Statistical Principles in Experimental Design. New York, McGraw-Hill, 1962

Maurice I. Mendel

9
Electroencephalic Tests of Hearing

The idea of testing hearing in either infants or adults by monitoring stimulus-related changes in the electrical activity of the brain is certainly not a new concept. The initial efforts in this respect date from the early 1930s, but these first attempts were generally limited by the restricted technology of the times. Electroencephalic tests of hearing were of limited value until the development of the special purpose computer in the 1950s. For approximately the past 20 years, there has been a great deal of progress in this area of electric response audiometry (ERA) or electroencephalic audiometry (EEA).

Interest was first focused on what have come to be called the middle components of the auditory evoked potentials (AEP) (Fig. 9-1), that is responses with approximate latencies of 8–50 milliseconds. Because of a controversy concerning the origin of the middle components, this initial work was followed by a large number of studies of the late components or vertex potentials (50–500 milliseconds), and to a lesser extent for audiometric testing, the contingent negative variation (CNV) and P_{300} waves, latencies greater than 300 milliseconds. Since about 1968, there has been a great deal of effort expended on the direct recording of the compound action potential (AP) and cochlear microphonic (CM) of the eighth nerve (Fig. 9-2). This activity occurs within approximately 0–2 milliseconds following stimulus onset, and the general area has come to be known as electrocochleography (ECoG). Finally, the time domain between 2 and 8 milliseconds has been shown to reflect activity of the eighth nerve and successive brainstem auditory nuclei and tracts, and has come to be known as the early components (Fig. 9-1). The middle and late components are generally spoken of as the evoked cortical potentials, and the early components as the evoked brainstem potentials.

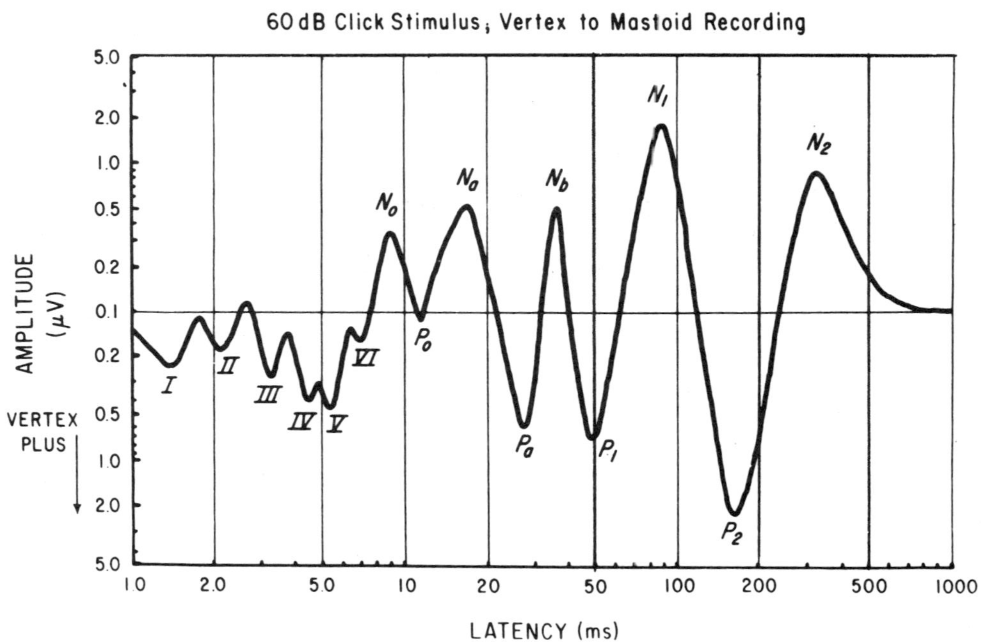

Fig. 9-1. Diagrammatic representation of the 15 individual waves of the auditory evoked potentials from eight subjects. Evoked brainstem potentials (1–8 milliseconds) are labeled with Roman numerals (I–VI), middle components (8–50 milliseconds) are labeled *No–Nb*, and the late components (50–500 milliseconds) are labeled P_1–N_2. Latency has been plotted on a logarithmic scale. (From Picton et al: EEG Clin Neurophysiol, 1974).

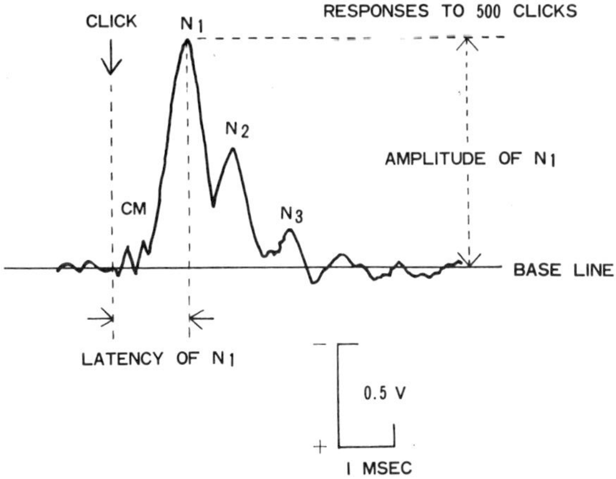

Fig. 9-2. A typical summed waveform of the AP in man recorded at the external acoustic meatus by a nonsurgical technique. Responses to 500 clicks with an intensity of 100-dB peak equivalent SPL, given at an interval of 160 milliseconds, were summed by an average response computer with an analysis time of 31.25 milliseconds. The vertical arrow in the upper left-hand corner of the figure indicates the moment of arrival of the stimulating click. The baseline is an ideal line drawn simply by visual interpolation through the tracing of spontaneous activity to represent zero level of the amplitude of the response. (From Yoshie and Ohashi; Acta Otol (Suppl) (Stockh) 252, 1969.)

Historically, the cortical potentials have received the most attention and occupy the greatest share of the literature, and thus are treated in this chapter first. Work on electrocochleography and the brainstem potentials is of more recent origin, but occupies more of today's research and clinical effort and thus is covered in the next two chapters. The general instrumentation used to record these various potentials, with the exception of electrodes, is similar and is treated in one section of this chapter, with specifics detailed for each time domain. These three chapters are organized largely on the basis of chronologic development, although an overall historical review precedes the specific consideration of the cortical potentials. Finally, much of the research with infants has used adults as subjects in order to compare electroencephalic responses with known behavioral results. Although the emphasis of this book is on audiometry with infants, it is necessary to document the development of these electroencephalic tests with adult subjects before describing their application to infants.

In chapters such as these, the greatest problem that arises is to define the material that will not be covered, since this cannot be a completely inclusive effort. Because of their limited audiometric utility, the CNV and P_{300} waves will not be considered in these chapters. For the interested reader who desires more general information on the evoked potentials, four texts are available: Regan, 1972; Shagass, 1972; Callaway, 1975; and Ruben et al., 1976. A recent book by Reneau and Hnatiow (1975) provides an annotated bibliography of the late components of the auditory evoked potentials. In addition, several recent review articles (Eggermont et al., 1974; Hecox, 1975; Hood, 1975; Price, 1975; Simmons and Glattke, 1975; Picton et al., 1977; and Skinner and Glattke, 1977) provide coverage of differing aspects of the auditory evoked potentials in both infants and adults. Finally, a monograph by Davis (1976b) describes the principles of electric response audiometry as they have been seen and developed by the man who has probably had more influence on this area of investigation than any other person.

HISTORIC CONSIDERATIONS

The Early Period

The recording of the electrical activity of the brain, the electroencephalogram or EEG, has a long and fascinating history. An excellent account of the early history of electrophysiology is provided by Brazier (1959), while Lindsley (1969) gives a personal view of the development of the evoked potentials. Although numerous investigators working in many different countries contributed to the eventual understanding of the EEG, the landmark discoveries of four of these individuals deserve attention.

du Bois-Reymond, of Germany, working with frogs, demonstrated in 1848 that activity in a peripheral nerve was accompanied by an electrical change, a negative variation in the standing potential between the cut end of the nerve and its longitudinal surface. He wrote, "If I do not greatly deceive myself, I have succeeded in realizing in full actuality . . . the hundred years' dream of physicists and physiologists, to wit, the identity of the nervous principle with electricity" (Brazier, 1959). This negative variation is what is now known as the action potential, and its discovery led directly to the discovery of the electrical activity of the brain.

The cerebral counterpart of du Bois-Reymond's action potential in nerve was first reported by Richard Caton in England in 1875, from his work with rabbits, and later with monkeys. He noticed that when both electrodes were on the cortical surface, there was a continuous waxing and waning of the potential which disappeared when he eliminated all experimental stimulation of the animal. He called these potentials the "electric currents of the brain," and demonstrated them to the British Medical Association in 1875 and the International Medical Congress in Washington, D.C. in 1887. In spite of the prominent groups before whom Caton gave his demonstrations, and the fact that his discovery appeared in journals in three countries, his work received little attention at the time.

In 1890, Adolf Beck in Poland, who was ignorant of Caton's work, also set out to look for signs of action potentials in the brain. Working with dogs, he independently discovered the electrical waves of the brain. Although other investigators became interested in changes in the electrical activity of the brain in response to sensory stimulation, the idea of a continuously fluctuating electrical potential intrinsic to the "resting" brain was a novel concept, and remained of interest primarily to Caton and Beck. Although the EEG from animals was recorded by many investigators—for example, Lindsley (1969) lists 28 papers published between 1875 and 1933—there were no reports of the EEG being successfully recorded from the intact scalp of humans until 1929, and very little attention was paid to this fact in the United States until about 1935.

The monumental first communication in 1929 and subsequent publications over the next eight years by Hans Berger of Jena gave us much of the basic information that we have, even today, about the spontaneous electrical activity of the brain. Berger made unpublished studies of the electrical activity of the brain in animals as early as 1902, and extended this work to humans for at least five years before his first publication in 1929. He studied and named the electroencephalogram (EEG) in normal man, and found the two major rhythms, alpha and beta, that had been found earlier in dogs. The first published human EEG was taken from Berger's son. Berger is generally recognized as the founder of clinical electroencephalography.

Development in the United States

It took some time before Berger's discoveries were generally recognized in the United States. However, the publications by Gibbs, Davis, and Lennox, and by Jasper and Carmichael, both in 1935, set the stage for a series of extensive investigations of the human EEG in America. The instrumentation for recording the EEG was relatively simple and inexpensive, and the procedures could be quickly carried out on the intact scalp with no danger to the subject. Electroencephalography was a promising tool for many disciplines, with investigators relating the EEG to perception, pathology, and personality. Early research was directed to finding the source and significance of the electrical activity of the brain.

The effects of sensory stimulation on the EEG were observed from the beginning. Caton had attempted to localize cortically the sensory modalities as early as 1875, but his most successful experiments dealt with the area of the brain concerned with vision (Schoenberg, 1974). Beck, in 1890, also localized the visual and auditory cortex in rabbits and dogs, and recorded responses to stimulation of the skin. Berger described the effects of sensory stimulation on the human EEG in 1929.

Berger also showed that the EEG was affected by hypoxia and anesthesia, as well as being changed during sleep. The remarkable changes that take place in the EEG comparing the awake record to various stages of sleep had been noted from the earliest days (Loomis et al., 1935). In awake subjects, a brief change in the ongoing EEG was described as the effect of sudden auditory stimulation (Gibbs et al., 1935). However, the idea of testing hearing by observing changes in the ongoing EEG activity evoked by the presentation of auditory stimuli during sleep dates from about 1939 (Davis et al.). The difficulty of conducting this type of test, and the fact that a sound repeated within three or four seconds after a previous stimulus usually failed to evoke a second response, was made clear by these investigators. It was generally recognized that the response to sound was not always identifiable in the background EEG activity.

The Use of Ongoing EEG

This early interest in the EEG was interrupted by World War II, and very little progress was made for about 10 years. Doerfler (1948) compared four neurophysiologic measures which could be used to assess hearing, and concluded that the EEG was complex and unwieldy, required excess analyses, and did not yield reliable threshold measures. He considered electrodermal audiometry as a more promising testing technique. Marcus, Gibbs, and Gibbs (1949) were the first to report the use of the EEG to measure the reaction to sound of young children during barbiturate-induced sleep. They encountered problems in obtaining proper records when using an audiometer because the circuit interfered with the EEG due to improper shielding and grounding, and it became necessary to use loud and frightening sounds. It was not possible to determine threshold with these sounds, and many children could not be satisfactorily tested.

The earliest reported attempt to measure a pure tone audiogram using changes in the EEG was published by Gidoll in 1952. His preliminary report described the use of an audiometer to stimulate an 18-month-old infant with suspected hearing loss during barbiturate-induced sleep. Because the audiometer was grounded, artifacts in the EEG were avoided, but this study reported the findings for only one case, and no follow-up is provided. This preliminary report was followed in 1953 by a study by Perl, Galambos, and Glorig of 66 adults with normal and impaired hearing. This study represents the first successful use of the EEG techniques to measure hearing thresholds in adults, and it was reported that the thresholds established with the EEG for deaf subjects corresponded reasonably well with conventional testing. When testing the effects of faint sounds, the drowsy state provided the most clear responses.

Many of the remaining studies of changes in the ongoing EEG in response to sound published in the 1950s dealt with attempts to standardize response scoring, and reflect the influence of either Derbyshire or Goldstein. In a series of papers (e.g., Derbyshire et al., 1956; Norkus et al., 1960; Withrow and Goldstein, 1958) attempts were made to more precisely define the major components of the EEG response to sound, to find more accurate measurement techniques such as zero axis crossings and area measurements, and to make scoring techniques more objective. Derbyshire et al. (1956) found an 18-dB average deviation between behavioral tests and changes in the ongoing EEG during sleep. Thresholds within 10 dB of behavioral audiometry were reported by Withrow and Goldstein (1958) for hearing-impaired school children using EEG audiometry. Nevertheless, EEG techniques, compared to conventional behavioral audiometry, required complex instrumentation, exacting procedures, and difficult scoring maneuvers. Few laboratories were equipped to offer such testing.

The Averaged Response

The use of changes in the ongoing EEG in response to acoustic stimulation as a testing technique probably would have remained a very minor specialty, except for two important developments.

Even though the potentials evoked by sensory stimulation were the first electrical phenomena of the brain to be observed in animal studies by Caton and Beck, they remained difficult to record from the scalp of man because they are obscured by the oscillations of the ongoing EEG and because early equipment could not reproduce their more rapid components. A technique of photographically superimposing responses evoked by stimulation of a peripheral nerve was first reported by Dawson in 1947. He averaged numerous traces on an oscilloscope following application of a sensory stimulus by superimposing them one on another. This technique showed that a waveform, representing the evoked potential, time-locked to the presentation of each stimulus, could be detected against the background EEG activity, whose temporal distribution was random in time. The use of Dawson's photo superimposition technique to describe the evoked potential in the human brain to auditory stimuli was reported by Abe in Japan in 1954, and was used with children by Itakura (1955) and Suzuki and Asawa (1957). This technique, however, quickly became outmoded and was soon replaced by various electromechanical and electronic devices for automatic summation of the evoked potentials (Brazier and Barlow, 1956; Barlow, 1957; Clark, 1958).

The development of the general purpose digital computer vastly simplified the technique of response averaging and a paper by Geisler, Frishkopf, and Rosenblith in 1958 marks the beginning of the modern era of evoked potential audiometry. Specialized laboratory computers, which made averaging extremely simple and accessible, were introduced about 1960; and this development was followed by widespread use of the method of recording sensory evoked potentials. Recordings from an atypical subject whose auditory responses stand out from the background EEG, as well as the averaged responses, are shown in Fig. 9-3. Commercially available evoked potential audiometers have been in use for about 10 years.

INSTRUMENTATION

Although the specific equipment used for recording the auditory evoked potentials (AEP) varies among laboratories, the general needs are similar and may be summarized as follows: signal presentation system, recording system, averaging system, and response storage system. The block diagram of the laboratory shown in Fig. 9-4, which I developed at the University of Iowa, may be used for illustrative purposes. A system such as this could be used, with appropriate electrodes, to record the evoked cortical potentials, brainstem potentials, or cochlear potentials.

Signal Presentation System

The acoustic stimuli used when recording the evoked potentials must be controlled in terms of duration, rise-decay time, intensity, frequency, and rate of presentation. Stimuli may take the form of tone or noise bursts, tape recorded signals, or computer generated tones or speech. As shown in Fig. 9-4A signal generators are used in combination with appropriate electronic timers and switches, or alternatively, electronic gates and filters. The generator produces pure tone signals that are shaped by the appropriate gates into pulsed signals which can be phase-locked to stimulus onset. The intensity of the pulsed signal is controlled by an attenuator which precedes final amplification. Signals may be presented from a loudspeaker, as shown, or earphones may be used. For the various evoked potential time domains, signals ranging in duration from clicks of a few microseconds to tone bursts from three or four milliseconds to 500 milliseconds have been used. The spectral characteristics of the stimuli, of course, depend on the rise-fall times chosen, as well as the overall duration of the pulse. In some cases, an audiometer is used to produce the acoustic stimuli.

Another important component shown in Fig. 9-4A, is the pulse generator, which serves as the master clock for the entire system. Trigger

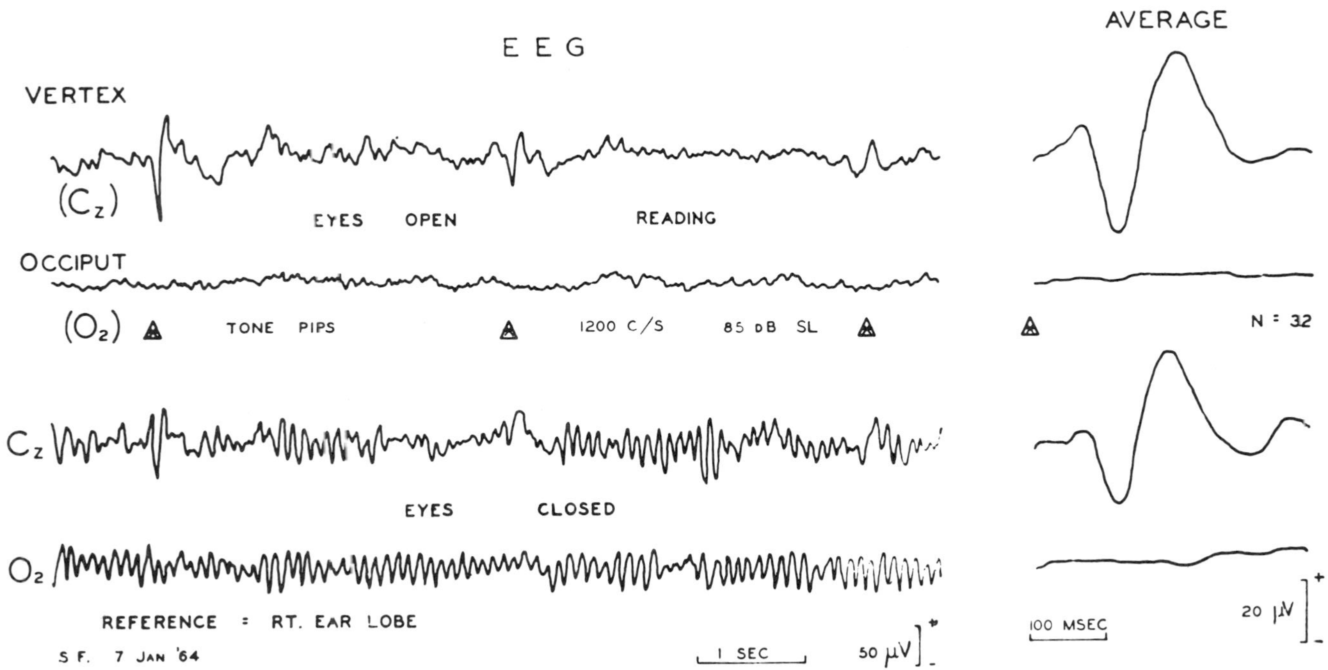

Fig. 9-3. Auditory evoked responses. The EEG was recorded from vertex and from occiput with eyes open and with eyes closed while tone pips were delivered by loudspeaker at intervals of 3.2 seconds (as indicated by the triangles). Upward deflection indicates vertex more positive, both in the raw EEG and in the average response. Average responses were collected simultaneously from vertex and occiput. Stimuli were tone pips at 1200 Hz at a level 85 dB above the subject's threshold. (From Zerlin and Davis; by permission of the Editor of *Electroencephalogr Clin Neurophysiol* 1967)

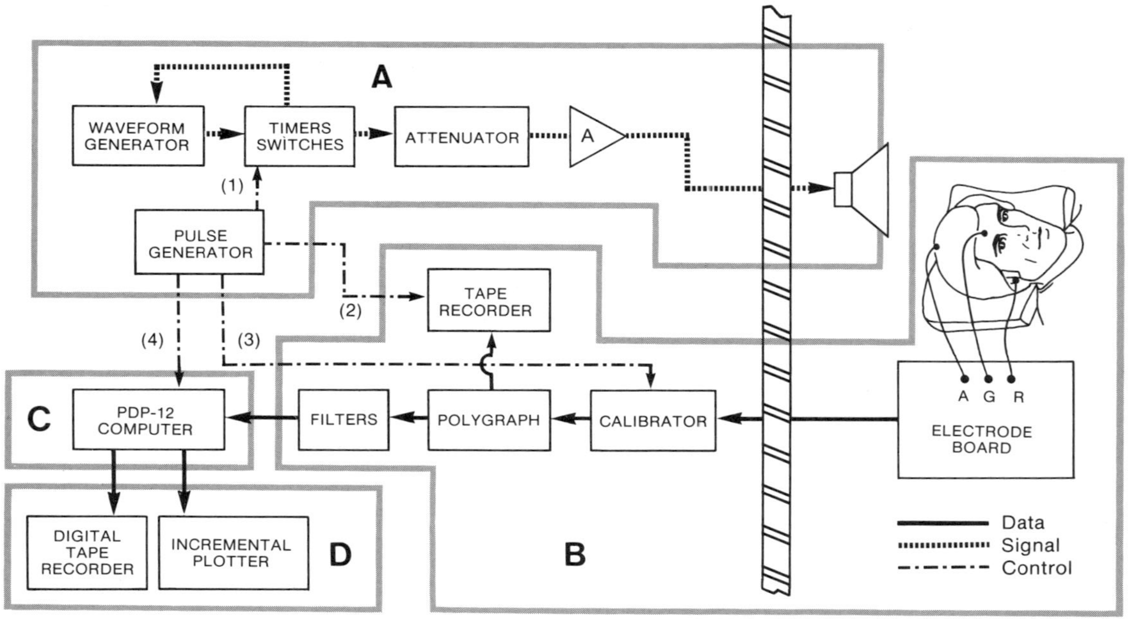

Fig. 9-4. Equipment used to record the auditory evoked potentials at the University of Iowa. A. The signal presentation system. B. The recording system. C. The averaging system. D. The storage system. The subject is shown with an active electrode on the vertex referred to an earlobe electrode (R), with a ground electrode (G) attached to the forehead. The acoustic signal is shown with a dashed line, the EEG signal from the subject with a solid line, and the control signal from the pulse generator with a broken line (1–4).

pulses from the pulse generator serve to control the timing of the acoustic stimuli (1), the triggering channel on the FM tape recorder (2), the triggering of the calibrator (3), and the onset of each sweep of the computer (4). The rate of signal presentation is thus set by the pulse generator.

Recording System

While recording the evoked potentials, the subject is seated comfortably in an electrically shielded room, or in the case of an infant, is usually tested while lying in a crib. An electrical potential can be measured at a given point only with reference to a second point. Thus, it is necessary to have two electrodes to record the evoked potentials. As Goff (1974) has shown in an extensive review, the characteristics of differential amplifiers are such that the amplifier output is the algebraic difference of all electrical activity occurring at the two electrodes connected to its input. Therefore, the placement of both electrodes is very important to the recording of the evoked potentials. For the evoked cortical and brainstem potentials, the active electrode is usually placed at the vertex (the top of the head), with the reference electrode located on the earlobe or mastoid area. A controversy exists as to whether this is in fact a ''monopolar'' recording scheme, since the inactivity of the reference electrode site has been questioned. Attempts have been made to use the chin, nose, linked ears, and such noncephalic locations as the sternum as a more inactive reference site, but the earlobe or mastoid is generally used. For electrocochleography, the active electrode is commonly placed on the promontory of the stimulated ear, with a reference electrode on the ipsilateral earlobe. For both cortical and cochlear recording, the ground electrode is usually attached to the forehead. In Fig. 9-4B, the subject is shown in a prone position, with an active electrode (A) on the vertex referred to the earlobe (R), and a ground electrode (G) attached to the forehead for recording one channel of EEG activity.

The ongoing EEG is picked up by the electrodes, led through an electrode board to a calibration system which superimposes a reference signal of known voltage, and then amplified in two stages by the polygraph. Both the preamplifier and power or driver amplifier are located in the polygraph. The amplitude range in the normal EEG may be from 5 to over 100 μV; therefore voltage amplification between 10,000 and 200,000 is required to achieve a nominal 1 V signal level. To amplify the low level brain stem potentials, with amplitudes in the nanovolt range, additional gain of a factor of 10 is necessary.

The amplifying system must also have extremely broad-band frequency response characteristics from almost a DC range to an upper limit of about 10,000 Hz. In order to band-limit the EEG for the different time-domain responses, a filter may be placed between the amplifiers and the computer. Several studies (e.g., Dawson and Doddington, 1973; Lane et al., 1974; Desmedt et al., 1974) have shown that the introduction of analog filters into the system may produce unwanted distortion (seen as a phase or latency shift) of the evoked potentials. Although the use of filters is very common, caution must be exercised in their application. Finally, as shown in Fig. 9-4B, an FM tape recorder may be used to store the ongoing EEG activity for off-line analyses.

Averaging System

The heart of the auditory evoked potential laboratory, the averaging or summing computer, is shown in Fig. 9-4C. With the exception of only one or two systems, most computers do not average the evoked potentials, since the term ''average'' implies first summing the responses and then dividing by the number of sweeps. Instead, most computers are summing devices which, through a process of algebraic addition, extract the time-locked electrical activity and reduce the amplitude of the more random ongoing activity. To accomplish this, the computer discretely samples across time the voltage of the EEG trace and stores it in hundreds of continuous memory locations, called bins. Each bin represents a specific time period following the onset of the stimulus. Each successive sweep of the computer is then subdivided into each of the sequential bins. At the end of the data collection period, the averaged response is shown as the sum of the voltage present in each successive bin. Activity which is time-locked to the presentation of the stimuli tends to add up in time, while random activity is cancelled. Since the final summed response is scaled by some factor for display purposes, it is, in effect, almost an average. More detailed descriptions of the averaging process are provided by Buchsbaum (1970) and McCandless (1971).

Response Storage System

The averaged response produced by the computer is usually displayed on an oscilloscope. Permanent storage of each response may be accomplished, as shown in Fig. 9-4D, through the use of a plotter, or in the case of a general purpose computer, on digital magnetic tape or a disc file. Responses which are stored on digital magnetic tape may be called up off-line for further processing or for automatic analyses.

It should be pointed out that the laboratory illustrated in Fig. 9-4 was developed solely for the purpose of research and clinical studies of the auditory evoked potentials. It was, thus, elaborate and, unfortunately, expensive. Less expensive, but unfortunately less flexible, total systems are available commercially and are shown in Fig. 9-5. Some features of the clinical

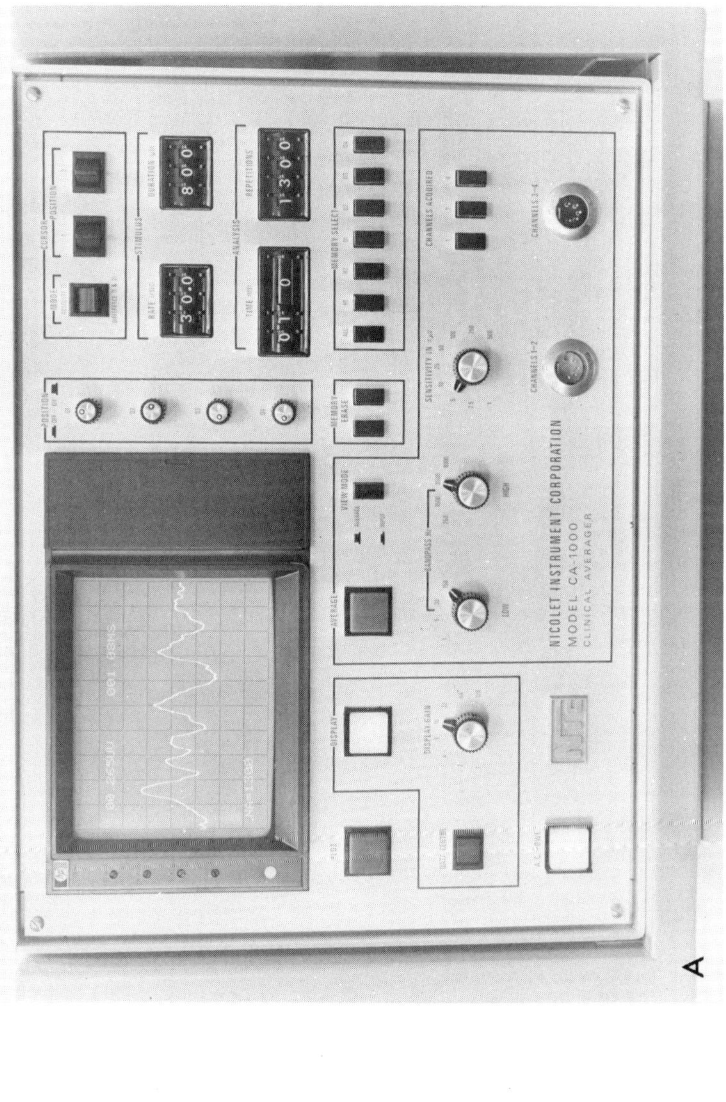

A

Fig. 9-5A. Example of electric response audiometer system. (Courtesy of Nicolet Instrument Corporation.)

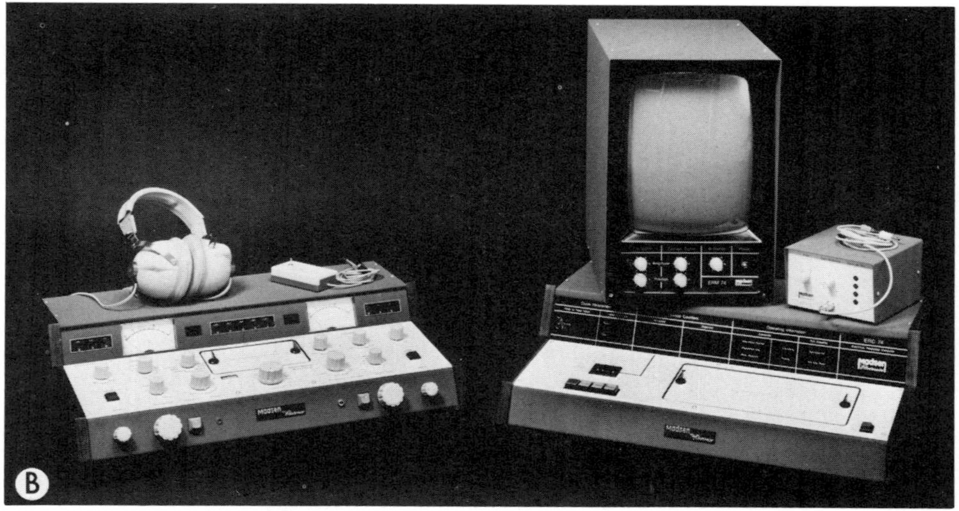

Fig. 9-5B. Example of electric response audiometer system. (Courtesy of Madsen Electronic.)

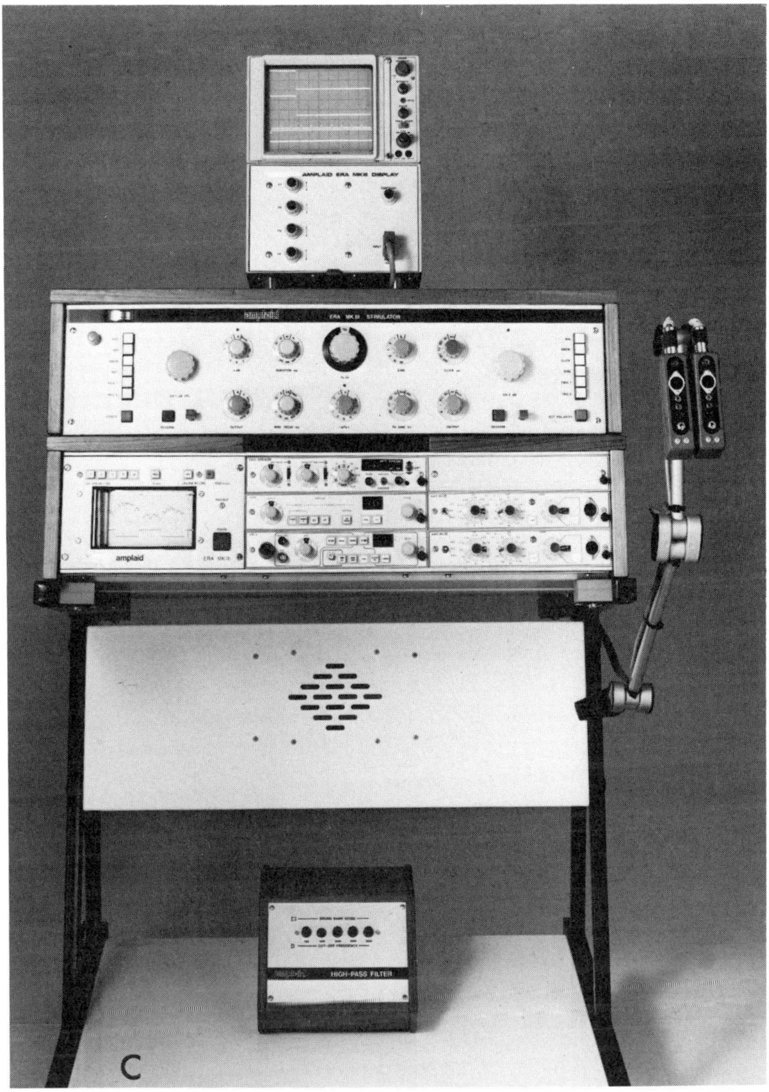

Fig. 9-5C. Example of electric response audiometer system. (Courtesy of Amplaid USA, Inc.)

laboratory shown in Fig. 9-4, for example, multichannel recording and analysis, and magnetic storage of the averaged response, are not available in commercial units.

EVOKED CORTICAL POTENTIALS

Late Components

Although the middle components of the auditory evoked potentials were the first computer averaged responses to be reported from the human scalp (Geisler, Frishkopf and Rosenblith, 1958; Lowell et al., 1960, 1961), the vast majority of the papers on electric response audiometry have dealt with the late components. As shown in Fig. 9-6, the late components are labeled P_1, N_1, P_2, N_2, and occur between about 50 and 300 milliseconds after the onset of the stimulus. The late components can be recorded widely over the frontal and central scalp areas, but as Davis and Zerlin (1966) have shown, they are maximal at the vertex with a reference on the mastoid or earlobe. The late components have also been called the *V* or vertex potentials (Bancaud et al., 1953) because of their maximal amplitude distribution, or the slow potentials because of their latency distribution. First described by P. A. Davis in 1939, the late components are a polysensory response that are generally assumed to represent activity occurring simultaneously in the primary auditory cortex, the temporal auditory association cortex, and the frontal association areas (Picton et al., 1974). Responses in this time domain may be elicited with auditory, visual, or tactile stimuli, but the auditory evoked potentials demonstrate the shortest latencies (Fig. 9-7). In general, modality specific patterns may be seen with auditory, tactile, electric shock, or visual stimuli. This chapter, however, concentrates on the response to auditory stimulation.

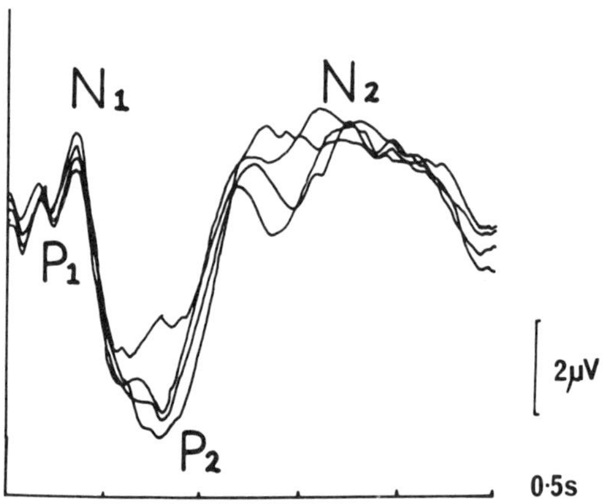

Fig. 9-6. Late components of the auditory evoked potentials to 60-dB SL clicks presented monaurally at a rate of 1/second. Each tracing represents the average of 1024 responses from vertex-mastoid electrodes. Each latency division represents 100 milliseconds. (From Picton et al: EEG Clin Neurophysiol 1974.)

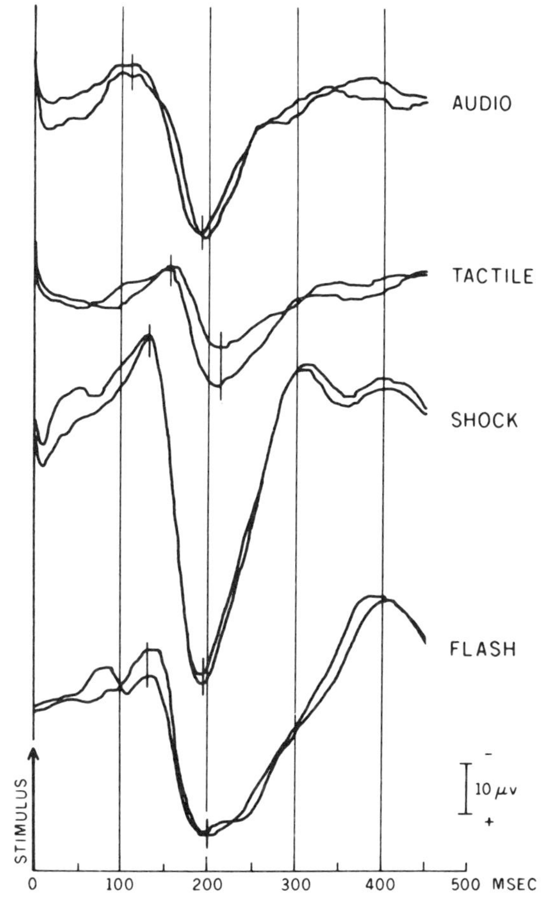

Fig. 9-7. Superimposed tracings of late components evoked by stimuli in different modalities. The latencies of the first (N_1) wave in audio and tactile (vertical lines) are no longer than average in this subject. Stimuli were: audio, 1200-Hz tone pips to the left ear; tactile, vibration of left middle finger; shock, percutaneous stimulation of left median nerve at wrist; flash, binocular view of a Grass photostimulator. All stimuli were comfortably strong. Vertex-negative is upward. (From Davis et al: Electroencephalogr Clin Neurophysiol 1972, by permission.)

General Findings in Adults

The late components have peak-to-peak amplitudes (this is the measurement most often reported in the amplitude domain) of about 5–20 μV. Narrow bandpass filters, for example, 2–10 Hz, are used with the late components, and these responses may be obtained with as few as 30–50 stimulus presentations. The refractory period of the late components is fairly long (Fig. 9-8); the amplitude of the response increases as inter-stimulus interval is increased from 1 to 10 seconds (Davis et al., 1966; Nelson and Lassman, 1968). Optimum interstimuli intervals for the awake state are about 1 or 2 seconds, with slightly longer intervals required during sleep. Most research (e.g., Skinner and Jones, 1968; Onishi and Davis, 1968; and Ruhm and Jansen, 1969) has shown that the late components can be elicited optimally with pure tones having rise-fall times of 20 milliseconds, and a duration of 20 milliseconds. Although pure tones between 250 and 8000 Hz may be used as stimuli, the largest and clearest responses are found at 1000 and 2000 Hz (Antinoro, Skinner, and Jones, 1969; Evans and Deatherage, 1969; Rothman, 1970; and Henderson, 1972). McCandless and Rose (1970) reported

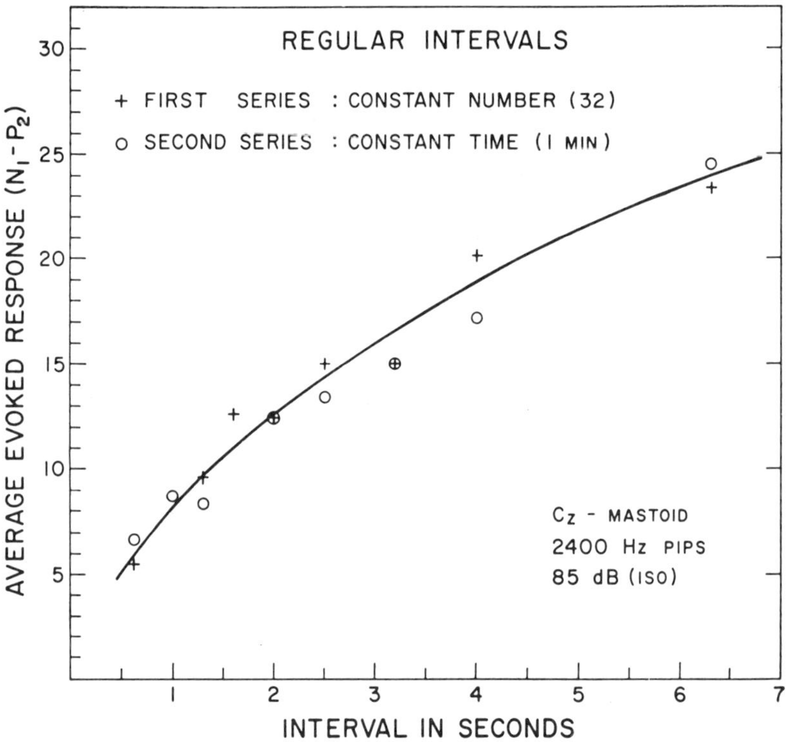

Fig. 9-8. Relative amplitude of N_1–P_2 of the late components as a function of interstimulus interval. Each point represents the average for six subjects. The voltages were normalized to the value of 15 at ISI = 3.2 seconds before averaging. In the first series a constant number of responses (32) was summed. In the second series the stimulation continued for one minute, regardless of the interstimulus interval. (From Davis et al: Electroenephalogr Clin Neurophysiol 1966, by permission.)

that a change in stimulus parameters, that is, frequency, intensity, ear stimulated, would elicit the late components.

The amplitude of the late components generally increases with increasing stimulus intensity up to moderate levels (Fig. 9-9) (Davis and Zerlin, 1966; Beagley and Knight, 1967). At high intensity levels (70–80 dB and above), some individuals show further increases in amplitude with increasing intensity, while others saturate (amplitude is unchanged) at high levels (Moore and Rose, 1969; Picton, Goodman, and Bryce, 1970; Beagley and Kellogg, 1970; Khechinashvili et al., 1973). Latency, on the other hand, decreases with increasing intensity. This effect is relatively small at moderate levels, but becomes quite pronounced near threshold.

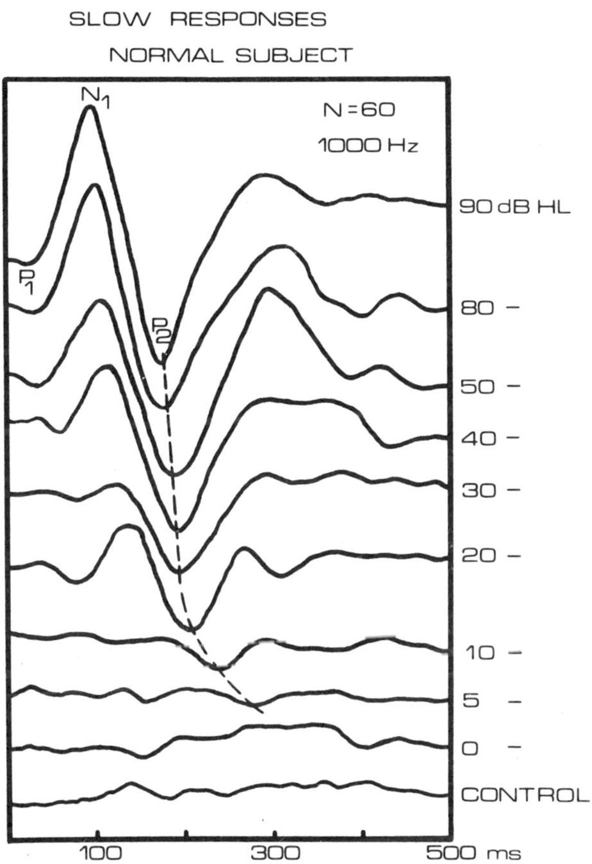

Fig. 9-9. Amplitude and latency of the late components as a function of stimulus intensity. As stimulus level decreases (top to bottom), amplitude decreases while latency increases. (From Madsen Clin Manual, 1974.)

The use of the late components as a measure of threshold in awake adults has been reported in several studies. Most of these studies report thresholds determined with the late components agree with behavioral threshold within° 20 dB (McCandless and Best, 1966; Price et al., 1966; Cody et al., 1967; Davis et al., 1967; Beagley and Kellogg, 1969). In a more recent study (Mendel et al., 1975), using a predetermined latency and voltage criterion scoring system, the median threshold level for 28 normal-hearing awake adults was 30 dB SL.

The late components demonstrate variability associated with changes in subject awareness, attention, or state of consciousness. The level of attention with which subjects attend to the auditory task can change the amplitude of the late components (Davis, 1964; Keating and Ruhm, 1971; Picton and

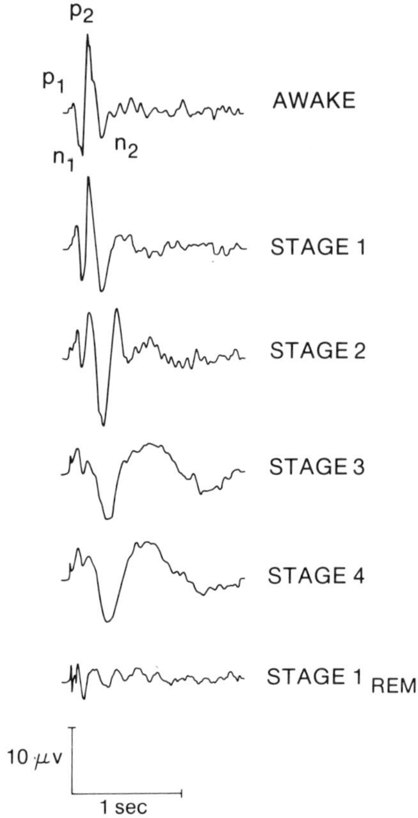

Fig. 9-10. Late components of the auditory evoked potentials to clicks as a function of the EEG stage of sleep from which they were evoked. Each tracing represents the average of 100 responses from vertex-occiput electrodes. (From Williams, Tepas, and Morlock: Science, 1962.)

Hillyard, 1974). The effect of sleep (Fig. 9-10) also contributes to the variability of the waveform, latency, and amplitude of the response. Although first reported by Williams, Tepas, and Morlock (1962), it has been shown repeatedly that the late components in sleep differ from those in the waking state, and that these differences are related to depth of sleep (Weitzman and Kremen, 1965; Cody, Klass, and Bickford, 1967; Ornitz et al., 1967; Anch, 1971; Rapin, Schimmel, and Cohen, 1972; Scott, 1973; Osterhammel et al., 1973; Mendel et al., 1975). In particular, latency and amplitude of the N_2 component increase as subjects progress through deeper stages of sleep, while earlier peaks became smaller. During rapid eye movement (REM) sleep the amplitude of the late components is considerably smaller than during the other sleep stages or the waking state, and often is unidentifiable. In sleeping adults, the late components can be recognized only at intensities of 30 dB hearing level (HL) or above (Cody et al., 1967; Osterhammel et al., 1973; Mendel et al., 1975). In addition, sedation used to put subjects to sleep may cause further variability in the late components (Skinner and Shimota, 1975; Hosick and Mendel, 1975).

The late components of the auditory evoked potentials have received more attention than any other components. A major problem with these responses is their variability both between and within subjects. Most recent reports, however, are pessimistic, as they call attention to the repeated failures in the clinical use of the late components. Roeser et al. (1971) stated that the efficacy of the late components was inversely related to the diagnostic need. Rose et al. (1971, 1972) concluded that the late components should be used cautiously as a clinical tool until more reliable and valid scoring procedures were developed. With careful techniques, however, the late components can contribute useful clinical information.

Application to Infants

Although many of the general findings surveyed in the previous section on adults have been replicated in children, this section deals primarily with findings obtained from infants. Normative studies have been reported on infants with presumed normal hearing. The first of these, published by Goodman et al. (1964) was devoted largely to a description of instrumentation and techniques. Two other studies of the response of normal-hearing infants to clicks were published in 1965 (Barnet; Barnet and Goodwin), in which the amplitude of the late components was related to the intensity of the stimulus.

Many studies have been reported on infants and young children in which changes in the late components have been related to changes in the depth of sleep. The two stages of sleep generally observed in the newborn and in early infancy are active-REM-sleep and quiet sleep (Anders, Emde, and Parmelee,

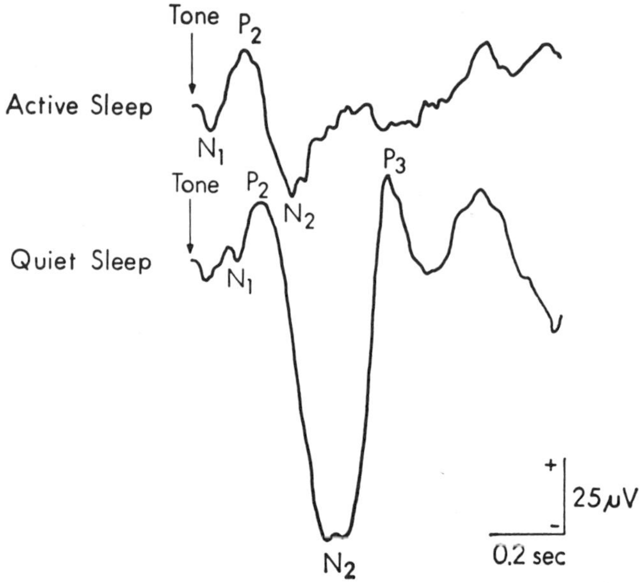

Fig. 9-11. Influence of the stage of sleep upon the late components of the auditory evoked potentials in a normal 6-month-old infant. Each trace is the average of 100 responses from left parietotemporal-ear electrodes to 1000-Hz tone pips at 101 dB SPL. Note the shorter latency and smaller amplitude during active sleep. (From Rapin and Graziani: Neurology, 1967.)

1971). In infants, the most important maturational change within the sleep cycle is an increase in the amount of quiet sleep (QS) in relation to active sleep (AS). The cycle is about equally divided between QS and AS in the newborn, but by three months of age the proportion of QS is twice that of AS (Parmelee, 1969). Since the late components have a larger amplitude in QS than AS (Rapin and Graziani, 1967; Akiyama et al., 1969; and Ellingson et al., 1974) (Fig. 9-11), and since there is a shift in the proportion of QS to AS during this time, an important change takes place in the late components in the first few months of life.

In general, the pattern of the late components in infants changes in form, amplitude, and latency with change in the stages of sleep (Weitzman, Fishbein, and Graziani, 1965; Ferriss et al., 1967; Suzuki and Taguchi, 1968; Taguchi et al., 1969; Davis and Onishi, 1969; and Ohlrich and Barnet, 1972). During similar sleep stages the latency of the response in infants is 40 to 150 milliseconds greater than in adults (Weizman, Fishbein, and Graziani, 1965), but as maturation progresses, there is a decrease in latency of the major negative and positive peaks (Graziani et al., 1968; Weitzman and Graziani,

1968). Barnet and Goodwin (1965) found that the depth of sleep in newborn infants influenced the late component response. Deep sleep was associated with responses of larger amplitudes and longer latencies than those elicited during lighter sleep.

Changes in the late components have also been reported in children older than a few months, characterized by variability of a given peak by as much as 100 milliseconds for different stages of sleep (Rapin and Bergman, 1969) or by the appearance of a large negative peak (N_2) at about 300 milliseconds (Price and Goldstein, 1966). Tanguay, Lee, and Ornitz (1973) report a negative peak at 80 milliseconds typically found in stage 2 sleep, but present only 50% of the time in REM sleep in children aged 27–60 months. While Ornitz et al. (1967) and Ritvo, Ornitz, and Walter (1967) reported a consistent enhancement of the late components within 10 minutes of sleep onset, McCandless (1967) found the characteristic pattern was often absent or modified as a child began to drowse or fall asleep. Late components collected during REM sleep in children from 2 to 68 months gave rise to significantly more equivocal response judgments than any other sleep stage (Cohen et al., 1971). Changes in the amplitude and latency of the late components, consistent with the oscillations of a basic rest activity cycle of the nervous system in children and adults, have been shown by Tanguay et al., 1973.

Other studies with normal-hearing infants have attempted to establish threshold measures using the late components. Response thresholds from 40 to 80 dB above adult threshold have been reported from infants by Barnet (1965), Barnet and Goodwin (1965), Appleby (1965), Rapin and Graziani (1967), Engel and Young (1969), Hrbek et al. (1969), and Lenard, von Bernuth, and Hutt (1969). Comparisons of threshold measures with the late components and by behavioral audiometry in normal and hearing-impaired infants have been reported by Suzuki and Origuchi (1969) and by Tyberghein and Forrez (1971). Results generally agreed within ± 10 dB, but differences as large as ± 30 dB were found. Most of the studies noted above, as well as those reported by Weitzman and Graziani (1968), Taguchi et al. (1969), and Monod and Garma (1971) have found late component patterns from infants similar to those from adults, but usually displaying longer latencies.

Changes in the late components in infants and children brought about by the use of drugs to induce sleep have been discussed by Davis (1973) and by Skinner and Shimota (1975). General agreement on one or more drugs which can be used to induce sleep without bringing about changes in the late components has not yet been achieved. It is difficult to separate out changes in the late components brought about by sleep itself from those which result from the use of drugs to induce sleep.

Several studies have been reported which attempted to use the late components to diagnose hearing loss in infants. Barnet and Lodge (1966) first reported on the use of the late components to test the hearing of infants suspected of being congenitally deaf. Evoked potential and behavioral results correlated highly, but there is no longitudinal validation of the results. Other studies by Davis et al. (1967), McCandless (1967). Rapin et al. (1970), Taguchi et al. (1970), Lentz and McCandless (1971), Barnet (1971a and b), and Morgon et al. (1971) have explored the diagnostic value of the late components in infants. None of these studies reports test-retest reliability across frequency in clinical populations. The reliability and validity of the late components in young children suspected of hearing loss was examined by Goodhill, Lowell, and Lowell (1970). Their sample of 129 children was tested with the late components at 500 Hz only and followed at 6-month intervals until they were old enough to be tested with behavioral audiometry. Test–retest correlations for the late components ranged from 0.72 to 0.87, and correlations between evoked potential and behavioral tests were as high as 0.94 at twelve months. However, they also found their results to be in error by an average of 30 dB in 20% of the cases. This finding raises questions as to the clinical usefulness of the late components in infants.

As noted in this section, and in the previous section on adults, the major problem that still besets the late components is that of variability. Variability is seen both between and within subjects, brought about by changes in stimulus, subject, and recording parameters. The use of the late components as a diagnostic tool seems to be of limited value until a methodology can be developed that effectively reduces the variability brought about by sleep, drugs, pathology, maturation, and psychological states. However, since the late components represent the functioning of the ear, as well as the integrity of the entire auditory pathways in the central nervous system, the effort is certainly necessary.

Middle Components

As stated previously, the middle components were first recorded by Geisler, Frishkopf, and Rosenblith in 1958. As shown in Fig. 9-12, the middle components are labeled N_o, P_o, N_a, P_a, and N_b, and occur between about 8 and 50 milliseconds after the onset of the stimulus. The middle components are recorded maximally at the vertex with a reference on the earlobe or mastoid (Picton et al., 1974), and are widely and symmetrically distributed lateral to the midline (Peters and Mendel, 1974).

At the time of their discovery, the existence of activity earlier than 8 milliseconds was unknown. Therefore, in articles published between 1958 and about 1974, the activity in the time domain from 8 to 50 milliseconds was called early components. Since that time (Picton et al., 1974), however, activity from 0 to 8 milliseconds has been described as the early components,

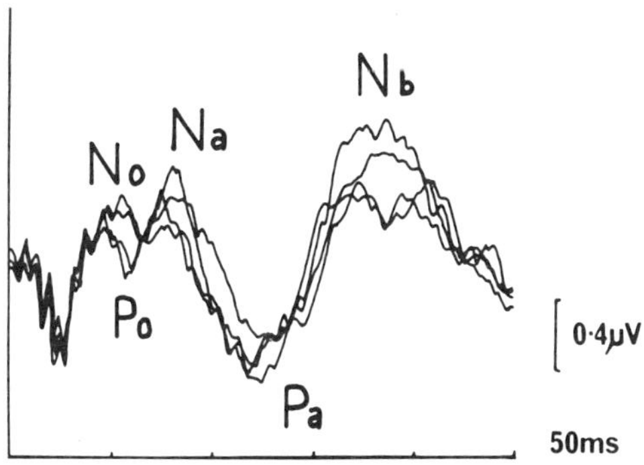

Fig. 9-12. Middle components of the auditory evoked potentials to 60-dB SL clicks presented monaurally at a rate of 1/second. Each tracing represents the average of 1024 responses from vertex/mastoid electrodes. Each latency division represents 10 milliseconds. (From Picton et al: EEG Clin Neurophysiol, 1974.)

while the 8–50 millisecond domain is known as the middle components. To avoid confusion, it is necessary to examine the time domain described in the older literature, and disregard the term early components. It should also be noted that all of the dividing lines in the time domains are strictly arbitrary, and have been used for convenience rather than on the basis of strict anatomical or morphological evidence. The later waves of the early components and the earliest waves of the middle components, for example, may overlap in time. These waves, in fact, may reflect activity of the same neural generator (or generators), and may look different due to differences in recording instrumentation and filter bandwidth. Of course, the same argument holds true for the artificial distinction at 50 milliseconds between the middle and late components.

When Geisler, Frishkopf, and Rosenblith (1958) first reported the recording of the middle components from the human scalp, they suggested that the short-latency components were cortical in origin. This interpretation of the neurogenic (from the brain) origin of the response was challenged by Bickford, Jacobson, and Cody (1964) and others who attributed activity in the 8–50 millisecond time domain to myogenic origins from the muscles of the head and neck. Bickford, Jacobson, and Cody have shown that myogenic responses occur with high level auditory stimulation (perhaps as great as 135 dB). These myogenic responses could be enhanced or diminished by manipulating the tension on the postural muscles of the head and neck, or abolished by muscle paralysis with curare. Bickford et al. have argued that all responses in the middle component time domain are myogenic in origin. The myogenic-neurogenic argument over the origin of the middle components has raged ever since (Borsanyi, 1964; Mast, 1965; Horwitz et al., 1966; Ruhm et al., 1967; Yoshie and Okudaira, 1969; Celesia and Puletti, 1969; Vaughn and Ritter, 1970; Bickford, 1972; Picton et al., 1974; Goff et al., in press) with no clear solution in sight.

The middle components as I have recorded them from relaxed, sleeping (natural or drug-induced), or paralyzed subjects, adults or infants, in response to moderate level stimuli, are neural in origin. For the determination of threshold, the question of the origin of the middle components is moot. If this is an accurate technique to assess threshold, it makes no difference whether the response comes from the thalamus or the scalp musculature, as long as the auditory information has been transmitted through the cochlea and into the auditory pathway. For the study of the underlying mechanisms of hearing, however, the origin of the middle components is important; and, for moderate level stimuli, apparently it is neural.

General Findings in Adults

The middle components have peak-to-peak amplitudes of about 0.5–2.0 μV, an order of magnitude smaller than the late components. Bandpass filters set at 25–175 Hz are used for the middle components and these responses may be obtained with about 400–500 stimulus presentations. One study (McFarland et al., 1975) reports identifiable and repeatable responses with as few as 128 stimuli. Although cleaner (less noisy) responses can be obtained by increasing the number of stimulus presentations per average, a simple doubling of the number of sweeps/average does not necessarily improve the signal-to-noise ratio by one-half, because of the nonstationarity of the background electrophysiologic noise (Vivion et al., 1977; Thornton et al., 1977). The rate of stimulus presentation (see Fig. 9-13) has almost no effect on response amplitude between one and 16 stimuli/second (Goldstein, Rodman, and Karlovich, 1972; Picton et al., 1974; McFarland et al., 1975). Most studies have used rates of about 5 or 10 stimuli/second. Although all of the initial studies of the middle components used clicks as stimuli, it has recently been shown that tone pips, tone bursts, or filtered clicks may be used as stimuli, and thus frequency-specific audiometric results can be obtained (Zerlin, Mowry, and Naunton, 1971; Zerlin, Naunton, and Mowry, 1973; and Zerlin and Naunton, 1974; Kupperman and Mendel, 1974; McFarland, Vivion, and Goldstein, 1974; Thornton et al., 1977). The effects of rise-time, duration, and spectrum on the middle components have been studied (Lane et al., 1971; Skinner and Antinoro, 1971; Beiter and Hogan, 1973), and it is probable that rise-time is the most influential of these three parameters (Kupperman, 1970). Tone bursts having rise-fall times of about 2.5 milliseconds, and a duration of about 2 milliseconds appear to be ideal. We have produced these stimuli by gating electronic timers and switches, and Zerlin et

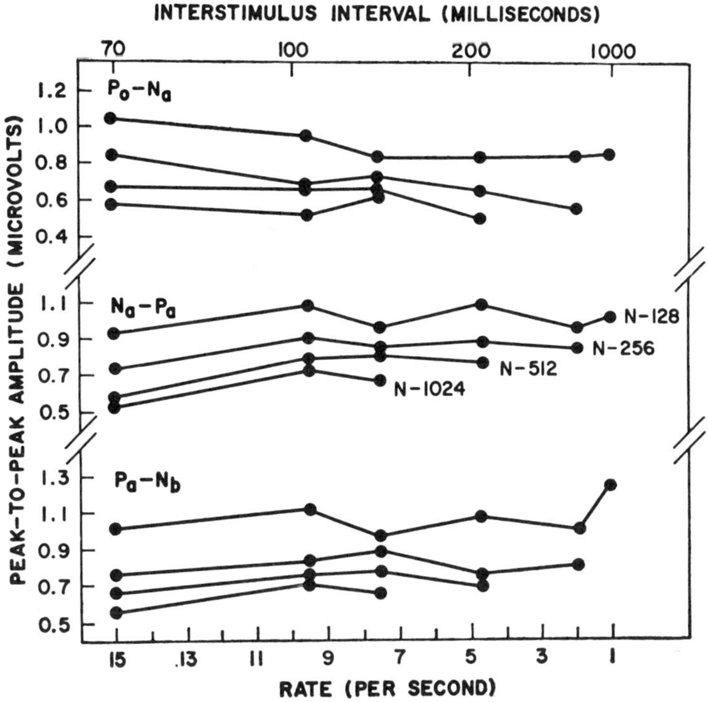

Fig. 9-13. Mean peak-to-peak amplitudes of the middle components for 12 subjects, two trials and both sides of head combined, for six rates and increasing numbers of stimuli. (From Goldstein, Rodman, and Karlovich: J Speech Hear Res 1972.)

al. have advocated the use of third-octave filtered clicks. While the spectrum of the gated tone burst is constant regardless of center frequency, the spectrum of the filtered click is set by the center frequency at one-third octave. There remains some doubt as to which of these methods of generating tone bursts is actually best at different frequencies. As with the late components, the largest and clearest responses appear to be elicited at a center frequency of 1000 Hz (Kupperman and Mendel, 1974; Thornton et al., 1977).

The amplitude of the middle components increases and latency decreases slightly with increasing stimulus intensity (Fig. 9-14) up to moderate levels of about 50 to 60 dB SL (Madell and Goldstein, 1972; Mendel, 1974). At high intensity levels (70–80 dB SL) a different response (myogenic in origin?) may occur from some subjects (Thornton, 1975). Thresholds determined with the middle components in adults, whether awake or asleep agree with behavioral threshold within 10 to 20 dB (Mendel and Goldstein, 1971; Mendel, 1974; McFarland, et al., 1974; Mendel et al., 1975).

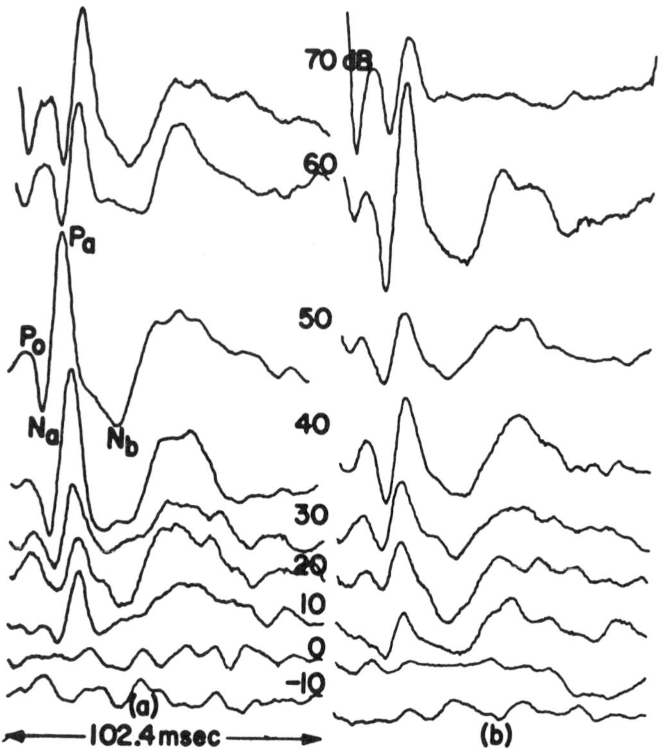

Fig. 9-14. Amplitude and latency of the middle components as a function of stimulus intensity. Each tracing represents the average of 1536 responses to clicks at a rate of 9.6/second from vertex-earlobe electrodes. Parts (a) and (b) show examples of intertrial consistency from one subject. (From Madell and Goldstein: J Speech Hear Res 1972.)

Unlike the late components, the middle components remain remarkably stable during changes in subject state. The effects of attention have not been thoroughly explored with the middle components. In the three studies dealing with the effects of attention, Mendel and Goldstein (1969a) found no significant differences in the middle components caused by changes in test conditions (sitting in the dark with eyes closed, sitting quietly in a lighted room with eyes open, or reading); while Thompson (1972) and Picton and Hillyard (1974) found no effect of attention on the amplitude of the middle components. These responses show long-term stability when tested at three-hour intervals for a 24-hour sleepless period (Mendel and Goldstein, 1969b), and remain quite stable during overnight sleep (Mendel and Goldstein, 1971). Responses obtained during REM sleep are repeatable and similar to those obtained during the other stages of sleep (Mendel and Kupperman, 1974).

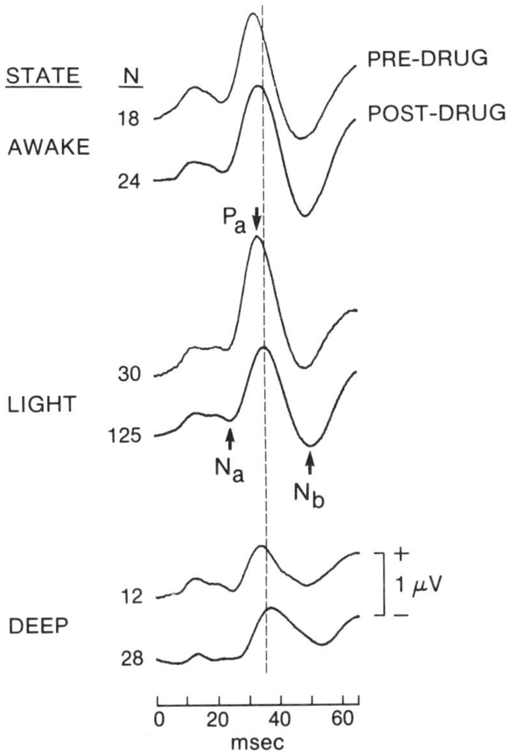

Fig. 9-15. Middle components of the auditory evoked potentials as a function of the state from which they were obtained, preceding and following the intravenous administration of secobarbitol. Responses from one subject from the awake, light sleep (stages 2 and REM), and deep sleep (stages 3 and 4) states are shown pre- and post-drug administration. An averaged response consisted of 512 presentations of 1000-Hz tone pips at 40 dB SL at a rate of 9/sec. In this figure, composite responses of the number of individual responses in the N column are shown. For example, the predrug awake waveform includes a total of 9216 (18 × 512) stimuli, while the postdrug awake waveform includes 12,288 (24 × 512) stimuli. (From Mendel and Hosick: Rev Laryngol 1975.)

The middle components are unaffected by light sedation (Fig. 9-15) (Mendel and Hosick, 1975; Mendel et al., 1974), although at anesthetic levels of

total muscle paralysis with succinylcholine (Horwitz et al., 1966; Harker et al., 1977). Clinical patients, sedated with secobarbital, have been routinely tested for well over 2 years (Mendel, Pals, and Harker, 1976).

Although the middle components were the first averaged evoked potentials recorded from the human scalp, progress with these responses has been hindered by the lingering myogenic controversy. Considerable evidence now exists to support the neurogenic origin of the response for low and moderate level stimuli from relaxed subjects. Frequency specific information can be obtained at levels within 10–20 dB of behavioral threshold from adults who are awake, or in natural, or drug-induced sleep. These components seem to offer exciting possibilities for threshold evaluation at various frequencies, and may lend themselves conveniently to automated audiometry using predeterimined scoring criteria (Mendel et al., 1975), complex template matching routines (McFarland et al., 1974), or machine scoring (Schimmel, Rapin, and Cohen, 1975).

Application to Infants

The middle component responses of infants have received relatively little attention. In an early paper, Engel (1971) studied the middle and late components in sleeping neonates. He reported the presence of late component responses in all 24 babies tested, but identified middle components in only eight. In contrast, McRandle et al. (1974) in an initial report on 10 neonates, and more recently (Goldstein and McRandle, 1976) in 22 additional neonates, elicited repeatable and stable middle component waveforms from the sleeping babies. The waveforms of the neonates, one to three days of age, resemble those of adults tested under similar conditions. Although the late components were also obtained, McRandle et al. (1974) found their identification was more dependent on the sleep stage of the infant, and the responses in some cases were obscured by large amplitude, low frequency components.

In a recent study (Mendel et al., 1977), the middle components were recorded from 18 infants; six each at one, four, and eight months of age (see Fig. 9-16). We found middle component responses in all of the infants tested during natural sleep with tone bursts centered at 1000 Hz presented at 60 dB HL. The amplitude of the responses was somewhat smaller than that found with adults tested under similar circumstances, and interestingly, latencies were shorter in infants than in adults. In contrast, both the early and late components show decreasing latencies with increasing age. We found (like Goldstein and McRandle, 1976) little activity takes place beyond 50 milliseconds in the responses from infants; adults show a later wave (P_c–N_c) between about 50 and 80 milliseconds.

Although Davis and Hirsh (1973) report difficulty with the middle components in their experience with young children in the hearing clinic, we (Mendel et al., 1976) have now successfully used these responses for clinical

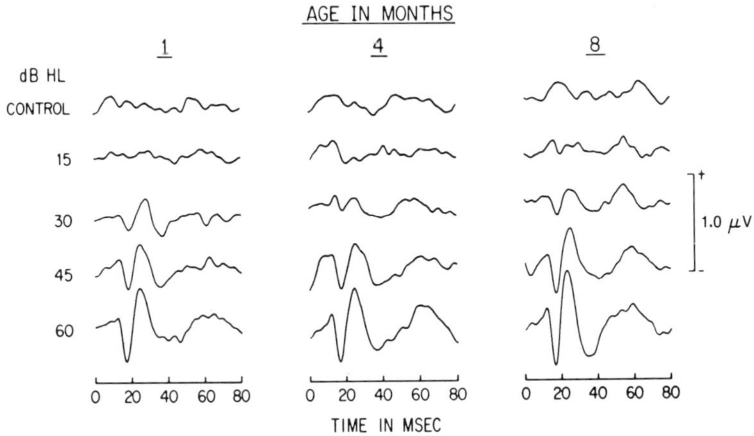

Fig. 9-16. Composite middle components from six infants each at 1, 4, and 8 months of age during natural sleep. Tone bursts centered at 1000 Hz were presented at 15, 30, 45, and 60 dB (re: normal adult threshold) and in a no stimulus control condition. (From Mendel, Adkinson, and Harker: Ann Otol Rhinol Laryngol, 1977.)

testing for over two years. Infants less than one year of age were tested during natural sleep, while older infants and children were tested during sleep induced with an intramuscular injection of secobarbital. Of the 28 infants from 1 month to 2 years of age referred, a period of sleep adequate for our clinical determination of threshold was accomplished in all but one.

Davis (1976a) has reviewed four electrophysiologic time domains for electric response audiometry in young children who require sedation. After weighing the relative merits and difficulties of electrocochleography, the brainstem response, the muscle reflexes, and the middle components, he concludes that the middle components are good candidates, but that they have not yet been adequately validated in the clinic. Based on clinical experience with the middle components, I agree with Davis and feel that these responses offer the best means of evaluating thresholds at various frequencies.

Since many references in this chapter are repeated in the next two chapters, all references are given at the end of Chapter 11.

Maurice I. Mendel

10
Evoked Cochlear Potentials

The previous chapter in this tripartite section of the book dealt with electroencephalic audiometry, that is, the recording of the electrical activity of the brain from electrodes on the scalp. This chapter, in contrast, deals with electrocochleography, the recording of the electrical activity of the peripheral auditory system from an electrode placed near the cochlea. Primary attention is focused on the recording, in humans, of the responses of the cochlea and the eighth nerve, the cochlear microphonic (CM), and the action potential (AP). While electrodes placed on the vertex and earlobe (or mastoid) yield patterns like those shown in Fig. 9-1 (which are called the evoked brainstem potentials, and are discussed in the next chapter), electrodes on the promontory of the middle ear or in the external auditory meatus near the tympanic membrane and the earlobe yield patterns like those of Fig. 9-2. This is confusing, since both patterns occur in approximately the same time domain of 0 to 8 milliseconds, and wave I of Fig. 9-1 and peak N_1 of Fig. 9-2 represent the same activity. However, the difference in the location of the recording electrodes yields this apparent distinction in the pattern of the response, as well as real differences in response amplitude.

The evoked potentials generated at the level of the cochlea can be divided into three categories: the cochlear microphonic (CM), the summating potential (SP), and the compound (or whole nerve) action potential (AP) (Fig. 10-1). The CM is linearly related to the amplitude of displacement of the cochlear partition over a considerable frequency and intensity range. Its waveform reflects the waveform of the acoustic stimulus—being in phase with the amplitude of the movement of the cochlear partition and occurring nearly instantaneously after stimulus onset—much like the output of a microphone. The SP is a direct current (DC) shift that continues throughout the presentation of a stimulus. The magnitude and polarity of the DC shift are dependent on the recording site, stimulus frequency, and stimulus intensity. Dallos (1973) distinguishes between a differential SP, measured between scala vestibuli and scala tympani, and an average SP between the average of the two scalae and a distant reference point. The SP has not been thoroughly studied as an index of hearing in the literature of electrocochleography (ECoG) from humans. Eggermont (1976) has shown that, with proper stimulating and recording techniques, the SP can be recorded from humans. However, diagnosis of different types of hearing loss is not yet possible with the SP alone. The main index of ECoG has been the AP of the whole auditory nerve. It results from the nearly simultaneous discharge of many individual nerve fibers in an all-or-none fashion in the production of a neural spike in the auditory branch of the eighth nerve. The major advantage of the AP as an index of peripheral auditory function, therefore, is that while the CM and SP reflect activity at the level of the hair cell, the AP reflects not only the transmission of energy to the hair cell, but also the transduction of this energy in the auditory nerve. It has been suggested (Sohmer and Pratt, 1976; Naunton and Zerlin, 1976a) that the relation between the CM and the AP might allow qualitative differentiation to be made between pathology from the hair cell (sensory) and the nerve (neural).

HISTORICAL CONSIDERATIONS

While studying electrical potentials recorded from the auditory nerve of laboratory animals, Wever and Bray (1930) observed the curious phenomenon that if these amplified potentials were led to a loudspeaker, then words spoken into the animal's ear could be recognized. Although Wever and Bray thought they were recording the AP, Adrian (1931) felt that the electrical changes were generated in the cochlea and passively conducted by the nerve to the recording site. He further suggested that the potentials were due to some kind of microphonic action of the inner ear, hence the name cochlear microphonic. It soon became clear, however, that this Wever-Bray effect consisted of a mixture of the AP and the CM. Various authors at that time speculated about the genesis site of the CM, but these arguments concerning the source of the CM are still not completely settled (Dallos, 1973). A few years later, 1935, the application of cochlear recording techniques was extended to human subjects by Fromm, Nylen, and Zotterman.

Other studies were undertaken in animals to separate the two electrical responses—the AP and the CM—and to improve recording techniques (Saul

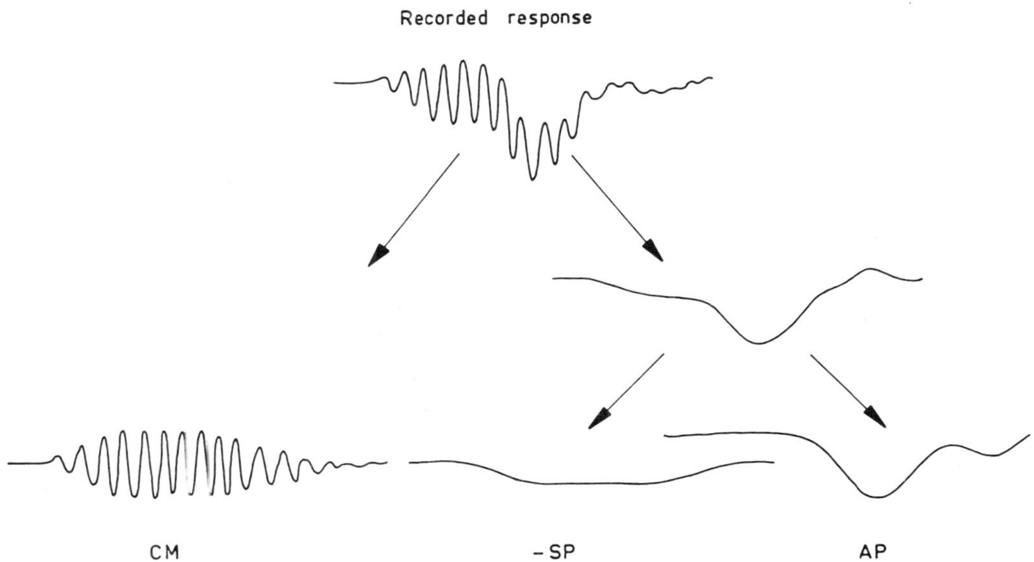

Fig. 10-1. Stimulus-related potentials in the cochlea. In response to short tone-bursts three stimulus-related potentials can be recorded from the cochlea. These potentials, that is, CM, SP, and AP, appear intermingled in the recorded response. By presenting the stimulus alternately in phase and counterphase and averaging the recorded response, a separation can be obtained between CM on the one hand and AP and SP on the other. High-pass filtering provides a separation between SP and AP. This can also be obtained by increasing the repetition rate of the stimuli, which results in an adaptation of the AP but leaves the SP unaltered. (From Eggermont et al: Acta Otolaryngol (Suppl) (Stockh) 316, 1974.)

and Davis, 1932; Davis et al., 1934; Hallpike and Rawdon-Smith, 1934). Davis et al. (1949) introduced localized differential electrodes to separate these responses. Using this approach, they were able to study the two potentials independently. Davis et al. (1950) used tone pips to show that another response could be recorded in the cochlea—the SP. They believed that the SP was a response to the stimulus envelope, rather than to the instantaneous variations contained therein.

Although round-window recordings of the CM from humans with large perforations of the tympanic membrane were first reported by Fromm, et al., (1935), the responses were small and not as clear as those recorded by the authors from cats. Similar results were obtained in Russia by Andreev, Arapova, and Gersuni (1939) in the vicinity of the round window from patients who also had perforations of the tympanic membrane. These investigators were the first to publish a graphic record of the CM from humans. Perlman and Case (1941) were the first Americans to record the CM in humans. They carried out extensive investigations with rabbits and monkeys prior to employing the technique on human subjects with perforated tympanic membranes. Perlman and Case reported unsuccessful attempts to record the CM from normal human subjects with the electrode against the intact tympanic membrane. Further attempts to record the CM from humans were not reported for another six years. Lempert et al. (1947) were interested in developing ECoG for both general diagnostic purposes and for surgical guidance during middle ear explorations in humans. They proposed the term cochleogram, and suggested (1950) the placement of a needle electrode through the intact tympanic membrane onto the promotory at the time of surgery as a recording technique.

No more papers were published on electrocochleography in humans for the next nine years. Interest in this area was revived by Ruben and his colleagues (1959, 1960), who described surgical procedures for recording the cochlear potentials from the round window niche. Ruben et al. were the first to obtain clear CM responses from the round window, as well as recording the AP at high click levels (1961, 1962, 1963). They found that the first peak in the AP, N_1, was of greater amplitude than the other peaks (N_2 and N_3). Ruben and colleagues developed a technique that separated the AP from the CM by changing the phase of the signal. The CM, because it is sensitive to phase shifts, was effectively cancelled when the signal was alternately reversed. This basic technique is widely used today to record the AP without the interference of the CM (Fig. 10-2). In a summary of this work, Ruben (1967) suggested the use of electrocochleography to investigate and differentiate conductive, cochlear, and neural lesions in an operating room technique. Ronis (1966) refined this surgical procedure by employing computer averaging techniques, which set the stage for rapid developments of ECoG.

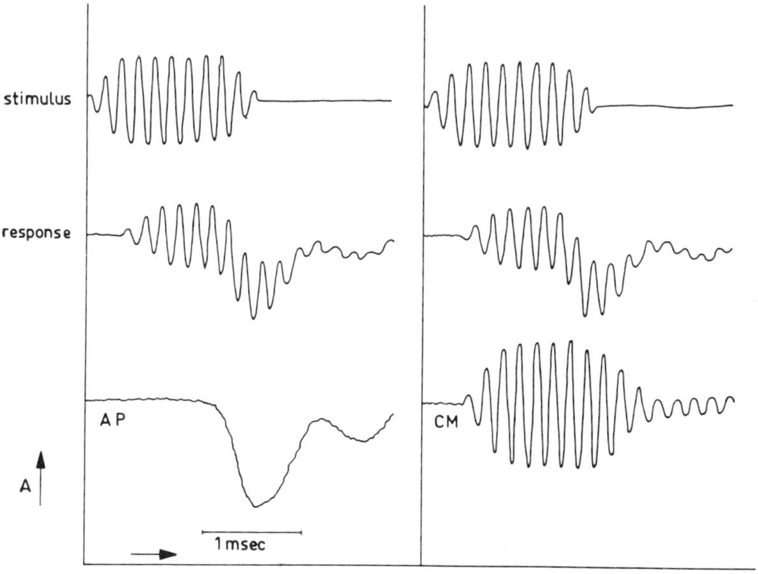

Fig. 10-2. Commutator action. Odd and even stimuli have opposite phase. In the responses the AP have the same phase; the CM are in opposite phase. During the averaging process the CM is cancelled in one channel by simple summation of all responses. The AP is cancelled simultaneously in the other channel, because the phase of the even responses is reversed before the summation. (From Spoor in Eggermont et al: Acta Otolaryngol (Suppl) (Stockh) 316, 1974.)

The modern era in ECoG began in 1967 with the simultaneous publication by three groups of investigators (Yoshie et al.; Portmann et al.; and Sohmer and Feinmesser) of computer averaging techniques to record the AP from the promontory, external ear canal, and earlobe. The latter two recording sites, the external ear canal and earlobe, allow ECoG to be carried out as a nonsurgical procedure. Although many investigators have reported on the CM, the vast majority of studies in clinical ECoG deal with the AP of the eighth nerve.

CLINICAL ELECTROCOCHLEOGRAPHY

As shown in Fig. 9-2, the cochlear evoked potentials are divided into the CM, occurring almost instantaneously after the onset of the stimulus, and the subsequent AP, labeled N_1, N_2, and N_3 and occurring within about the next 3 milliseconds. Many studies have been published showing the effects of re-

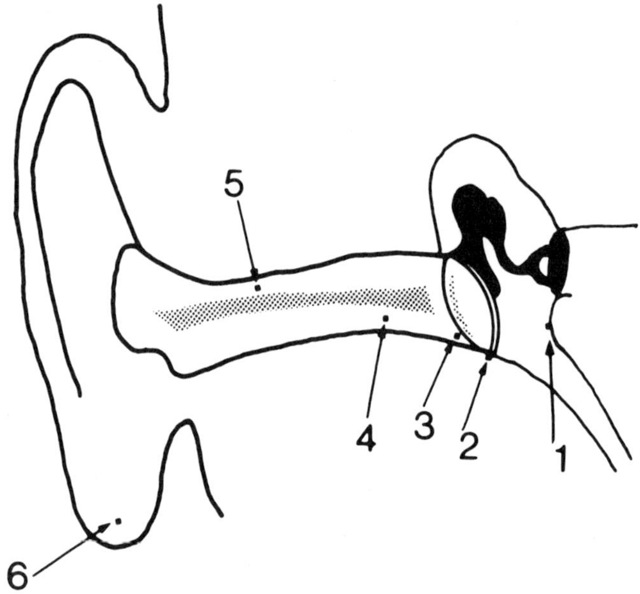

Fig. 10-3. Examples of recording locations used in electrocochleography. These have included the promontory and round window (1); the annulus and posterior-inferior quadrant of the tympanic membrane (2); the posterior canal wall (3,4,5); and the earlobe (6). Representative studies based on these sites are: Aran (1971), Portmann and Aran (1971), Yoshie and Ohashi (1969) for the round window or promontory; Cullen et al. (1972) and Yoshie (1968) for the tympanic membrane; Coats and Dickey (1970) and Yoshie (1968) for the external canal; Moore (1971) and Sohmer and Feinmesser (1967) for the earlobe. Site comparison data include those of Simmons (1972) and Yoshie and Ohashi (1969). (From Simmons and Glattke, in Bradford L (ed): *Physiological Measures of the Audio-Vestibular System*. New York, Academic, 1975.)

cording the AP from the three sites mentioned above (Fig. 10-3). It has been shown that electrodes closest to the cochlea provide the clearest records (AP of about 10 μV at 90 dB SL), but this technique requires penetrating the tympanic membrane. This transtympanic recording site (Figs. 10-4 and 10-5) was first reported by Portmann, LeBert, and Aran (1967), and subsequently used by Aran and LeBert, 1968; Aran et al. 1969, 1971, 1972; Aran, 1971, 1973; Aran and Portmann, 1972; Aran and Negrevergne, 1972; Portmann and Aran, 1971a, b, c; Yoshie and Ohashi, 1969, 1971; Yoshie, 1971, 1973; Eggermont et al., 1974; Simmons, 1974, 1975; Naunton and Zerlin, 1976a; and by Yanz, 1976. Recordings from the tympanic membrane are smaller than those from the promontory (about 3 μV at 90 dB SL), while those from

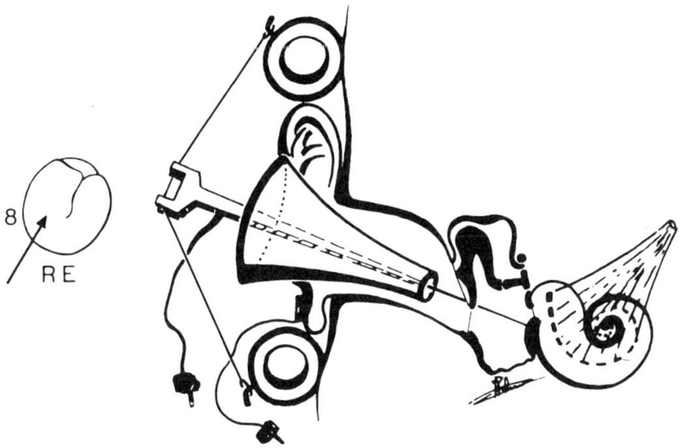

Fig. 10-4. The transtympanic recording technique as devised by Portmann and Aran. The active needle electrode penetrates the tympanic membrane and is embedded in the promontory. The reference electrode is shown on the earlobe. A doughnut cushion surrounds the ear, supporting the active electrode in place with an elastic band. (From Aran: Adv Otorhinolaryngol 1973.)

the canal wall are further diminished (about 1 μV at 90 dB SL). These recording sites on or near the tympanic membrane have been reported by Coats and Dickey (1970, 1972); Coats (1974); Cullen et al. (1972); while the canal wall location has been used by Sohmer and Feinmesser (1967); Yoshie et al. (1967); Yoshie (1968); Salomon and Elberling (1971); Elberling and Salomon (1971); Khechinashvili et al., (1974); Khechinashvili and Kevanishvili (1974); Montandon et al. (1975a,b). The smallest AP responses (about 0.3 μV at 90 dB SL) are recorded from the surface of the earlobe, using either earclip or needle electrodes (Sohmer and Feinmesser, 1967, 1970; Hood, 1970; Moore, 1971; Thornton, 1975a–c, 1976). Comparisons of the records obtained from the various recording sites which document the generalizations included above have been made by Yoshie and Ohashi, 1969; Eggermont and Odenthal, 1974c; and Simmons, 1975. All of these studies have shown that the largest and clearest AP recordings are obtained from an electrode placed directly on the promontory of the stimulated ear (Fig. 10-6). Recordings of this type are made by passing a small gauge needle through the tympanic membrane until it comes to rest against the promontory. Although the outer end of the electrode is usually fixed in place according to the techniques developed by Portmann and Aran (1971b), one recent study (Yanz, 1976) used a free-floating needle electrode in an attempt to use earphones to develop

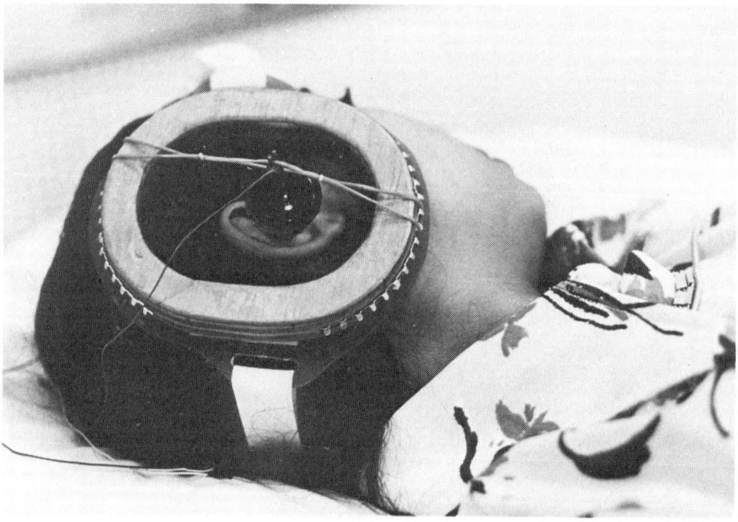

Fig. 10-5. A patient with electrode in place for transtympanic electrocochleography. (Photo courtesy of Dr. R. Naunton and University of Chicago Publications.)

a closed acoustic stimulating system. Transtympanic ECoG is generally carried out in infants and children under general anesthesia, while the electrode is placed in adults under a local anesthetic. In the laboratory at the University of Iowa, an otolaryngologist administers a topical anesthetic (4% xylocaine) iontophoretically (Medical Systems, Ltd., Model 22) after clearing the external auditory canal of wax. After the anesthetic takes effect (about 10 minutes), the electrode is inserted painlessly through the tympanic membrane and moved medially until the point is embedded in the bony wall of the promontory (Yanz, 1976). In a recent survey, Crowley, Davis, and Beagley (1975) have shown that this transtympanic promontory electrode technique has been used successfully on a worldwide basis on over 2100 patients ranging in age from 1 day to 79 years. In this total population of 2110 cases, there were three instances of problems arising from the placement of the electrode, and 45 cases of difficulty from the use of anesthesia. However, most of the problems associated with the use of anesthesia appear to have been overcome with experience. Therefore, the transtympanic recording technique appears to be the optimal approach for clinical ECoG, and appears to be a safe and efficient procedure in experienced hands.

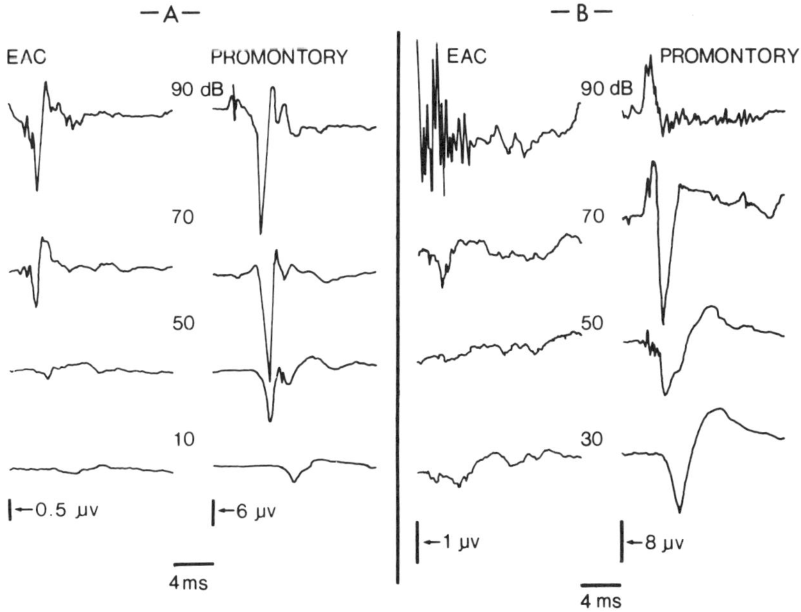

Fig. 10-6. Examples of external auditory canal (EAC) and promontory recordings from two subjects (A) and (B). The recordings in (A) were taken from an individual who showed remarkable sensitivity at both recording locations. Those in (B) are more typical, in the sense that EAC thresholds were elevated and high-intensity stimulation resulted in serious contamination of the response with microphone-like artifacts. Stimulus levels are shown in dB re normal perceptual threshold for the click stimulus. (From Simmons and Glattke, in Bradford L (ed): *Physiological Measures of the Audio-Vestibular System*. New York, Academic, 1975.)

General Findings in Adults

As previously mentioned, the AP can be recorded from a variety of locations between the earlobe and the promontory. For the optimal recording site on the promontory, an N_1 amplitude [which may be measured from the tip of the N_1 peak to an arbitrary baseline, to the first positive peak following N_1, or to the most positive point following N_1 (Fig. 10–7)] of about 10–20 μV is found for stimuli of 60–70 dB SL. Broad bandpass filters, for example, about 100–4000 Hz, are used to record the AP; and these responses from the promontory may be obtained with as few as 64 to 100 stimulus presentations. When recording with the active electrode on the earlobe, as many as 256 to

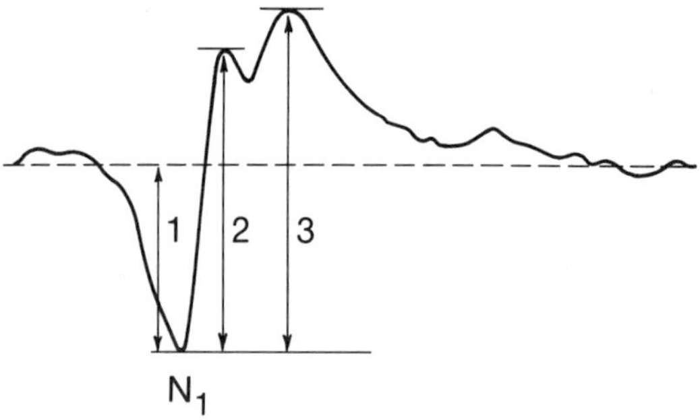

Fig. 10-7. Different techniques used for measuring the N_1 amplitude of the AP.

1536 stimulus presentations may be necessary in order to elicit a clear AP (Sohmer et al., 1974; Moore, 1971). Like the late components, the AP is sensitive to the rate of signal presentation (Fig. 10-8). The amplitude of the N_1 peak increases as interstimulus interval is increased from 8 to 512 milliseconds (Eggermont and Odenthal, 1974a). Optimum interstimulus intervals are about 100 milliseconds. Like the middle components, initial studies of the AP used clicks as stimuli; while more recently tone pips, tone bursts, or filtered clicks have been used (Fig. 10-9) (Yoshie, 1971, 1973; Eggermont and Odenthal, 1974b; Odenthal, Eggermont and Hermans, 1974; Elberling, 1974; Mouney et al., 1976; Naunton and Zerlin, 1976b; Eggermont, Spoor and Odenthal, 1976; Yanz, 1976). While most authors agree that high-frequency stimuli—for example, 2000, 4000, and 8000 Hz—yield clear frequency specific responses from the basal turn of the cochlea, serious doubts have been raised over the use of low frequency stimuli (250, 500, and 1000 Hz) for both electrocochleography and the brainstem potentials covered in the next chapter (Davis and Hirsh, 1976; Davis, 1976a and b). Davis (1976b) points out that the AP response to a 500 Hz tone pip seems to be initiated by stimulation of the basal turn of the cochlea by the low-frequency transient, and therefore is of limited usefulness for audiometric testing. The answer to this problem, however, may be provided ultimately by the derived responses of the selective masking techniques first described by Teas, Eldredge, and Davis (1962). Brief tone bursts of about 4–6 milliseconds total duration appear to be ideal stimuli. Unlike the middle and late components, where the optimal stimulus frequency is 1000 Hz, the largest and clearest AP responses appear to be elicited at center frequencies of 4000 or 8000 Hz.

As shown in Fig. 10-10, the latency of the N_1 peak varies regularly from about 4 milliseconds at 20 dB HL to about 1.2 milliseconds at 85 dB HL in

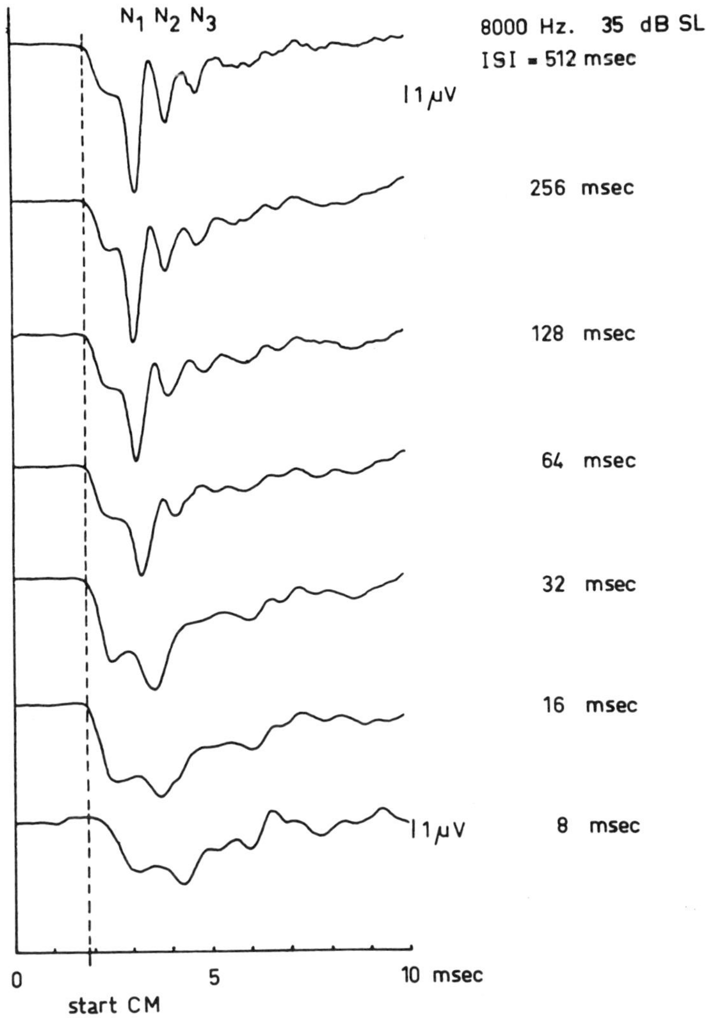

Fig. 10-8. Changes in the waveform of the final-value AP as a function of the interstimulus interval (ISI). In the unadapted AP (ISI = 512 milliseconds) at least three negative deflections ((N_1, N_2, *and* N_3) are clearly visible. When adaptation occurs (lower ISI values), first the N_3 (ISI = 64 milliseconds) and then the N_2 (ISI = 32 milliseconds) disappears. The early negative deflection is a summating potential. (From Eggermont and Odenthal in Eggermont et al. Acta Otolaryngol (Suppl) (Stockh) 316, 1974.)

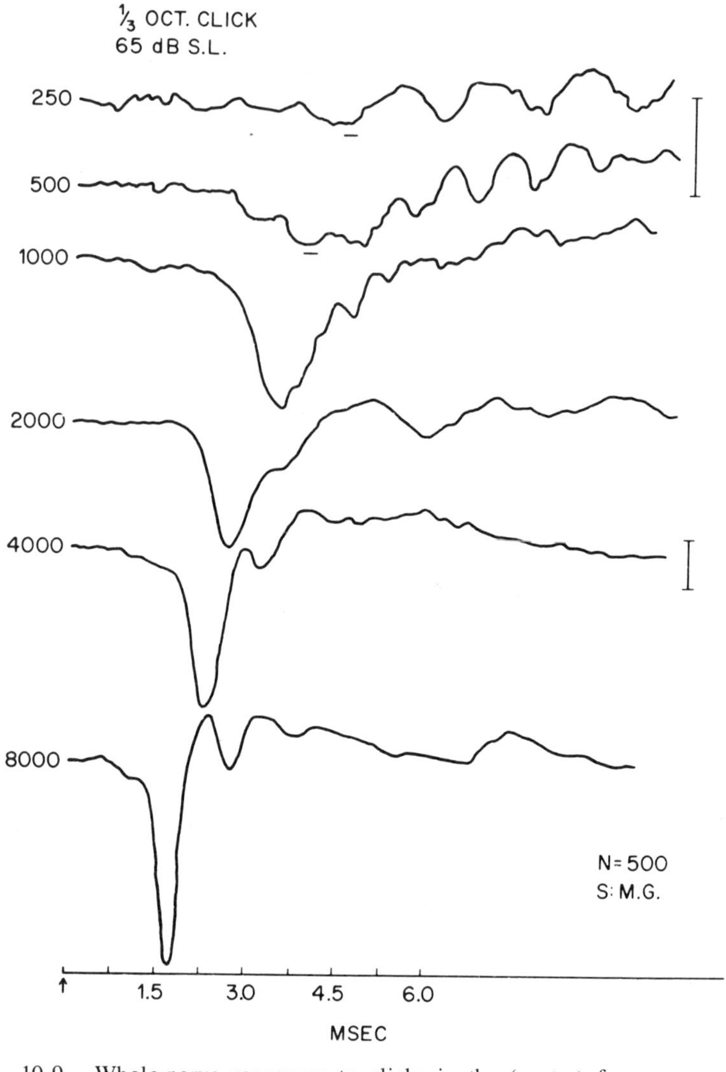

Fig. 10-9. Whole-nerve responses to clicks in the (center) frequency range, 250–8000 Hz. The vertical calibration lines equal 1 μV: the three upper traces are referenced to the upper vertical, the lower three traces to the lower vertical. (From Zerlin and Naunton in Ruben, Elberling, and Salomon (eds): University Park Press, 1976.)

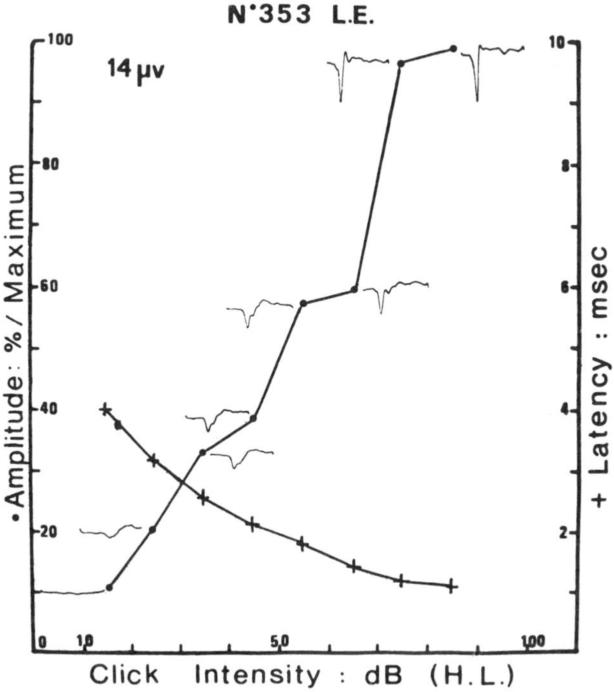

Fig. 10-10. Normal electrocochleographic recordings from the left ear of a 3-year, 5-month-old child who did not give consistent responses during classical testing. The features which correspond to the normal responses are: (1) a progressive decrease of the latency from around 4.0 milliseconds at threshold; (2) the L and H parts of the amplitude curve, with the plateau around 50 dB HL; (3) the diphasic response near threshold and monophasic pattern of 85 dB HL. On this figure the amplitude is expressed in percent of the maximum amplitude indicated in the top left-hand corner of the graph. The traces are such that a downward deflection corresponds to the promontory negative with respect to the ear lobe. Trace duration (window) is 10 milliseconds. Beginning of the trace is 1 millisecond before the arrival of the click at the ear, the latency is measured from this point to the trough of N_1. (From Portmann, Aran, and Lagourgne: Ann Otol Rhinol Laryngol, 82:36–43, 1973.)

response to click stimuli. The amplitude of the response increases gradually from low intensity levels up to about 50–60 dB HL. At higher levels, the amplitude increases much more rapidly up to about 80 dB, where it flattens out. Yoshie (1968) called the low intensity range the L-curve and the higher intensity range the H-curve, and the interpretation was soon offered that there were two populations of auditory units which caused these two curves, the outer and inner hair cells. An alternative explanation has been proposed by Elberling (1974) and by Eggermont et al. (1974) that the two populations are the hair cells located in the middle turn and the basal turn of the cochlea respectively. As shown by Davis (1976b), this problem, as well as the relation of outer to inner hair cells, has not been finally resolved. Thresholds determined with the AP are dependent upon the location of the active electrode. Eggermont and Odenthal (1974c) give the following threshold values:

round window	0 dB SL
promontory	5 dB SL
annulus tympanicus	10 dB SL
external ear	30 dB SL

Since the AP is strictly a monaural response, with no contribution or interaction from the opposite ear, masking of the opposite ear is not necessary in ECoG.

Like the early and middle components, the AP response remains remarkably stable during changes in subject state. To the best of my knowledge, there are no studies of the effect of attention on the AP. However, since this is an onset response of the cochlea and eighth nerve, I think we can safely predict that selective attention would have no effect on the AP. This response remains quite stable during sleep, and as I mentioned in the previous section, is usually elicited during general or local anesthesia. Zvonar, Zvonar-Kuhndl, and Odenthal (1974) and Crowley, Davis, and Beagley (1975) point out that, in children less than eight years of age, ketamine hydrochloride (Ketalar) has most frequently been used as a general anesthetic. Zvonar et al. (1974), however, point out that the use of ketamine has certain disadvantages. This method of anesthesia causes excessive swallowing action and minor movements of the patient, which produce electrical and mechanical artifacts in the recording. Because of these problems, they have begun to use inhalation anesthesia for testing children, while Innitzer and Schmid (1975) have attempted to alleviate this problem by preceding the administration of ketamine with an injection of droperidole and fentanyl (Thalamonal). Just as the services of an otolaryngologist are necessary for electrode placement with this technique, it should be obvious that the services of an anesthesiologist are also necessary with infants and children. This is not a testing technique which can be used by an audiologist working alone.

Simmons and Glattke (1975) describe the three principal characteristics—latency, amplitude, and shape—of the AP in the following manner. The latency of the AP, they suggest, is a clue to the frequency region of the cochlea contributing to the response. The amplitude of the AP is a reflection of the number of active elements contributing to it and the syn-

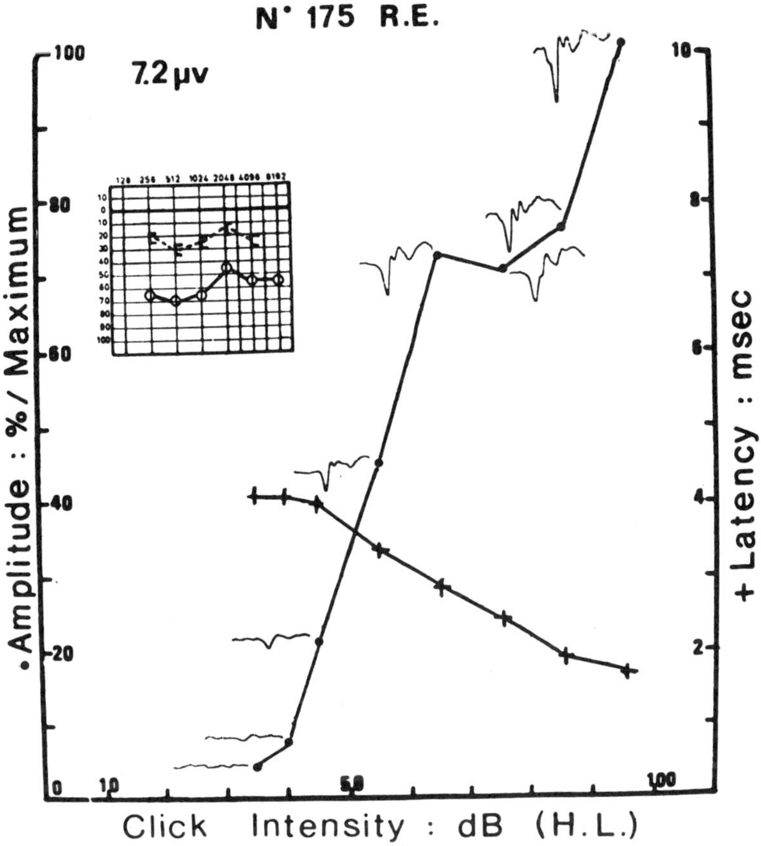

Fig. 10-11. Responses recorded from the right ear of a 48-year-old male with conductive hearing loss. The features of the responses are similar to the normal, but the threshold and curves are shifted to the right by an amount of 35 dB, which measures the conduction loss. Note latency threshold is still 4 milliseconds. (From: Portmann, Aran, and Lagourgne: Oral Rhinol Laryngol 1973.)

chrony of their discharges. The shape of the response, finally, is the result of a compromise between the electrical fields of neurons which have discharged and are refractory and neurons which are discharging at a given moment. While the plot of the N_1 peak latency and relative amplitude is used to develop the cochleogram shown in Fig. 10-10, the relation of all three measures (latency, amplitude, and shape) is taken into account to describe abnormal hearing.

In the simplest case where no AP can be found at any stimulus intensity, the interpretation is easy: the cochlea is nonfunctional for hearing. In cases of conductive hearing loss, the cochleogram is identical in configuration to that of normal, with both an L- and H-curve, but it is shifted to a higher intensity (Fig. 10-11). Therefore, it is mainly the threshold value that differs in conductive hearing loss, the shape of the AP response and the input-output relations are normal. In cases of sensory-neural hearing loss with recruitment, the cochleogram differs in configuration from that of normals (Fig. 10-12). The L-curve may be missing entirely, the threshold value is shifted to a higher value, and a rapid increase of amplitude is seen at intensity values just above threshold. The H-curve in a few cases reaches normal or supranormal values, which is indicative of the recruitment phenomenon. When the amplitude-intensity data are plotted on a logarithmic scale, the slope of the H-curve is twice as steep as the normal curve, and shows roughly a tenfold amplitude increase for a 10-dB intensity increase (Odenthal and Eggermont, 1974). This recruiting cochleogram may exist with loudness recruitment, but it has also been found in persons whose behavioral loudness recruitment studies are totally negative. Another type of abnormal cochleogram is the double-peaked or dissociated pattern (Fig. 10-13). The characteristic features of the dissociated cochleogram are: (1) a threshold that may be normal or moderately elevated; (2) a normal or slower than normal amplitude growth immediately above threshold; (3) an abrupt change in both the waveform and latency of the AP as the stimulus intensity is increased further; and (4) a response amplitude maximum that may be less than normal. This pattern is associated with hearing loss of cochlear origin which is not uniformly distributed along the cochlea (Simmons and Glattke, 1975).

Another consideration is the use of the AP in the diagnosis of acoustic neuroma, which was suggested by Aran (1971), and discussed more recently by Brackmann and Selters (1976) and Odenthal and Eggermont (1976). Although unusual appearing AP responses were seen in some patients with acoustic neuromas, these investigators, so far, have been unable to define a pattern which is indicative of acoustic neuroma.

The cochlear evoked potentials have received a great deal of attention in the European literature as a diagnostic test, and are now receiving more attention in the United States. There are several advantages to the clinical use of these responses. First, their source is known to be the cochlea and the auditory nerve. Second, although not reviewed in this chapter, a large volume of data has been accumulated on cochlear potentials in animals, representing many different stimulation and recording techniques. Some of these techniques, such as single unit recordings, are not possible with human subjects. Third, since the responses do reflect activity of the peripheral system, they may be valuable in the differential diagnosis of peripheral auditory defects.

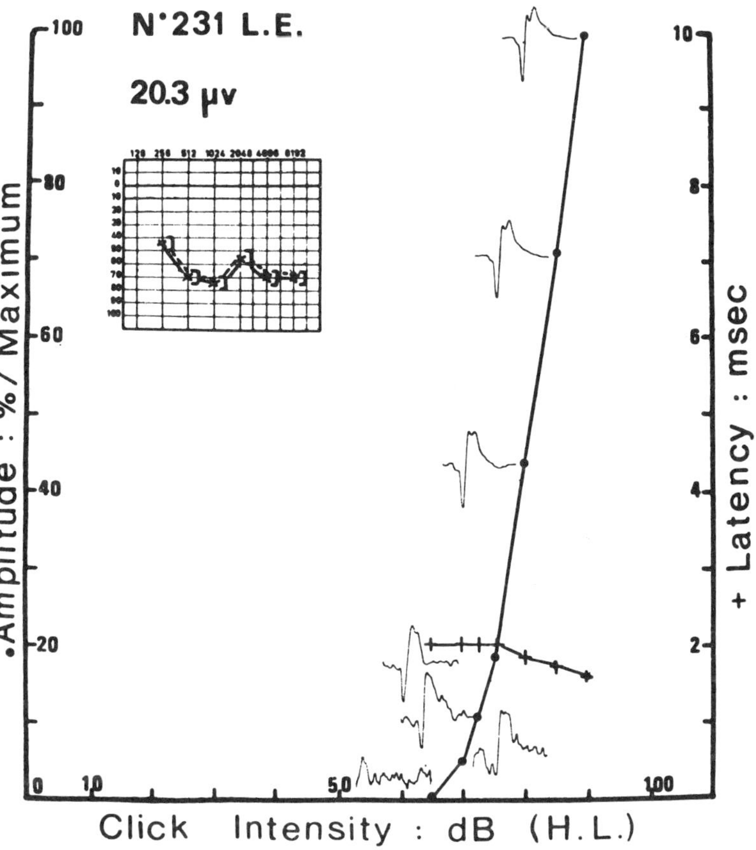

Fig. 10-12. Responses recorded from the left ear of a 39-year-old male with sensorineural deafness (recruitment was not tested). Note the characteristics of what we call the recruiting response: (1) the short latency at the threshold (2 milliseconds); (2) the high value of the amplitude at 90 dB HL; (3) the very fast diphasic pattern of the responses. (From: Portmann, Aran, and Lagourgne, Ann Otol Rhinol Laryngol 1973.)

Although most work on these potentials has focused on the AP, recent studies (Sohmer and Pratt, 1976; Naunton and Zerlin, 1976a) have reiterated the value of the CM in separating sensory and neural hearing losses. Finally, when recorded from the promontory using clicks or high-frequency tone bursts, the AP can be measured in response to stimuli which are within about 5 dB of behavioral threshold.

Two drawbacks limit the use of this technique. First, at low frequencies such as 250 and 500 Hz, the amplitude of the responses is small, frequency

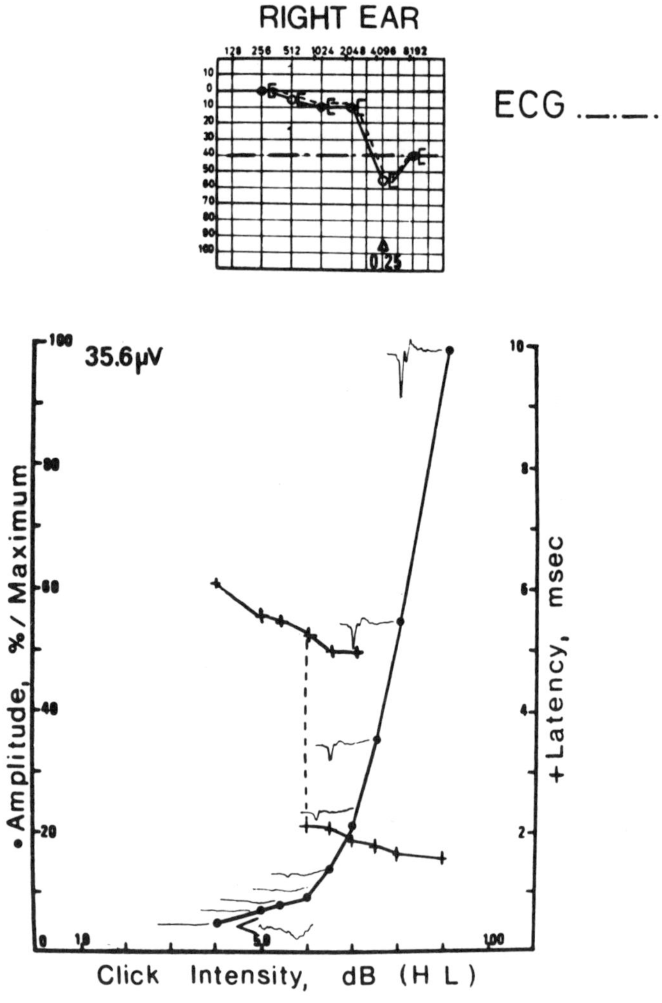

Fig. 10-13. Patient (34 years). We note, for the right ear, the typical dissociated responses at low and high click intensities; the latencies of the late response and of N_1 could be measured simultaneously at 60, 65, and 70 dB. We note on the audiogram that the hearing loss is restricted to the high frequencies. For the left ear there are only two

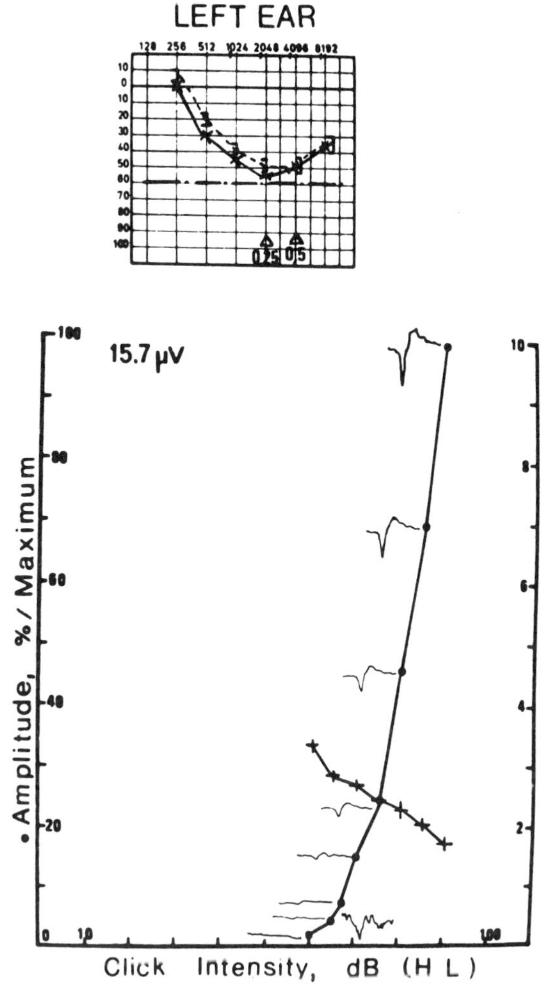

characteristics of the recruiting responses: diphasic patterns and fast increase of the amplitude, but the latency varies from 3.2 to 1.7 milliseconds. This could be due to the better hearing thresholds both for low frequencies. (From: Aran: Otorhinolaryngol 1973.)

selectivity is poor, and threshold detection is unreliable. Second, this is a surgical technique when a promontory electrode is used. The services of an otlogist are always necessary, and when used with infants and children, an anesthesiologist is also required.

Application to Infants

Like the middle components, the evoked cochlear potentials in infants have received relatively little attention. Because ECoG with a promontory electrode is a surgical procedure requiring general anesthesia in children, it is understandable that normative studies with infants have not been reported. Most of the studies reviewed in this section were carried out on infants suspected of hearing impairment, usually after routine behavioral measures failed to give satisfactory results.

ECoG with infants and children has been reported primarily by three laboratories: that of Portmann and Aran in Bordeaux, that of Berlin and Cullen in New Orleans, and that of Sohmer and Feinmesser in Jerusalem. While a promontory electrode has been used routinely in Bordeaux, the New Orleans group usually records with an electrode at or near the tympanic membrane in the external auditory canal, and work in Jerusalem was all accomplished with surface electrodes on the earlobe and scalp.

In a series of related papers, the Bordeaux group (Aran, 1971; Portmann and Aran, 1971a and b; and Portmann et al., 1974) has shown that the AP can be reliably elicited in most newborns and infants. By 1974, they had tested 220 patients under three years of age, which was 32% of their total population of 692 cases tested with ECoG. Infants and babies were tested under light general anesthesia induced by intravenous or intramuscular ketamine following premedication with an atropine-like drug. Results in the 220 babies ranged from normal hearing to profound deafness. However, no systematic comparison is given in any of these papers of the "normal" responses from babies to normal adult responses. Using the techniques of Portmann and Aran, Sudaka and Chaperon (1972) have tested 15 infants with ECoG, and report similar results.

Three recent papers (Berlin, 1976; Berlin and Gondra, 1976; and Cullen et al., 1976) review the clinical experience of the New Orleans group with ECoG, including applications to infants and children. In a summary of 121 cases, Berlin and Gondra tested 47 children less than 10 years of age. Ketamine anesthesia was used in 83% of these children. They found that 20 of the 47 children showed no acoustic reflex and no N_1 response of the AP. Twelve of the children yielded normal N_1 responses, but showed no response to sound. In another study, Cullen et al. provide follow-up information on 35 children who were tested with extratympanic ECoG.

The Jerusalem group also published a series of related papers on the AP elicited with surface electrodes from infants (Sohmer et al., 1972; Leiberman et al., 1973a,b; Sohmer and Feinmesser, 1974; Sohmer et al., 1974) and more recently, a paper on the CM with surface electrodes (Sohmer and Pratt, 1976). Although case reports are included in these papers, the total number of subjects tested to date is not given. By 1973, Leiberman et al. had tested 12 infants from 2 to 12 months of age and 19 neonates from one to seven days old for AP responses. Infants were tested under sedation with chloral hydrate or Trichloryl, while neonates were studied during natural sleep. A trend was seen toward longer latencies in neonates than in adults, with the largest waves seen in the responses of infants. The average threshold in the infant group was 28 dB HL (re: normal adult threshold), and in neonates it was 45 dB HL, compared to 35 dB HL in 10 normal-hearing adults. Like adults, the neonates and infants display increased latency and decreased amplitudes in response to decreases in stimulus intensity. Unfortunately, data derived from wave 1, the AP, are not always separated from the remaining waves for threshold determination.

From these studies from three laboratories, it would appear that the following generalizations may be made about ECoG in infants—the AP exhibits prolonged latency, diminished amplitude, and elevated thresholds as compared to the adult AP. These responses become more like those of adults sometime during the first year of life. However, a great deal of information exists on ECoG in adults and from animal experiments, so that clinical information derived with ECoG from infants would seem to have firm theoretical and experimental grounding.

Since many references in this chapter are duplicated in the preceding and following chapters, all references are given at the end of Chapter 11.

John N. Gardi
and Maurice I. Mendel

11

Evoked Brainstem Potentials

The final chapter in this tripartite section of the book again deals with electroencephalic audiometry, that is, the recording of the electrical activity of the brain with electrodes on the vertex and earlobe (or mastoid). This chapter, however, focuses on the surface recorded activity in the time domain between 2 and 8 milliseconds which reflects activity of the auditory nuclei and tracts—the early components of the auditory evoked potentials or the evoked brainstem potentials (Fig. 9-1).

As shown in the previous chapter, the evoked cochlear potentials, the cochlear microphonic and the compound action potential of the auditory nerve, can be recorded in approximately the same time domain as the brainstem potentials (Fig. 9-2). In humans, the evoked cochlear potentials are recorded most efficiently with an electrode placed through the tympanic membrane onto the promontory of the middle ear. In addition, electrodes on the vertex and the earlobe can be used to record activity in later time domains, the middle and late components of the auditory evoked potentials (Fig. 9-1).

HISTORIC CONSIDERATIONS

Evoked brainstem potentials were first reported by Sohmer and Feinmesser in 1967. They were not aware that they had recorded unique potentials; in fact, the multiple waveforms which they recorded were thought to be repetitive firings of the auditory nerve. Jewett and his colleagues, in a series of papers (Jewett, 1969, 1970; Jewett et al., 1970; Jewett and Williston, 1971; and Jewett and Romano, 1972), first recognized that a unique response, different from the repetitive firing of the VIIIth nerve, could be recorded using averaging techniques from cats, rats, and humans. Jewett and colleagues proposed that these volume conducted signals generated within classical auditory structures could be recorded from diverse areas distant to known auditory neural centers. They differentially recorded volume conducted signals from an electrode stereotaxically placed in the large, nonauditory, caudate nucleus of the basal ganglia and a reference electrode attached to the cat's tongue. They observed four or five monophasic, positive waves with latencies of 2 to 7 milliseconds and peak amplitudes of 1–4 μV evoked by click stimuli.

In their later studies, Jewett and colleagues successfully recorded these far-field brainstem potentials from a human population. These waveforms were termed-far-field potentials because similar waveforms could be recorded from numerous locations on the scalp and head, and because the recording electrodes were distant from the source of the electrical activity. Electrodes positioned over vertex and mastoid, or over vertex and earlobe, gave the best recordings. The electrodes were grounded on the opposite earlobe or mastoid. Five to seven monophasic waves were typically recorded in man with peak latencies between 2 and 7 milliseconds.

In the years following Jewett's first publications, brainstem potentials evoked by click stimuli or high frequency tone bursts were recorded by numerous investigators: Lev and Sohmer, 1972; Leiberman et al., 1973; Sohmer and Feinmesser, 1973; Martin and Coats, 1973; Amadeo and Shagass, 1973; Plantz et al., 1974; Picton et al., 1974; Picton and Hillyard, 1974; Gerull et al., 1974; Hecox and Galambos, 1974; Hecox, 1975; Terkildsen et al., 1973, 1974, 1975a,b; Stein, 1975; Thornton, 1975a, b; Thornton and Coleman, 1975; Bochenek and Bochenek, 1975; Buchwald and Huang, 1975; Goldenberg and Derbyshire, 1975; Blegvad, 1975; Ornitz and Walter, 1975; Salamy et al., 1975; Salamy and McKean, 1976, 1977; Starr and Achor, 1975; Starr and Hamilton, 1976; Starr et al., in press; Starr, 1976, 1977; Schulman-Galambos and Galambos, 1975; Hyde et al., 1976; Hecox et al., 1976; Zöllner et al., 1976; Berry et al., 1976; Mokotoff et al., 1977.

Other investigators appreciated the need for a frequency specific response. Aware of the synchronous volley activity of cat medullary neurons to low frequency stimuli, Moushegian et al. (1973) recorded electrical activity which was synchronous with auditory stimuli for frequencies below 2 kHz from the scalp of humans. These early responses became known as the frequency following responses (FFR) and have since been investigated by numerous authors: Marsh et al., 1975; Smith et al., 1975; Gerken et al., 1975; Terkildsen et al., 1975; Stilman et al., 1976; Daly et al., 1976; Glaser et al., 1976; Suter et al., 1976; Davis, 1976a,b; and Davis and Hirsh, 1976.

The brainstem potentials, therefore, fall into two distinct types based on stimulus characteristics. The onset responses—referred to in the literature as: (1) far field potentials (Jewett and Williston, 1971), (2) surface recorded electrocochleography (Thornton, 1975a,b), (3) far field electrocochleography (Terkildsen et al., 1975), (4) brainstem auditory evoked responses (Hecox and Galambos, 1974), and (5) transient responses (Picton et al., 1977)—are produced by brief acoustic transients, usually less than 1 millisecond in duration (Fig. 11-1). The frequency specific responses—referred to in the literature as: (1) far field recorded frequency following response (Marsh et al., 1975), (2) early tone evoked responses (Stillman et al., 1976), (3) frequency following responses (Glaser et al., 1976), (4) brainstem responses to low frequency sounds (Davis and Hirsch, 1976), and (5) sustained responses (Picton et al., 1977)—are produced by low-frequency tone pips or tone bursts greater than 2–3 milliseconds in duration (Fig. 11-2).

Davis and Hirsh (1976) distinguish between the two responses. They state that both are brainstem potentials. One type, the onset (Fig. 11-1), arises from multiple locations in the brainstem. At slow repetition rates and at moderate intensities the onset potentials are typified by a characteristic wave pattern of five to seven waves, the fifth and most prominent wave having a latency of approximately 6 milliseconds. The other, the frequency following response (FFR) (Fig. 11-2), is a frequency specific response that is thought to

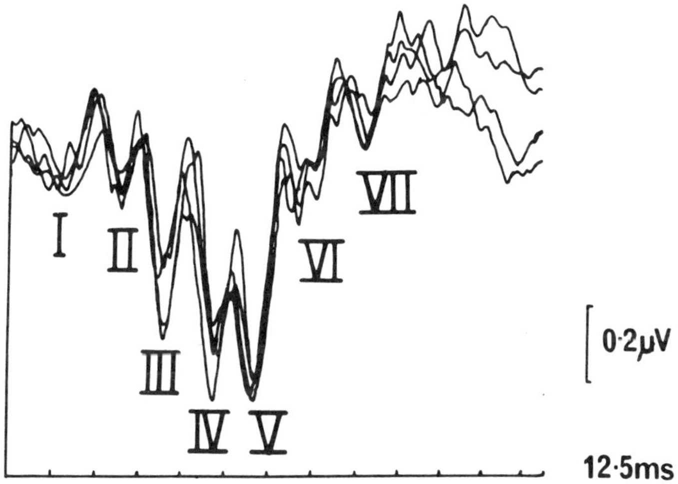

Fig. 11-1. Evoked onset brainstem potentials to 60-dB SL clicks presented monaurally at a rate of 1/second. Each tracing represents the average of 1024 responses from vertex-mastoid electrodes. Each latency division represents 1 millisecond (From: Picton et al: EEG Clin Neurophysiol 1974.)

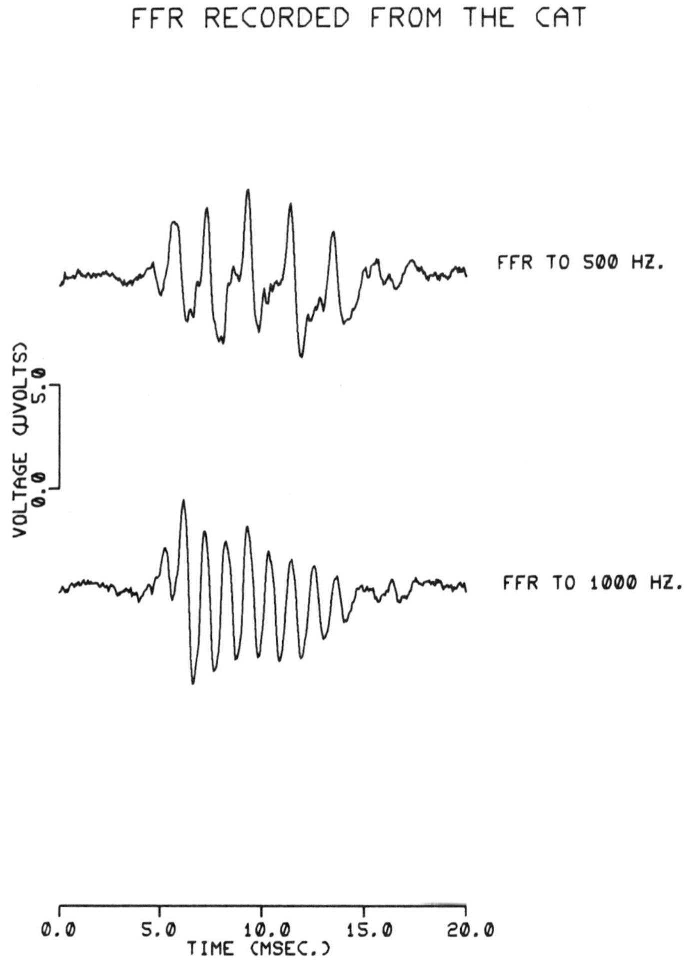

Fig. 11-2. Two examples of frequency following are shown. The top trace is FFR recorded from the cat to a 500-Hz, 11-msec tone burst. The bottom trace is a FFR from the same cat to a 1000-Hz tone burst. Stimulus intensity is 50-dB SPL. There is a 2 msec acoustic delay in the delivery system.

be elicited by synchronous slow wave dendritic activity in the auditory brainstem. It is most prominent when a low frequency, moderately intense tone burst is used as the stimulus. In the interest of clarity, the onset potentials are considered first in this chapter, followed by a brief review of the frequency following response.

CLINICAL APPLICATIONS: ONSET POTENTIALS

Neural Generators

The neural loci responsible for the generation of the onset potentials (Fig. 11-1) have not been completely identified. Investigators have concluded that the whole nerve action potential is responsible for producing wave I (Fig. 11-1) which is similar to, although smaller than, that recorded directly from the promontory, and the cochlear nuclear complex is always associated with the production of wave II (Jewett, 1970; Lev and Sohmer, 1972; Buchwald and Huang, 1975; Goldenberg and Derbyshire, 1975; and Starr and Hamilton, 1975). Considerations of the origins of the electrical activity responsible for the production of waves III, IV, and V in animal and human research, and waves VI and VII in human research, have generated much more controversy. In animal research, wave III is associated with activity generated in the region of the superior olivary complex (Jewett, 1970). Lev and Sohmer (1972) associated wave III production with activity of the lateral superior olive, while Buchwald and Huang (1975) associated wave III production with activity of the medial superior olive. In humans, Starr and Hamilton (1976) found that waves II and III reflected activity of the cochlear nuclear complex, trapezoid body, and superior olivary complex. Wave IV was localized by Jewett (1970) to the structures between the nuclei of the lateral lemniscus and the brachium of the inferior colliculus. Lev and Sohmer (1972) found wave IV to be associated with structures in the general area of the inferior colliculus. Buchwald and Huang (1975) found wave IV to be associated with activity from the ventral nucleus of the lateral lemniscus. Wave V was associated with the inferior colliculus in studies by Jewett (1970), Lev and Sohmer (1972), and Buchwald and Huang (1975). Goldenberg and Derbyshire (1975), however, found no change in the onset potential waveform upon bilateral aspiration of the inferior colliculi. In human studies, Starr and Hamilton (1976) reported that waves IV and V, which most often appear as a prominent complex (IV-V complex), reflected activity of the lateral lemniscus and inferior colliculus. Waves VI and VII, which appear frequently in human studies, have not been studied and their presence in the onset potential waveform can only be assumed to be due to activity further up the auditory pathway or due to repetitive firing of neurons in lower brainstem auditory centers.

Electrode Position

The scalp distribution of onset brainstem potentials was investigated in man by Picton et al. (1974). Wave I was found to be maximally negative at the earlobe or mastoid ipsilateral to acoustic stimulation. Waves II and III were negative at the ear or mastoid and positive on the contralateral mastoid or earlobe. Waves IV and V were recorded as positive over wide areas of scalp, with a maximal response recorded at the vertex.

Terkildsen et al., (1974) recorded from active electrodes placed on vertex, nose, ipsilateral and contralateral mastoids, and homolateral positions on the neck (overlying sternocleidomastoid) and from a reference electrode placed on the left third sternocostal joint of the thorax. They stated that the most well defined onset potentials were seen with vertex-thorax recordings. In a second experiment, an active electrode was attached to the vertex, while reference electrodes were attached to both neck positions. Waves I, II, IV, V, and VI were of higher amplitude with homolateral-vertex records than with contralateral-vertex recording.

Investigators with primary interest in wave I, then, usually record the onset brainstem potentials with an active electrode on the vertex and a reference on the ipsilateral mastoid; whereas wave V is best recorded using the vertex and ipsilateral neck positions. Either the forehead or opposite mastoid or neck is used for the ground.

General Findings in Adults

The onset brainstem potentials are smaller in amplitude than the evoked cortical potentials described in Chapter 9, or the evoked cochlear potentials described in Chapter 10. The late components of the AEP and the AP recorded from the promontory have peak-to-peak amplitudes of about 5–20 μV. The middle components of the AEP have peak-to-peak amplitudes of about 0.5–2.0 μV. In contrast, peak-to-peak amplitude values for the brainstem potentials are usually reported in the nanovolt range, an order of magnitude smaller than the middle components. Bandpass filters set at 100 to 3000 Hz are usually used to record the brainstem potentials. However, a low frequency setting as high as 300 Hz is preferred by some investigators, while the high frequency setting may be extended to 10,000 Hz by others. The number of stimulus presentations necessary to obtain the onset brainstem potentials also varies considerably. Most investigators use 2000 or more stimulus presentations to elicit a clear response, but one study (Salamy and McKean, 1977) reports identifiable and repeatable responses with only 256 trials.

Changes in the rate of stimulus presentation bring about differential effects within the waveform morphology of the brainstem potentials which can be seen in Fig. 11-3. As repetition rate increases, waves I through IV become less distinct and lower in amplitude (Jewett and Williston, 1971; Hyde et al., 1976). Wave V, however, maintains its amplitude and may even increase in amplitude at higher repetition rates. At very high repetition rates,

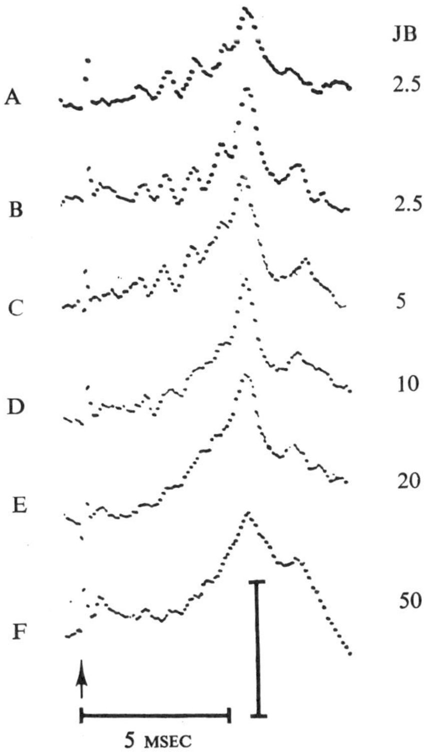

Fig. 11-3. Effect of repetition rate on the auditory onset brainstem potentials recorded at the vertex. Numbers at right indicate the repetition rate in stimuli/sec. Click stimulus delivered at the arrow. A. Recording at 2.5 stimuli/second recorded 6 months before B. B–F. Recordings from the same recording session at different stimulus repetition rates. Vertical calibration: A. 0–7 μV; B–F, 1–0 μV. Note the loss of definition of the wave components as stimulus rate increases. The height of wave I decreases with increasing rate while wave V increases in amplitude (comparing B and E). From Jewett and Williston: Brain 1971.)

80 to 100 stimuli/second, however, wave V decreases in amplitude and increases in latency (Terkildsen et al., 1975a; Zöllner et al., 1976).

Most studies have used rates of about 10–33 stimuli/second. Like the evoked cortical and cochlear potentials, initial studies of the onset brainstem potentials used clicks as stimuli, usually 200 μsec or less in duration. More recently, high frequency tone pips, tone bursts, or filtered clicks have been used as stimuli. As discussed earlier in this chapter, a different response, the frequency following response (FFR), is elicited by the use of low frequency tone pips or tone bursts. The FFR is described separately later in this chapter. Tone burst stimuli in the 2000–8000 Hz region appear to elicit frequency specific onset brainstem potentials (Terkildsen et al., 1975a), and therefore yield important high frequency audiometric information. A recent report by Hecox et al., (1976) showed that changes in stimulus duration and rise-fall time had an effect on response latency of wave V. As shown in Fig. 11-4, response latency increases as burst duration and rise time increase. Variations in fall time did not effect response latency. Ornitz and Walter (1975) found differences in some subjects when response latencies to

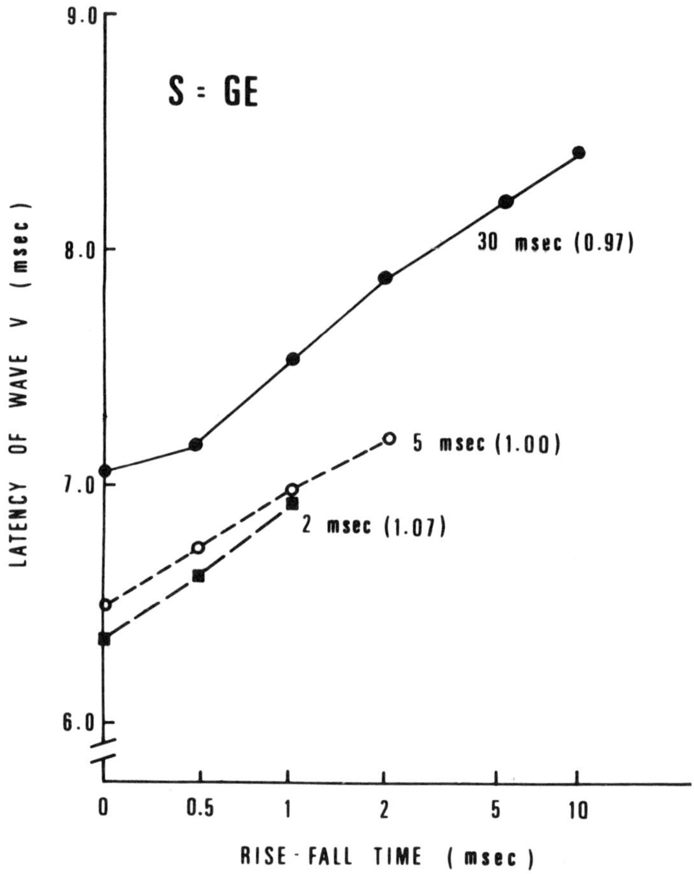

Fig. 11-4. The latency of wave V as a function of rise-fall time with duration as a parameter. Each point represents the mean of three replications. The rise-fall times are plotted on a logarithmic scale to facilitate comparisons of the slopes at each duration. The stimulus in each case was a monaural 75-dB SPL noise burst presented 16 times/second. (From Hecox, Squires, and Galambos: J Acoust Soc Am 1976.)

rarefaction clicks were compared to those obtained with condensation clicks. In most studies which use alternating positive and negative pulses, results are examined only in the averaged response to all pulses combined.

As stated by Picton et al. (1977), "The most striking characteristic about the brainstem auditory evoked potentials is their latency sensitivity to the intensity of the stimulus." Latency values of the various peaks reported by various investigators are remarkably similar, and are shown in Table 11-1. For click stimuli, the latency of wave V in adults increases from 5.5 to 9.0 milliseconds as stimulus intensity decreases from 90 dB sensation level to threshold (Hecox and Galambos, 1974; Starr and Achor, 1975). This latency-intensity function for wave V is highly replicable within and across subjects as well as among laboratories, and is shown in the left portion of Fig. 11-5 for normal-hearing listeners. For a detailed description of wave V latency determinants, the reader is referred to Picton et al. (1977).

The amplitude of the onset brainstem potentials varies as a function of stimulus intensity, inter-stimulus interval, and mode of presentation (monaural or binaural). Individual wave amplitude is not measured by the same method by all investigators. Peak amplitude, measured from peak to following trough, has been reported by Starr and Achor (1975) to vary between 40 and 350 nV, depending on stimulus intensity and which waveform is being measured. Amadeo and Shagass (1973) measured amplitude from baseline to peak amplitude. Using binaural stimulation they found peak amplitudes to vary between 0.4 and 1.6 μV for a 60 dB SL signal.

Table 11-1.
Latencies to Each Wave of the Onset Brainstem Potentials as Reported by Various Investigators

	I	II	III	IV	V	VI
Jewett and Williston (1971) 60–75-dB click	1.5*	2.6	3.5	4.3	5.1	6.5
Lev and Sohmer (1972) 65-dB click	1.5	2.5	3.5	5.0	6.7	
Amadeo and Shagass (1973) 60-dB click	1.6	2.8	3.7	5.6		
Picton et al. (1974) 60-dB click	1.5	2.6	3.8	5.0	5.8	7.4
Starr and Achor (1975) 65-dB click	1.6	2.8	3.8	4.8	5.5	7.1

*All latencies are in milliseconds.

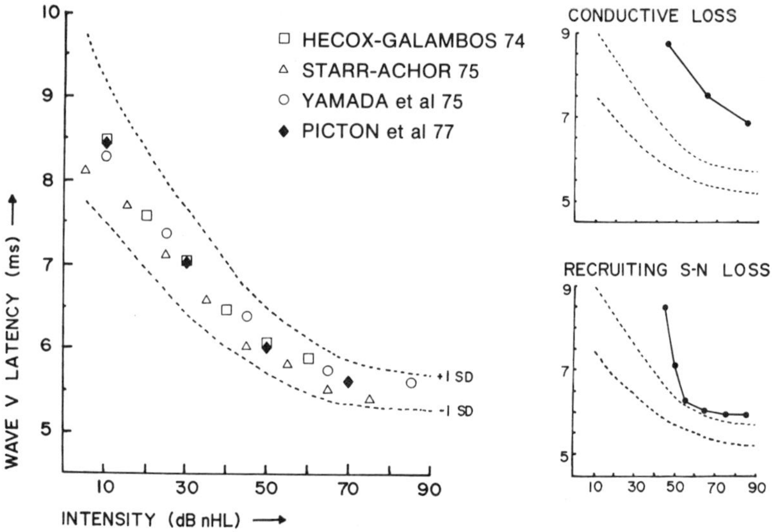

Fig. 11-5. The effect of stimulus intensity on the peak latency of wave V of the onset brainstem potentials reported from several laboratories. Wave V latency-intensity curves are shown for two patients on the right. (Modified from Picton et al: J Otolaryngol 1977.)

Blegvad (1975) and Møller and Blegvad (1976) showed that presentation of binaural stimuli produced onset potentials that had amplitudes 60% greater than corresponding monaural left or right stimulation. This effect was found over an 80 dB stimulus intensity range. Binaural stimulation has not been shown to affect onset potential latencies. Thresholds determined with the onset brainstem potentials agree with behavioral threshold to within 5 or 10 dB (Hecox and Galambos, 1974; Starr and Achor, 1975; Blegvad, 1975; and Davis, 1976b).

Like the middle components and the AP, the onset brainstem potentials remain remarkably stable during changes in subject state. Picton and Hillyard (1974) found no differences in the brainstem potentials when subjects were instructed either to read a book (ignore) or to listen for an occasional faint click (attend). These potentials are quite stable during changes in sleep stage (Fig. 11-6), with similar latency, amplitude, and waveform in the awake state, light and deep sleep, and during REM sleep (Amadeo and Shagass, 1973). Like the AP, the brainstem potentials are unaffected by sedation (Fig. 11-7) (Starr and Achor, 1975).

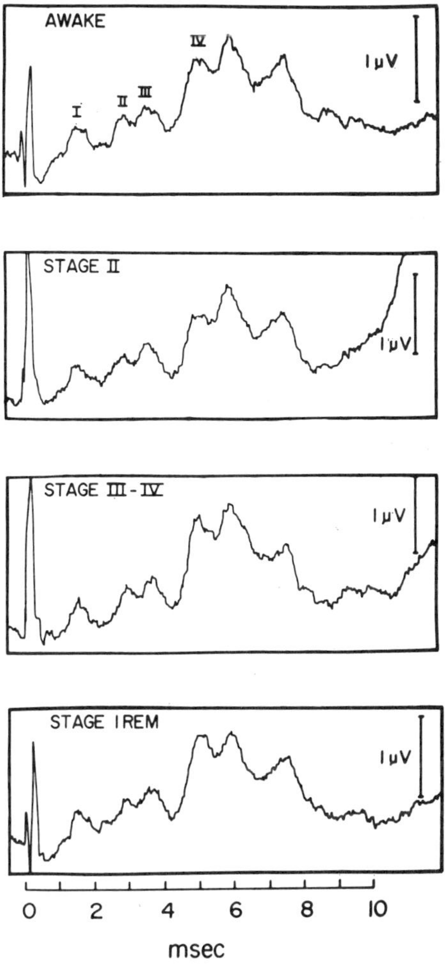

Fig. 11-6. Onset brainstem potentials to clicks as a function of sleep stage. Each tracing represents the average of 2000 responses to 60-dB SL clicks at 10/second from vertex-mastoid electrodes. (From Amadeo and Shagass: Psychophysiology 1973.)

Clinical Findings in Adults

The application of the onset brainstem potentials to clinical testing of adults has been based largely on the wave V latency–intensity curve first described by Hecox and Galambos (1974) and redrawn as shown in Fig. 11-5 by Picton et al. (1977). These clinical studies have used brief transients,

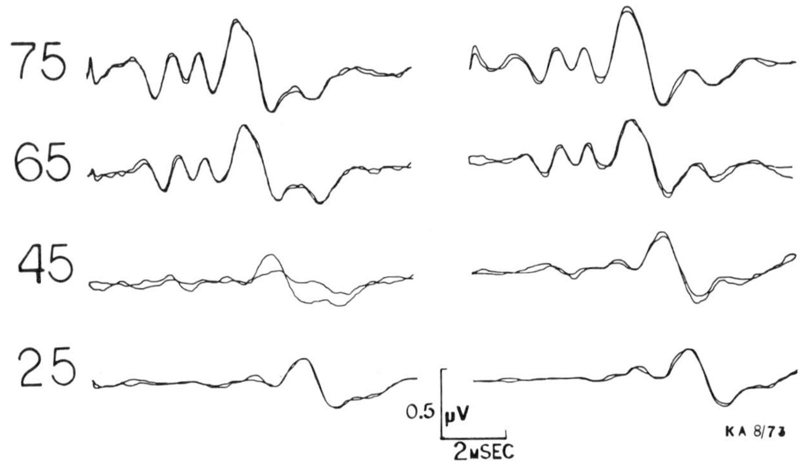

Fig. 11-7. Auditory brainstem potentials recorded from a patient in coma due to barbiturate overdosage (left) and again 5 days later after regaining consciousness (right). Binaural click signals were presented at varying intensities (25–75 dB SL). Note the remarkable similarity of the responses with regard to amplitude and latency in the two conditions. (From Starr and Achor: Arch Neurol 1975.)

usually 200 μsec clicks, as stimuli. The results of studies by Hecox and Galambos (1974), Starr and Anchor (1975), Yamada et al. (1975), and Picton et al. (1977) have been combined, and a normal latency-intensity curve, plus and minus 1 standard deviation, is shown within broken lines in the left portion of the figure. A patient whose results fall within this curve would be defined as having normal hearing. In a conductive hearing loss, there is a displacement of the latency-intensity relationship to the right by an amount equal to the hearing loss. This result is the same as the resultant shift in the cochleogram described for a conductive loss in the previous chapter, and shown in Fig. 10-11. A sensory-neural hearing loss with recruitment would display an abnormally rapid decline in the latency of wave V with increasing intensity. The threshold latency values would be higher than normal, but latency values would rapidly fall to near or within normal values at suprathreshold levels, as shown in Fig. 11-5. This pattern shows some similarity to the recruiting cochleogram shown in Fig. 10-12. Actual results obtained with the brainstem potentials in a patient with acoustic neuroma and another with sensory-neural hearing loss have been reported by Berry et al., (1976), but latency-intensity functions are not reported.

Because this clinical information is obtained with click stimuli, the latency-intensity relationship of the onset brainstem potentials reflects information primarily from the 2000 Hz region of the audiogram. In certain cases, e.g., with an abrupt sensory-neural hearing loss above 4000 Hz, results obtained with the brainstem potentials would be within normal limits. In addition, some of the latency-intensity functions display patterns which are difficult to interpret. However, the stability of the waveform, the similarity between individuals, and the characteristic latency-intensity functions from most hearing-impaired adults make the use of these potentials a powerful tool for electric response audiometry.

Application to Infants

The general findings of investigators interested in evaluating infants using the onset potentials are: (1) responses can be reliably obtained at moderate stimulus intensity levels, (2) latency values to peaks I and V are systematically reduced as a function of increasing age to about 12–16 months, and (3) most infants, especially the youngest tested, need no medication to insure subject cooperation.

The onset potentials have been studied by investigators interested in two different applications. One group (e.g., Jewett and Romano, 1972; Salamy et al., 1975; Salamy and McKean, 1976; Starr et al., in press; Hecox, 1975) has been concerned specifically with the use of the onset potential technique as a measure of auditory neural development, and more generally as a measure of human neural development. Another group (Hecox and Galambos, 1974; Schulman-Galambos and Galambos, 1975; Mokotoff et al., 1977) has been interested in using the onset potentials as an audiometric screening technique. Their efforts have been directed toward the construction of latency-intensity functions for various age groups and toward the development of a clinical test useful in the diagnosis of hearing loss in the young infant and child.

AUDITORY-NEURAL DEVELOPMENT

The definition of the onset potentials in infants has been investigated as an index of neural maturation. Various investigators (Hecox and Galambos, 1974; Hecox, 1975; Salamy et al., 1975; Starr et al., in press; Salamy and McKean, 1976) agree that newborns exhibit three waves (I, III, and V) in the onset potentials, in contrast to adults, who usually show six or seven waves (Fig. 11-8). There is, however, some disagreement about the configuration of the onset potentials in older infants as a function of stimulus repetition rate. Hecox (1975) found no differences in onset potential waveform with repetition rates from 20 to 66/second (Fig. 11-9). At these rates, waves I, III, and V were consistently identified. Salamy and McKean (1976) noted differences in waveform configuration at rates of 5 or 15 stimuli/second with more waves seen at the slower rate. Since the stimulus repetition rates employed by the

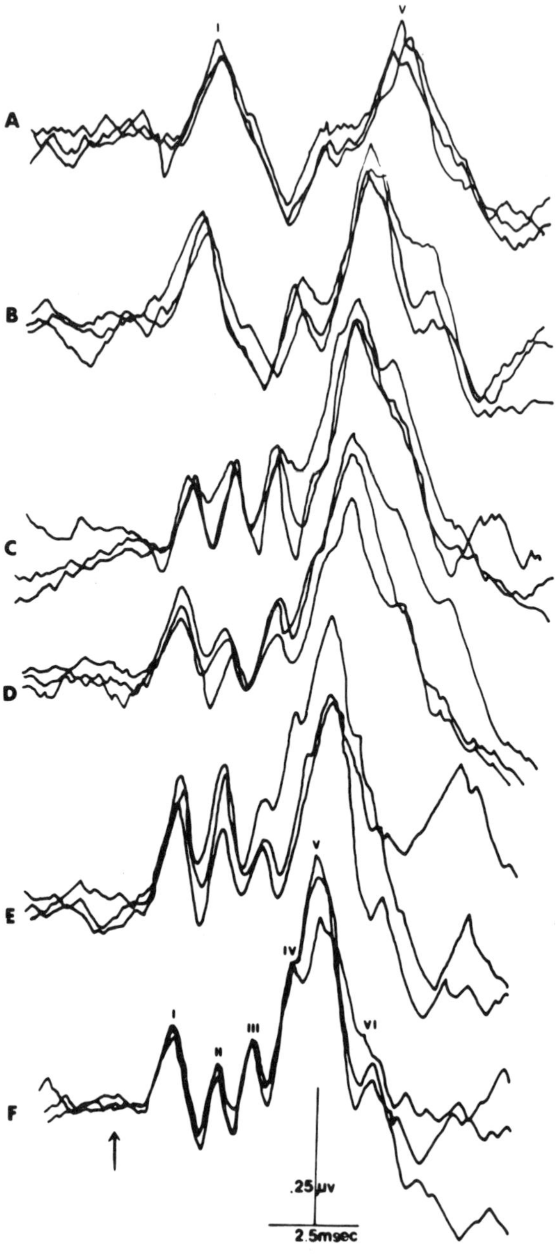
I
V
A
B
C
D
E
F
I
II
III
IV
V
VI
.25μv
2.5msec

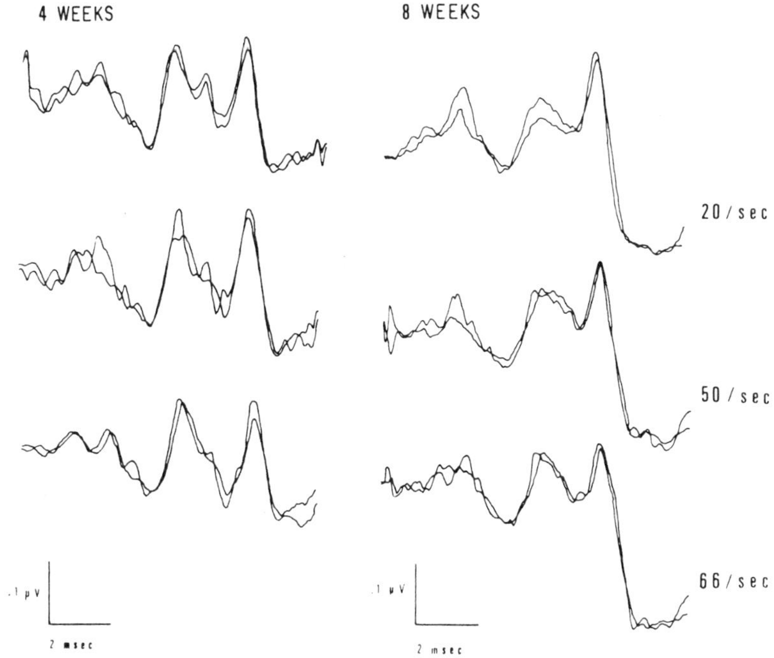

Fig. 11-9. Infant evoked brainstem potentials as a function of repetition rate. Evoked responses to a 50-dB SL monaural click are shown from two infants at three rates of presentation. Note that reliable recordings were obtained at all rates. Each of the superimposed tracings represents the summed response to 2048 stimuli. Positivity to the vertex is upwards. (From Hecox in Cohen and Salapatek: Academic, 1975.)

two research groups did not overlap, it could be concluded that repetition rates above 5/second decreased the individual clarity of the onset potential waveform. This observation is not surprising, since the use of repetition rates above 10/second frequently decreases individual wave clarity in adults. Hecox and Galambos (1974) showed that onset potential wave V latency decreased as a function of increasing age, up to about 16 months (Fig. 11-10). Salamy and McKean (1976) report similar findings, except that their cutoff

---

Fig. 11-8. Maturational changes in onset brainstem potential waveform as a function of age: A. Newborns. B. Six-week-olds. C. Three-month-olds. D. Six-month-olds. E. One-year-olds. F. Adults. Each trace represents an average of 2400 responses obtained from a different subject. Note also the obvious shifts (shortening) in peak latency with increasing age. Positivity at the active (Cz) electrode is indicated by an upward deflection. (From Salamy and McKean: EEG Clin Neurophysiol 1976.)

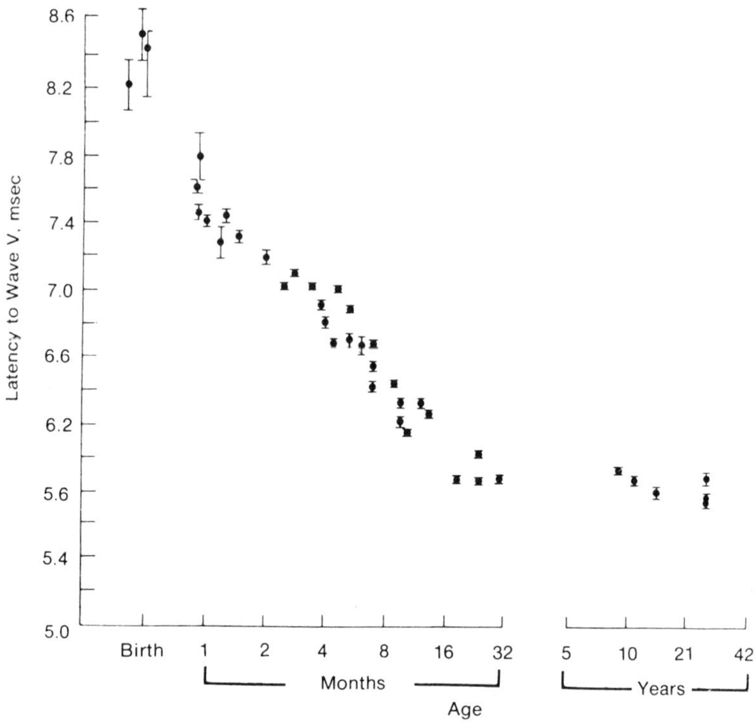

Fig. 11-10. Latency of the wave V response to 60-dB SL click as function of age of subject. Systematic decline from birth to 1–2 years is evident. Vertical bars enclose all measurements (at least three) made on given subject. (From Hecox and Galambos: Arch Otol 1974.)

age is closer to 12 months. These results suggest that the auditory system, through the level of the brainstem, has reached functional maturity by the first year of life. It also more loosely suggests that the entire neural function of the brainstem has reached maturity by this time because of the diffuse layout of auditory structures in the brainstem.

Salamy and McKean (1976) have derived separate measures for peripheral vs. central maturation in the auditory system. They took wave I latency to reflect peripheral conduction time and wave V latency minus wave I latency to reflect central transmission time. They showed (Fig. 11-11) that maturation of the peripheral organ, as reflected by wave I latency values, is complete by about 6 weeks after birth, and that maturation of the central auditory system to the level of the inferior colliculus seems to be a two step process. There are dramatic shifts in central transmission time between the

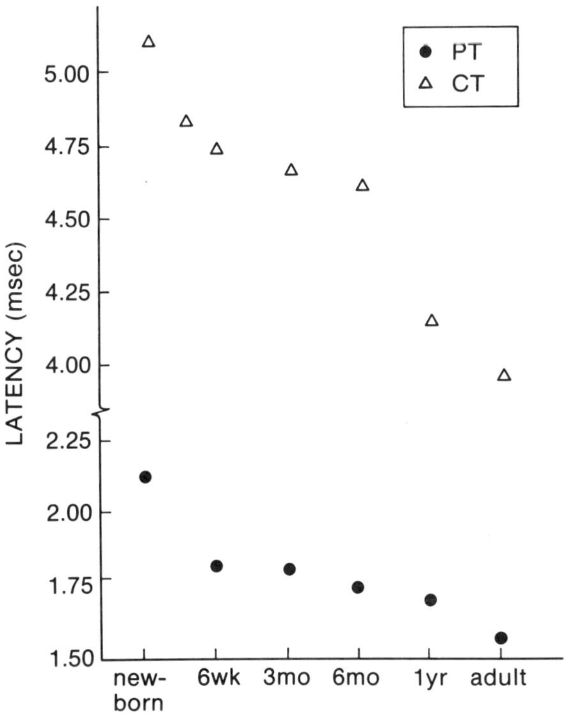

Fig. 11-11. Maturational trends for peripheral transmission (PT) and central transmission (CT). Each closed circle and square represents the mean latency (in msec) for PT and CT respectively for each age group. (From Salamy and McKean: EEG Clin Neurophysiol 1976.)

newborn and the 6-week-old infant and between the 6-month-old infant and the 12-month-old infant. The question still remains as to whether these physiologic changes reflect synaptogenesis or myelogenesis, and whether the changes have behaviorally defined correlates.

AUDIOMETRIC APPLICATIONS

Starr et al. (in press) recorded onset potentials from premature infants (33–41 weeks gestational age) to levels as low as 25 dB HL (referenced to six adults with normal hearing). Schulman-Galambos and Galambos (1975) recorded onset potentials at 30 dB HL from premature infants, 36–39 weeks gestational age. Hecox and Galambos (1974) recorded onset potentials at 20 dB HL for a group of 35 infants, ranging in age from three weeks to three years.

Only two studies have dealt directly with the use of the onset potentials as an aid in audiological evaluation. Stein (1975) reported the results of brainstem potential evaluations of 150 infants and children. Results from three illustrative cases were presented, but detailed information is not included in his report.

Mokotoff et al. (1977) tested 81 children ranging in age from 6 weeks premature to 15 years. Thirty-eight of the patients had undergone previous audiologic evaluations and were referred for brainstem potential testing because their initial behavioral results were inconclusive. Table 11-2 shows the audiologic questions asked and whether the results of the brainstem technique answered these questions. Of the 38 patients, 9 were suspected to have moderate to profound hearing impairment by the audiologist, but were found to have normal responses with the brainstem potential. Another group of 43 patients had been referred directly to the clinic without prior audiological evaluation. Of this group, 26 showed normal onset potential waveforms and 17 were identified as having abnormal peripheral auditory systems. Of the 17 patients who exhibited abnormal onset potential waveforms, 10 were successfully tested with impedance techniques. The results in all ten cases agreed with the onset potential tests. In five of the remaining seven cases, impedance measurements were not attempted due to the presumed extent of the loss (80 dB or more). In the remaining cases, impedance measurements were attempted unsuccessfully. Follow-up information on all patients is in the process of being acquired.

Table 11-2.
Questions Asked by Audiologists and Brainstem Response Answers

Audiological Question	Number of Children	BER Answer *Yes*	*No*	*No Answer*
1. Is HL near normal?	8	8	0	0
2. Is there significant hearing loss?	23	15	8	0
3. Is amplification needed?	5	4	1	0
4. Is there a retrocochlear lesion?	2	0	0	2

From Mokotoff B, Schulman-Galambos C, and Galambos, R Arch Otolaryng 1977

CLINICAL APPLICATIONS: FREQUENCY FOLLOWING RESPONSE

As discussed earlier in this chapter, the frequency following response (FFR) is a frequency specific response within 10–12 milliseconds of stimulus onset that is thought to be elicited by synchronous slow wave dendritic activity in the auditory brainstem. It is most prominent when a low frequency, moderately intense tone burst is used as the stimulus.

The literature dealing with origins of the FFR has been meager. Only one paper has been published dealing directly with this question. Smith et al. (1975) used a cryogenic probe to cool selected brainstem areas in the cat. They concluded that frequency specific responses were generated in the inferior colliculi. Recent experiments in the Coleman Laboratory (Gardi et al., 1977) contradict this conclusion. Bilateral aspiration of the inferior colliculi did not alter the frequency following waveform. The responses were virtually identical in waveform shape, amplitude, and latency.

Changes in FFR amplitude or latency due to different electrode position have not been investigated.

General Findings in Adults

Implicit in the recording of the FFR is the fact that it is observed using low frequency, continuous or pulsed, tone burst stimulation or pulsed noise bursts of rapid repetition rate. Recording conditions are essentially the same as those used for recording the onset brainstem potentials. Filter settings of 100–10,000 Hz are optimal, and the number of stimulus trials necessary to elicit a FFR is about 2000.

Changes in inter-stimulus interval have not been thoroughly investigated with the FFR. Stillman et al. (1976) showed that the FFR waveform is essentially unchanged as repetition rate is increased from 5 to 25 stimuli/sec (Fig. 11-12). A recent study by Suter et al. (1976) showed that the FFR could be obtained using rapidly presented clicks at rates of 100–500 stimuli/sec.

Tone bursts of 500 Hz have been used by most investigators to elicit the FFR, although Moushegian et al., (1973) have recorded FFR at frequencies up to 2000 Hz, and Glaser et al. (1976) have recorded FFR at frequencies as low as 70 Hz. In general, lower frequency stimuli produced greater amplitude FFR waveforms (Fig. 11-13).

Changes in FFR amplitude or latency due to variations in signal duration or rise-fall time have not been systematically investigated. Tone burst durations used by investigators have ranged from the short value of 2½ milliseconds (Terkildsen et al., 1975) to the longest value of 20 milliseconds

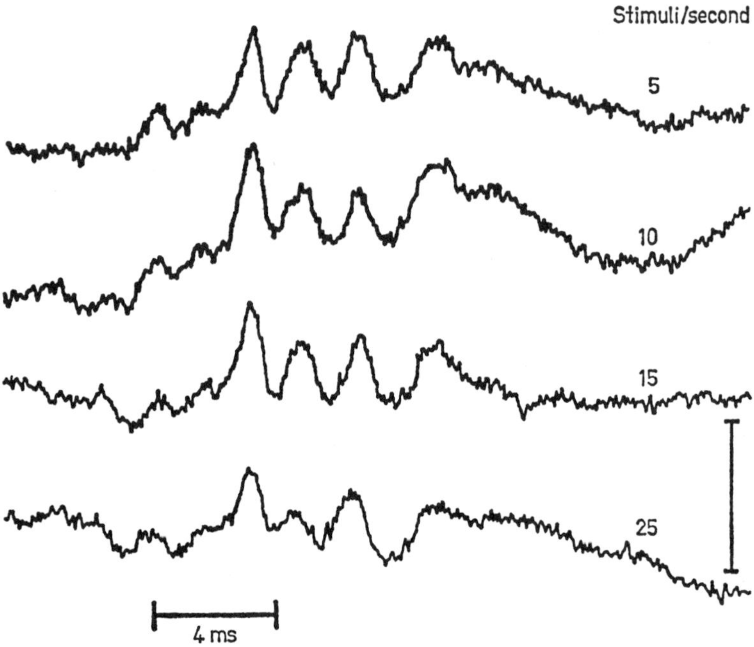

Fig. 11-12. Effect of stimulus presentation rate on the frequency following response. Each tracing represents the average of 3000 responses to 500 Hz tone bursts (rise-fall time–1 milisecond; duration–4 milliseconds) at 70-dB SL from vertex-earlobe electrodes. (From Stillman, Moushegian, and Rupert: Audiology 1976.)

(Marsh et al., 1975). Various other durations between these two extremes have been used as well as various rise times (1–5 milliseconds). Continuous tone stimulation has also been used (Glaser et al., 1976).

The amplitude of the FFR varies as a function of stimulus intensity. Marsh et al. (1975) and Glaser et al. (1976) have shown that, as stimulus intensity is increased, FFR amplitude also increases (Fig. 11-14). Latency to the first peak in the FFR decreases as stimulus intensity is increased. This function has been plotted for 16 normally hearing adults in Fig. 11-15. In general, the latency of wave V of the onset response is earlier and its latency–intensity function shows a more gradual slope than does the analogous function for FFR (compare with Fig. 11-5). Binaural presentation of stimuli increases FFR amplitude. However, no study has been published which quantifies the amount of improvement during binaural stimulation. FFR threshold varies widely from 20 dB SL (Stillman et al., 1976) to 50 dB SL

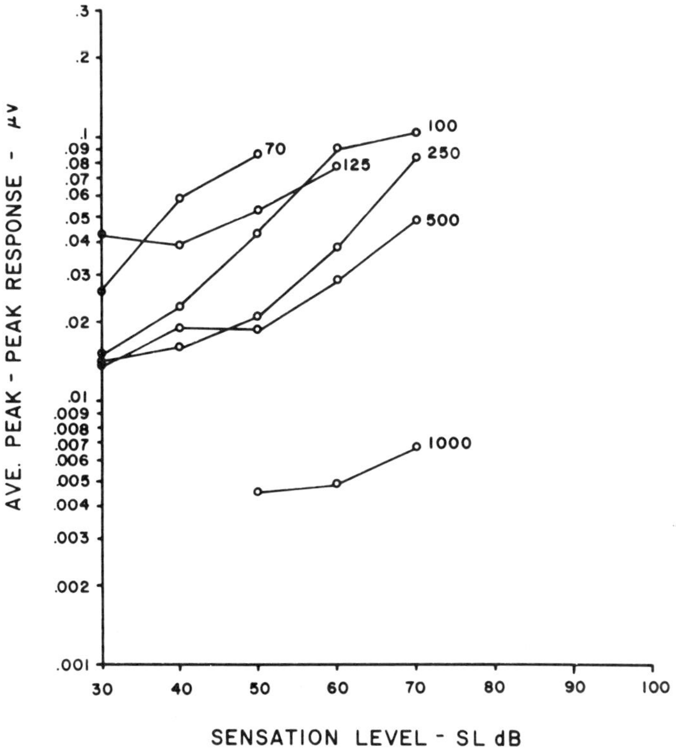

Fig. 11-13. The average peak-to-peak amplitude of the continuous frequency following responses at the different stimulus frequencies employed. The average is across all subjects. The responses are plotted as a function of sensation level (SL). The averages were measured from data filtered at the tone frequency by a band-pass filter centered at the tone frequency, f_0, and having a bandwidth of $0.4 f_0$. (From Glaser et al. EEG J 40, 1976.)

(Davis, 1976b). Most investigators agree that an easily identifiable response can be recorded at 45 dB SL.

Davis, in a recent series of papers (Davis, 1976a,b; Davis and Hirsh, 1976) summarized the effect of frequency, duration, rise-fall time, and threshold on the FFR. The use of click stimuli and tone pip (500 Hz, 2–4 msec duration, 1–2 msec rise-fall time) stimuli elicited complicated response waveforms at levels as low as 10 dB SL. Longer duration tone burst stimulation (500 Hz, 15–20 msec duration, 2–4 msec rise-fall time) elicited FFR waveforms that had moderate thresholds (40–50 dB SL), but clear frequency following phenomena.

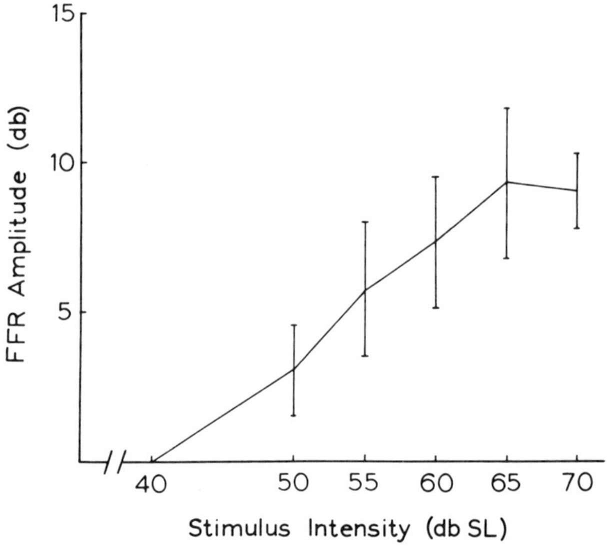

Fig. 11-14. Mean FFR amplitude gain with increases in stimulus intensity for eight subjects. The ordinate is the mean increment in FFR voltage ratio referenced to the response to the 40-dB SL stimulus, a level below which no FFR was observed. The vertical bars show one standard deviation above and below the mean. (From Glaser et al. Electroencephalogr Clin Neurophysiol 1976.)

The effects of attention, sleep, and drug-induced sleep have not been systematically explored with the FFR. However, various investigators have observed that these parameters do not change the FFR waveform (Glaser et al., 1976; Davis 1976b; Davis and Hirsh, 1976). In addition, the shape of the FFR waveform is stable over long periods of time (Fig. 11-16).

Clinical Findings in Adults

Hearing-impaired adults have been investigated with the FFR by Daly et al., (1976) and Stillman et al. (1976) using a low frequency tone burst (500 Hz). Subjects with profound hearing loss were tested by the first group of authors. Stimulus presentation to the impaired ear failed to elicit FFR recorded from either ear. Stimulus presentation to the unimpaired ear produced normal FFR waveforms recorded from either ear. Stimulus intensity was always kept below the bone conduction threshold, but above the FFR threshold. This value was usually 50 dB SL.

Stillman et al. (1976) used a 500-Hz short-duration tone burst to elicit

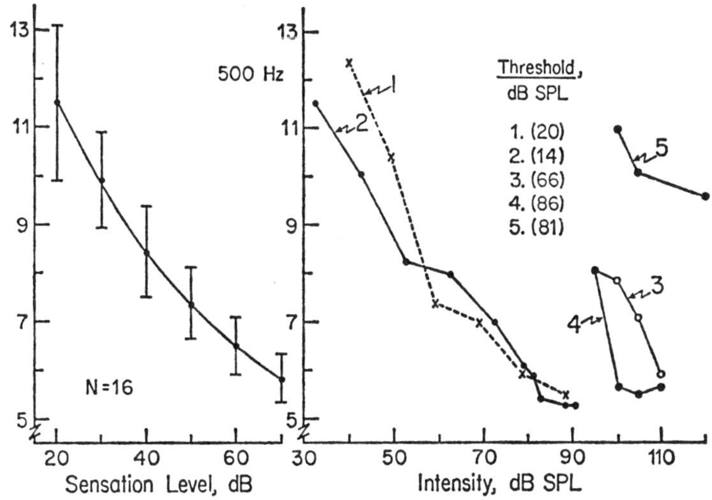

Fig. 11-15. A. Mean latency of the frequency following response as a function of sensation level in 16 normally hearing subjects. Brackets indicate = 1 SD. Latency measured from the peak of the first downward departure of the stimulus at the earphone to the first positive peak in the response. B. Curves 1 and 2 = latency-intensity functions for two normally hearing subjects; curves 3 and 4 = latency-intensity functions for two hearing-impaired subjects who did not exhibit a recruiting response. (From Stillman, Moushegian, Rupert: Audiology 1976.)

FFR from varied populations of normal subjects, hearing–impaired subjects, deaf-blind subjects and subjects exhibiting learning disorders and mild speech discrimination deficits. Normal-hearing adults produced FFR at 10 to 30 dB SL. Figure 11-15a shows the latency-intensity function for the normal adult listeners. Hearing-impaired subjects and deaf-blind subjects exhibited elevated FFR thresholds that corresponded to their varied behavioral thresholds. Figure 11-15b shows the latency-intensity graph for individual normal and hearing impaired subjects. The individual curves of hearing-impaired subjects do not conform to the curves seen in normals. FFR waveforms obtained from some of the hearing-impaired subjects did not show the characteristic frequency following peaks even at intense levels of stimulation (Fig. 11-17).

Application to Infants

To date, the FFR has not been studied in infants and young children. However, these responses offer possibilities for eliciting low frequency in-

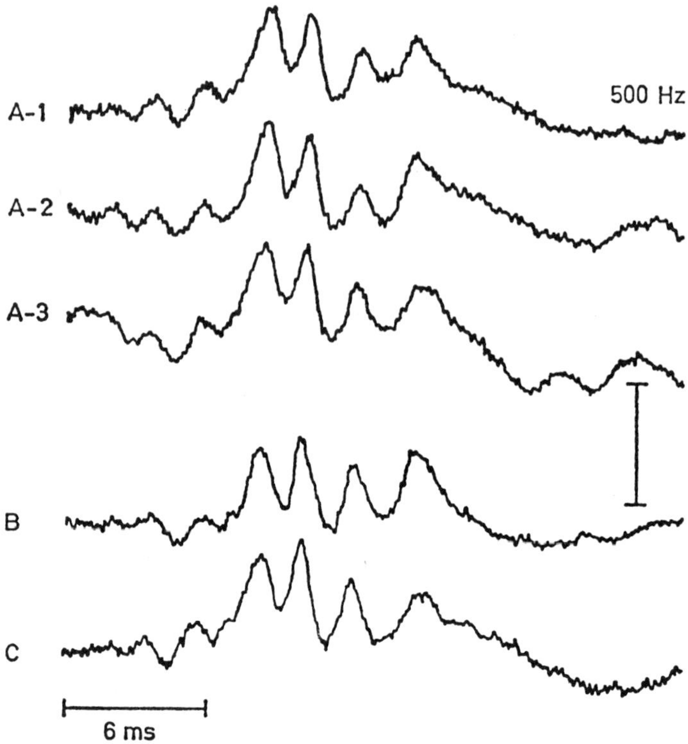

Fig. 11-16. Frequency following responses at 70 dB SL from one subject. Traces A-1 to A-3 were obtained at 30-minute intervals in one session. Trace B was obtained 1 week later and trace C, 1 month later. (From Stillman, Moushegian, and Rupert: Audiology 1976.)

formation within the earliest time domain of the evoked potentials in a non-surgical procedure.

In summary, the cortical and cochlear evoked potentials reviewed in these three chapters offer exciting possibilities for assessing various portions of the auditory pathway in infants and children. Information at various levels of the auditory pathway may be obtained with these techniques efficiently and in an increasingly reliable manner. Although current research tends to stress information derived from the exclusive use of any one time domain, the ultimate diagnostic power of the evoked potentials may be realized in the sequential or simultaneous collection of information within each time domain. In this manner, the auditory system may be sampled from the cochlea to the cortex and specific diagnostic information obtained from infants at any age.

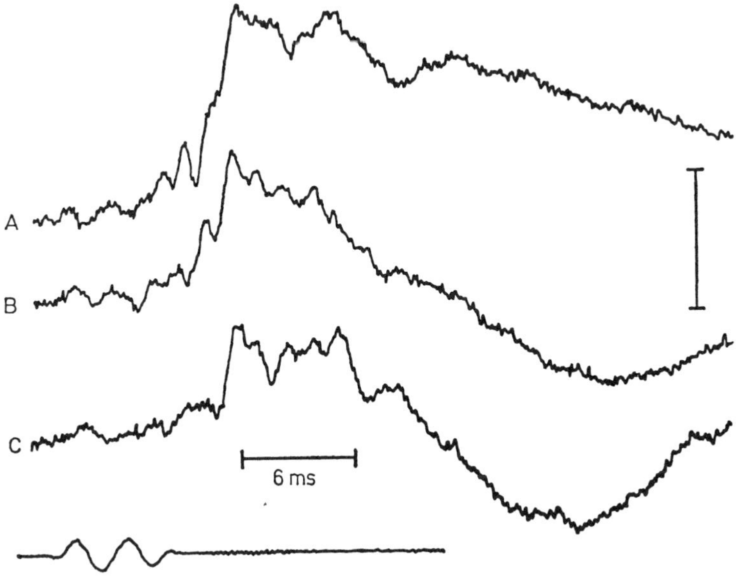

Fig. 11-17. Traces A–C: aberrant frequency following responses from 3 subjects at 70 dB SL. Hearing threshold of A = 18 dB SPL. B = 17 dB SPL, C = 18-dB SPL. Lowest tracing is an electrical artifact. Subjects B and C were dyslexic siblings. (From Stillman, Moushegian, and Rupert: Audiology 1976).

REFERENCES

Abe M: Electrical responses of the human brain to acoustic stimulus. Tohoku J Exp Med 60:47–58, 1954

Adrian E: The microphonic action of the cochlea in relation to theories of hearing, in Report of a Discussion of Audition, Physical Society of London, 1931

Akiyama Y, Schulte FJ, Schultz M, et al. Acoustically evoked responses in premature and full term newborn infants. Electroencephalogr Clin Neurophysiol 26:371–380, 1969

Amadeo M, Shagass C: Brief latency click-evoked potentials during waking and sleeping in man. Psychophysiology 10:244–250, 1973

Anch AM: The auditory evoked brain response during adult human sleep. Unpublished doctoral dissertation, St. Louis University, 1971

Anders T, Emde R, Parmelee A: A Manual of Standardized Terminology, Techniques and Criteria for Scoring of States of Sleep and Wakefulness in Newborn Infants. UCLA Brain Information Service/BRI Publications Office, Los Angeles, CA 1971

Andreev AM, Arapova AA, Gersuni GV: On electrical potentials in the human cochlea. J Physiol 26:205–212, 1939

Antinoro F, Skinner PH, Jones JJ: Relation between sound intensity and amplitude of the AER at different stimulus frequencies. J Acoust Soc Am 46:1433–1436, 1969

Appleby S: The slow vertex maximal sound evoked response in infants, in Davis H (ed): The Young Deaf Child: Identification and Management. Acta Oto–laryngol Suppl 206:146–152, 1965

Aran JM: Clinical measures of VIIIth nerve functions. Adv Oto Rhinol Laryngol 20:374–394, 1973

Aran JM: The electro-cochleogram: Recent results in children and in some pathological cases. Arch Klin Exp Ohren Nasen Kehlkopf 198:128–141, 1971

Aran JM, Delaunay J: Etude electrophysiologique de l'audition humaine. Rev Acoust 4:91–94, 1971

Aran JM, LeBert G: Les réponses nerveuses cochléaires chez l'homme image du fonctionnement de l'oreille et nouveau test d'audiométrie objective. Rev Laryngol 89:361–378, 1968

Aran JM, Negrevergne M: Clinical study of some particular pathological patterns of eighth nerve responses in the human being. Audiology I 12:488–503, 1973

Aran JM, Pèlerin J, Lenoir J, et al: Aspects théoriques et pratiques des enregistrements électro-cochléographique selon la méthode établie à Bordeaux. Rev Laryngol Suppl: 601–644, 1971

Aran JM, Portmann M: L'électro cochléogramme. J Fr Otol Rhinol Laryngol 21:211–221, 1972

Aran JM, Portmann C, Delaunay J, et al: L'Electrocochléogramme: Méthodes et premiers resultats chez l'enfant. Rev Laryngol 90:615–634, 1969

Aran JM, Portmann M, Portmann C, et al: Electrochochleography in adults and children: electrophysiological study of the peripheral receptor. Audiology 11:77–89, 1972

Bancaud J, Bloch V, Paillard J: Contribution EEG à l'étude des potentiels evoques chez l'homme au niveau du vertex. Rev Neurol 89:399–418, 1953

Barlow J: An electronic method for detecting evoked responses of the brain and for reproducing their average waveforms. Electroencephalogr Clin Neurophysiol 9:340–343, 1957

Barnet AB: Average evoked electroencephalographic responses to clicks in the infant, in Davis H (ed.): The Young Deaf Child: Identification and Management, Acta Otolaryngol Suppl 206:134–146, 1965

Barnet AB: Evoked response audiometry in 241 normal and hearing impaired children under three years. Arch Klin Exp Ohren Nasen Kehlkopf 198:154–157, 1971

Barnet AB: EEG and evoked response correlates of mental retardation. Clin Proc CAJ Child Hosp 94:250–260, 1971

Barnet AB, Goodwin RS: Averaged evoked electroencephalographic responses to clicks in the human newborn. Electroencephalogr Clin Neurophysiol 18:441–450, 1965

Barnet AB, Lodge A: Diagnosis of deafness in infants with the use of computer-averaged electroencephalographic responses to sound. J Pediatr 69:753–758, 1966

Beagley HA, Kellogg SE, A comparison of evoked response and subjective auditory thresholds. Int Audiol 8:345–353, 1969

Beagley HA, Kellogg SE: Amplitude of the auditory evoked response at high intensities. Sound 4:86–90, 1970

Beagley HA, Knight JJ: Changes in auditory evoked response with intensity. J Laryngol Otol 81:861–873, 1967

Beck A: Oznaczenie lokalizacyi w mozgu i rdzeniu za pomoca zjawisk elektry czynch. Krakow, Univ Jagiellonski, 1890

Beiter RC, Hogan DD: Effects of variations in stimulus rise-decay time upon the early components of the auditory evoked response. Electroencephalogr Clin Neurophysiol 34:203–206, 1973

Berger H: Über das Elektrenkephalogramm des Menschen. Arch Psychiatrie Nervenkrankheiten 87:527–570, 1929

Berlin CI: New developments in evaluating central auditory mechanisms. Ann Otol Rhinol Laryngol 85:833–841, 1976

Berlin CI, Gondra MI: Extratympanic clinical electrocochleography with clicks, in Ruben RJ, Elberling C, Salomon G (eds): Electrocochleography. Baltimore, Univ Park Pr, 1976

Berry H, Briant TD, Winchester BT: Electrophysiologic assessment of the lower portion of the auditory pathway in the human subject. J Otolaryngol 5:3–11, 1976

Bickford RG: Physiological and clinical studies of microreflexes. Recent Contributions to Neurophysiology, EEG Supplement 31:93–108, Elsevier, 1972

Bickford R, Jacobson J, Cody D: Nature of averaged evoked potentials to sound and other stimuli in man. Ann NY Acad Sci 112:204–223, 1964

Blegvad B: Binaural summation of surface-recorded electrocochleographic responses. Normal hearing subjects. Scand Audiol 4:233–238, 1975

Bochenek Z, Bochenek W: Early (12–16 ms) responses evoked by tones and clicks. Rev Laryngol 96:114–120, 1975

Borsanyi SI: Some aspects of auditory evoked potentials in man. Ann Otol Rhinol Laryngol 73:61–71, 1964

Brackmann DE, Selters WA: Electrocochleography in Ménière's disease and acoustic neuromas, in Ruben RJ, Elberling C, Salomon G, (eds): Electrochochleograpy. Baltimore, Univ Park Pr, 1976

Brazier M: The historical development of neurophysiology, in Field J, Magoun H, Hall V (eds): Handbook of Physiology. Section 1 Neurophysiology, Vol. 1. Baltimore, Williams and Wilkins, 1959

Brazier M, Barlow J: Some applications of correlation analysis to clinical problems in electroencephalography. Electroencephalogr Clin Neurophysiol 8:325–331, 1956

Buchsbaum M: Average evoked response: Techniques and applications. Schizophrenia Bull 3:10–18, 1970

Buchwald JS, Huang C-M: Far-field acoustic response: Origins in the cat. Science 189:382–384, 1975

Callaway E: Brain Electrical Potentials and Individual Psychological Differences. New York, Grune & Stratton, 1975

Caton R: The electric currents of the brain. Br Med J 2:278, 1875

Celesia GC, Puletti F: Auditory cortical areas of man. Neurology 19:211–220, 1969

Clark W Jr: Average response computer (ARC-1). Quarterly Progress Report, MIT Research Laboratory of Electronics, 1958, pp 114–117

Coats AC: On electrocochleographic electrode design. J Acoust Soc Am 56:708–711, 1974

Coats AC, Dickey JR: Nonsurgical recording of human auditory nerve action potentials and cochlear microphonics. Ann Otol Rhinol Laryngol 79:844–852, 1970

Coats AC, Dickey JR: Postmasking recovery of human click action potentials and click loudness. J Acoust Soc Am 52:1607–1612, 1972

Cody DTR, Klass DW, Bickford RG: Cortical audiometry: An objective method of evaluating auditory acuity in awake and sleeping man. Trans Am Acad Ophthalmol Otolaryngol 71:81–91, 1967

Cohen MM, Rapin I, Lyttle M, et al: Auditory evoked response (AER) —Consistency of detection in young sleeping children. Arch Otolaryngol 94:214–219, 1971

Crowley DE, Davis H, Beagley HA: Survey of the clinical use of electrocochleography. Ann Otol Rhinol Laryngol 84:297–307, 1975

Cullen JK, Berlin CI, Gondra MI, et al: Electrocochleography in children: A retrospective study. Arch Oto Laryngol 102:482–486, 1976

Cullen JK, Ellis MS, Berlin CI, et al: Human acoustic nerve action potential recordings from the tympanic membrane without anesthesia. Acta Oto-laryngol 74:15–22, 1972

Dallos P: The Auditory Periphery, Biophysics and Physiology. New York, Academic, 1973

Daly DM, Roeser RJ, Moushegian G: The frequency-following response in subjects with profound unilateral hearing loss. Electroencephalogr Clin Neurophysiol 40:132–142, 1976

Davis H: Enhancement of evoked cortical potentials in humans related to a task requiring a decision. Science 145:182–183, 1964

Davis H: Sedation of young children for evoked response audiometry (ERA). Summary of a symposium. Audiology 12:55–57, 1973

Davis H: Brain stem and other responses in electric response audiometry. Ann Otol Rhinol Laryngol 85:3–14, 1976a

Davis H: Principles of electric response audiometry. Ann Otol Rhinol Laryngol (Suppl 28) 85:1–96, 1976b

Davis H, Davis P, Loomis A, et al: Electrical reactions of the human brain to auditory stimulation during sleep. J Neurophysiol 2:500–514, 1939

Davis H, Derbyshire AJ, Lurie M, et al: The electric response of the cochlea. Am J Physiol 107:311–332, 1934

Davis H, Fernández C, McAuliffe DP: The excitatory process in the cochlea. Proc Natl Acad Sci 36:580–587, 1950

Davis H, Gernandt BE, Riesco-MacClure JS, et al: Aural microphonics in the cochlea of the guinea pig. J Acoust Soc Am 21:502–510, 1949

Davis H, Hirsh SK: Clinical trial of fast responses in ERA. Paper presented at the Third Symposium of the International Electric Response Audiometry Study Group, Bordeaux, 1973

Davis H, Hirsh SK: The audiometric utility of brain stem response to low-frequency sounds. Audiology 15:181–195, 1976

Davis H, Hirsh SK, Shelnutt J, et al: Further validation of evoked response audiometry (ERA). J Speech Hear Res 10:717–732, 1967

Davis H, Mast T, Yoshie N, et al: The slow response of the human cortex to auditory stimuli: recovery process. Electroencephalogr Clin Neurophysiol 21:105–113, 1966

Davis H, Onishi S: Maturation of auditory evoked potentials. Int Audiol 8:24–33, 1969

Davis H, Zerlin S: Acoustic relations of the human vertex potential. J Acoust Soc Am 39:109–116, 1966

Davis P: Effects of acoustic stimuli on the waking human brain. J Neurophysiol 2:494–499, 1939

Dawson G: Cerebral responses to electrical stimulation of peripheral nerve in man. J Neurol Neurosurg Psychiatry 10:134–140, 1947

Dawson WW, Doddington HW: Phase distortion of biological signals: extraction of signal from noise without phase error. Electroencephalogr Clin Neurophysiol 34:207–211, 1973

Derbyshire A, Fraser A, McDermott M, et al: Audiometric measurements by electroencephalography. Electroencephalogr Clin Neurophysiol 8:467–478, 1956

Desmedt JE, Brunko E, Debecker J, et al: The system bandpass required to avoid distortion of early components when averaging somatosensory potentials. Electroencephalogr Clin Neurophysiol 37:407–410, 1974

Doerfler LG: Neurophysiological clues to auditory acuity. J Speech Hear Disord 13:227–232, 1948

du Bois-Reymond E: Untersuchungen über thierische Elektricität. Berlin, Reimer, 1848

Eggermont JJ: Summating potentials in electrocochleography: Relation to hearing disorders, in Ruben RJ, Elberling C, Salomon G (eds): Electrocochleography. Baltimore, Univ Park Pr, 1976

Eggermont JJ, Odenthal DW: Electrophysiological investigation of the human cochlea: recruitment, masking and adaptation. Audiology 13:1–22, 1974a

Eggermont JJ, Odenthal DW: Frequency selective masking in electrocochleography. Rev Laryngol 95:489–496, 1974b

Eggermont JJ, Odenthal DW: Methods in electrocochleography, in Eggermont JJ, Odenthal DW, Schmidt PH, et al. (eds): Electrocochleography. Basic Principles and Clinical Application. Acta Oto-laryngol Suppl 316:17–24, 1974c

Eggermont JJ, Odenthal DW, Schmidt PH, et al (eds): Electrocochleography: Basic Principles and Clinical Application. Acta Otolaryngol (Suppl) (Stockh)316:1–84, 1974

Eggermont JJ, Spoor A, Odenthal DW: Frequency specificity of tone-burst electrocochleography, in Ruben RJ, Elberling C, Salomon G (eds): Electrocochleography. Baltimore, Univ Park Pr, 1976

Elberling C: Action potentials along the cochlear partition recorded from the ear canal in man. Scand Audiol 3:13–19, 1974

Elberling C, Salomon G: Electrical potentials from the inner ear in man, in response to transient sounds generated in a closed acoustic system. Rev Laryngol (Suppl) 691:707, 1971

Ellingson RJ, Danahy I, Nelson B, et al: Variability of auditory evoked potentials in human newborns. Electroencephalogr Clin Neurophysiol 36:155–162, 1974

Engel R: Early waves of the electroencephalic auditory response in neonates. Neuropädiatrie 3:147–154, 1971

Engel R, Young NB: Calibrated pure tone audiograms in normal neonates based on evoked electroencephalographic responses. Neuropädiatrie 1:149–160, 1969

Evans TR, Deatherage BH: The effect of frequency on the auditory evoked response. Psychon Sci 15:95–96, 1969

Ferriss GS, Davis GD, Dorsen M, et al: Maturation of the evoked response to auditory stimuli in human infants. Electroencephalogr Clin Neurophysiol 23:83, 1967

Fromm B, Nylen CO, Zotterman Y: Studies in the mechanism of the Wever and Bray effect. Acta Oto-laryngol 22:477–486, 1935

Gardi JN, McKean C, Merzenich M: Origins of brainstem frequency following response. Annual Convention, American Speech and Hearing Association, Chicago, 1977

Geisler C, Frishkopf L, Rosenblith W: Extracranial responses to acoustic clicks in man. Science 128:1210–1211, 1958

Gerken GM, Moushegian G, Stillman RD, et al: Human frequency-following responses to monaural and binaural stimuli. Electroencephalogr Clin Neurophysiol 38:379–386, 1975

Gerull G, Giesen M, Mrowinski D, et al: Properties of an early AER of 5–10 ms latency. Rev Laryngol 95:560–565, 1974

Gibbs FA, Davis H, Lennox W: The electroencephalogram in epilepsy and in conditions of impaired consciousness. Arch Neurol Psychiatry 3:1133–1148, 1935

Gidoll SH: Quantitative determination of hearing to audiometric frequencies in the electroencephalogram; Preliminary report. Arch Otolaryngol 55:597–601, 1952

Glaser EM, Suter CM, Dashieff R, et al: The human frequency-following response: Its behavior during continuous tone burst stimulation. Electroencephalogr Clin Neurophysiol 40:25–32, 1976

Goff W: Human average evoked potentials: Procedures for stimulating and recording, in Thompson R, Patterson M (eds): Bioelectric Recording Techniques, Part B. Electroencephalography and Human Brain Potentials. New York, Academic, 1974

Goff W, Allison T, Lyons W, et al: Origins of short latency auditory evoked response components in man, in Desmedt J (ed): Cerebral Evoked Potentials in Man. (in press)

Goldenberg RA, Derbyshire AJ: Averaged evoked potentials in cats with lesions of auditory pathway. J Speech Hear Res 18:420–429, 1975

Goldstein R, McRandle CC: Middle components of the averaged electroencephalic response to clicks in neonates, in Hirsh SK, Eldredge DH, Hirsh IJ, Silverman SR (eds): Hearing and Davis: Essays Honoring Hallowell Davis, St. Louis, Mo., Washington Univ Pr, 1976

Goldstein R, Rodman LB, Karlovich RS: Effects of stimulus rate and number on the early components of the averaged electroencephalic response. J Speech Hear Res 15:559–566, 1972

Goodhill V, Lowell EL, Lowell MO: Computerized objective auditory testing in infancy. Final report of project DHEW H-181, 1970

Goodman WS, Appleby SV, Scott JW, et al: Audiometry in newborn children by electroencephalography. Laryngoscope 74:1316–1328, 1964

Graziani LJ, Weitzman ED, Velasco MSA: Neurologic maturation and auditory evoked responses in low birth weight infants. Pediatrics 41:483–494, 1968

Hallpike CS, Rawdon-Smith A: The origin of the Wever-Bray phenomenon. J Physiol 83:243–254, 1934

Harker LA, Hosick E, Voots RJ, Mendel MI: Influence of succinylcholine on middle component auditory evoked potentials, Arch Otolaryngol 103:133–137, 1977

Hecox K: Electrophysiological correlates of human auditory development, in Cohen LB, Salapatek P (eds): Infant Perception from Sensation to Cognition, Vol. II. Perception of Space, Speech, and Sound. New York, Academic, 1975

Hecox K, Galambos R: Brain stem auditory evoked responses in human infants and adults. Arch Otolaryngol 99:30–33, 1974

Hecox K, Squires N, Galambos R: Brainstem auditory evoked responses in man. I. Effect of stimulus rise-fall time and duration. J Acoust Soc Am 60:1187–1198, 1976

Henderson D: Behavioral and human evoked response thresholds as a function of frequency. J Speech Hear Res 15:390–394, 1972

Hood DC: Central effects on the human peripheral auditory system. Unpublished doctoral dissertation, Northwestern University, 1971

Hood DC: Evoked cortical response audiometry, in: Bradford LJ (ed): Physiological Measures of the Audio-Vestibular System. New York, Academic, 1975

Horwitz S, Larson S, Sances A: Evoked potentials as an adjunct to the auditory evaluation of patients. Proc Symp Biomed Eng 1:49–52, 1966

Hosick EC, Mendel MI: Effects of secobarbitol on the late components of the auditory evoked potentials. Rev Laryngol 96:185–191, 1975

Hrbek A, Hrbkova M, Lenard H: Somato-sensory, auditory, and visual evoked responses in newborn infants during sleep and wakefulness. Electroencephalogr Clin Neurophysiol 26:597–603, 1969

Hyde ML, Stephens SDG, Thornton ARD: Stimulus repetition rate and the early brainstem responses. Br J Audiol 10:41–50, 1976

Innitzer J, Schmid E: General anesthesia in children—a modified ketamine hydrochloride application. Paper presented to the Biennial Meeting, International Electric Response Audiometry Study Group, London, 1975

Itakura S: Electroencephalography and sound stimulation. Folia Psychiatr Neurol Jpn 9:280–281, 1955

Jasper H, Carmichael L: Electrical potentials from the intact human brain. Science 81:51–53, 1935

Jewett DL: Averaged volume-conducted potentials to auditory stimuli in the cat. Physiologist 12:262, 1969

Jewett DL: Volume-conducted potentials in response to auditory stimuli as detected by averaging in the cat. Electroencephalogr Clin Neurophysiol 28:609–618, 1970

Jewett DL, Romano MN: Neonatal development of auditory system potentials averaged from the scalp of the rat and cat. Brain Res 36:101–115, 1972

Jewett DL, Romano MN, Williston JS: Human auditory evoked potentials: Possible brain stem components detected on the scalp. Science 167:1517–1518, 1970

Jewett DL, Williston JS: Auditory-evoked far fields averaged from the scalp of humans. Brain 94:681–696, 1971

Keating LW, Ruhm HB: Some observations on the effects of attention to stimuli on the amplitude of the acoustically evoked response. Audiology 10:177–184, 1971

Khechinashvili SN, Kevanishvili ZS: Experiences in computer audiometry (ECoG and ERA). Audiology 13:391–402, 1974

Khechinashvili SN, Kevanishvili ZS, Kajaia OA: Amplitude and latency studies of the averaged auditory evoked responses to tones of different intensities. Acta Oto-Laryngol Suppl 76:395–401, 1973

Khechinashvili SN, Kevanishvili ZS, Khachjdze OA, et al: Electrocochleographical studies in humans. Br J Audiology 8:6–13, 1974

Kupperman GL: Effects of three stimulus parameters on the early components of the averaged electroencephalic response. Unpublished doctoral dissertation, University of Wisconsin, Madison, 1970

Kupperman GL, Mendel MI: Threshold of the early components of the averaged electroencephalic response determined with tone pips and clicks during drug-induced sleep. Audiology 13:379–390, 1974

Lane RH, Kupperman GL, Goldstein R: Early components of the averaged electroencephalic response in relation to rise-decay time and duration of pure tones. J Speech Hear Res 14:408–415, 1971

Lane RH, Mendel MI, Kupperman GL, et al: Phase distortion of averaged electroencephalic response. Arch Otolaryngol 99:428–432, 1974

Leiberman A, Sohmer H, Szabo G: Cochlear audiometry (Electro-cochleography) during neonatal period. Dev Med Child Neuorol 15:8–13, 1973a

Leiberman A, Sohmer H, Szabo G: Standard values of amplitude and latency of cochlear audiometry (electrocochleography) responses in different age groups. Arch Klin Exp Ohren Nasen Kehlkopf 203:267–273, 1973b

Lempert J, Meltzer PE, Wever EG, et al: The cochleogram and its clinical applications. Concluding observations. Arch Otolaryngol 51:307–311, 1950

Lempert J, Wever EG, Lawrence M: The cochleogram and its clinical applications. A preliminary report. Arch Otolaryngol 45:61–67, 1947

Lenard H, von Bernuth H, Hutt SJ: Acoustic evoked responses in newborn infants: The influence of pitch and complexity of the stimulus. Electroencephalogr Clin Neurophysiol 27:121–127, 1969

Lentz WE, McCandless GA: Averaged electroencephalic audiometry in infants. J Speech Hear Dis 36:19–28, 1971

Lev A, Sohmer H: Sources of averaged neural responses recorded in animal and human subjects during cochlear audiometry. Arch Klin Exp Ohren Nasen Kehlkopf 201:79–90, 1972

Lindsley D: Average evoked potentials—Achievements, failures and prospects, in Donchin E, Lindsley D (eds): Average Evoked Potentials: Methods, Results, and Evaluations. Washington, D.C., National Aeronautics and Space Administration 1969

Loomis A, Harvey E, Hobart G: Potential rhythms of the cerebral cortex during sleep. Science 81:597–598, 1935

Lowell EL, Troffer C, Warburton E, et al: Temporal evannation: A new approach in diagnostic audiology. J Speech Hear Dis 25:340–345, 1960

Lowell EL, Williams CT, Ballinger RM, et al: Measurement of auditory threshold with a special purpose analog computer. J Speech Hear Res 4:105–112, 1961

Madell JR, Goldstein R: Relation between loudness and the amplitude of the early components of the averaged electroencephalic response. J Speech Hear Res 15:134–141, 1972

Marcus RE, Gibbs EL, Gibbs FA: Electroencephalography in diagnosis of hearing loss in the very young child. Dis Nerv Syst 10:170–173, 1949

Marsh JT, Brown WS, Smith JC: Farfield recorded frequency-following responses: Correlates of low pitch auditory perception in humans. Electroencephalogr Clin Neurophysiol 38:113–120, 1975

Martin JL, Coats AC: Short-latency auditory evoked responses recorded from human nasopharynx. Brain Res 60:496–502, 1973

Mast TE: Short-latency human evoked responses to clicks. J Appl Physiol 20:725–730, 1965

McCandless GA: Clinical application of evoked response audiometry. J Speech Hear Res 10:468–478, 1967

McCandless G: Electroencephalic audiometry, in Rose D (ed): Audiological Assessment. Prentice-Hall, Englewood Cliffs, N.J. 1971

McCandless GA, Best L: Summed evoked responses using pure-tone stimuli. J Speech Hear Res 9:256–262, 1966

McCandless GA, Rose DE: Evoked cortical responses to stimulus change. J Speech Hear Res 13:624–634, 1970

McFarland W, Vivion MC, Goldstein R: Middle components of the AER as a response index for threshold audiometry on normal and pathologic subjects. Annual convention, American Speech and Hearing Association, Las Vegas 1974

McFarland W, Vivion MC, Wolf KE, et al: Reexamination of effects of stimulus rate and number on the middle components of the averaged electroencephalic response. Audiology 14:456–465, 1975

McRandle CC, Smith MA, Goldstein R: Early averaged electroencephalic responses to clicks in neonates. Ann Otol Rhinol Laryngol 83:695–702, 1974

Mendel MI: Influence of stimulus level and sleep stage on the early components of the averaged electroencephalic response to clicks during all-night sleep. J Speech Hear Res 17:5–17, 1974

Mendel MI, Adkinson C, Harker L: Middle components of the auditory evoked potentials in infants. Ann Otol Rhinol Laryngol 86:293–299, 1977

Mendel MI, Goldstein R: The effect of test conditions on the early components of the averaged electroencephalic response. J Speech Hear Res 12:344–350, 1969a

Mendel MI, Goldstein R: Stability of the early components of the averaged electroencephalic response. J Speech Hear Res 12:351–361, 1969b

Mendel MI, Goldstein R: Early components of the averaged electroencephalic response to constant level clicks during all-night sleep. J Speech Hear Res 14:829–840, 1971

Mendel MI, Hosick EC: Effects of secobarbital on the early components of the auditory evoked potentials. Rev Laryngol 96:178–184, 1975

Mendel MI, Hosick EC, Adkinson C: Effects of diazepam on the middle components of the auditory evoked potentials: A preliminary report. Paper presented to the Combined Meeting of the Western Electroencephalography Society and the Central Association of Electroencephalographers. Denver, 1974

Mendel MI, Hosick EC, Windman TR, et al: Audiometric comparison of the middle and late components of the adult auditory evoked potentials awake and asleep. Electroencephalogr Clin Neurophysiol 38:27–33, 1975

Mendel MI, Kupperman GL: Early components of the averaged electroencephalic response to constant level clicks during rapid eye movement sleep. Audiology 13:23–32, 1974

Mendel MI, Pals L, Harker L: Two years' clinical experience with the middle components of the auditory evoked potentials. Paper presented to the American Speech and Hearing Association Annual Convention, Houston, 1976

Mokotoff B, Schulman-Galambos CA, Galambos R: Brain stem auditory evoked responses in children. Arch Otolaryngol 103:38–43, 1977

Møller K, Blegvad B: Brainstem responses in patients with sensorineural hearing loss; monaural versus binaural stimulation. The significance of the audiogram configuration. Scand Audiol 5:115–127, 1976

Monod N, Garma L: Auditory responsivity in the human premature. Biol Neonate 17:292–316, 1971

Montandon PB, Megill ND, Kahn AR, et al: Recording auditory-nerve potentials as an office procedure. Ann Otol Rhinol Laryngol 84:2–10, 1975a

Montandon PB, Shepard NT, Marr EM, et al: Auditory-nerve potentials from ear canals of patients with otologic problems. Ann Otol Rhinol Laryngol 84:164–173, 1975b

Moore EJ: Human cochlear microphonics and auditory nerve action potentials from surface electrodes. Unpublished doctoral dissertation, University of Wisconsin, Madison, 1971

Moore EJ, Rose DE: Variability of latency and amplitude of acoustically evoked responses to pure tones of moderate to high intensities. Int Audiol 8:172–181, 1969

Morgon A, Charachon D, Gerin P: Electro-encephalographic audiometry for young children. Arch Klin Exp Ohren Nasen Kehlkopf 198:144–150, 1971

Mouney DF, Cullen JK, Gondra MI, et al: Tone burst electrocochleography in humans. Trans Am Acad Ophthalmol Otolaryngol 82:348–355, 1976

Moushegian G, Rupert AL, Stillman RD: Scalp-recorded early responses in man to frequencies in the speech range. Electroencephalogr Clin Neurophysiol 35:665–667, 1973

Naunton RF, Zerlin S: Basis and some diagnostic implications of electrocochleography. Laryngoscope 86:475–482, 1976a

Naunton RF, Zerlin S: Human whole-nerve response to clicks of various frequency. Audiology 15:1–9, 1976b

Nelson DA, Lassman FM: Effects of intersignal interval on the human auditory evoked response. J Acoust Soc Am 44:1529–1532, 1968

Norkus FJ, Derbyshire AJ, Mills PJ et al: Frequency measure of the EEG. J Acoust Soc Am 32:1147–1150, 1960

Odenthal DW, Eggermont JJ: Clinical electrocochleography, in Eggermont JJ, Odenthal DW, Schmidt PH, Spoor A (eds): Electrocochleography. Basic Principles and Clinical Application. Acta Oto-Laryngol (Stockh) Suppl 316:62–74, 1974

Odenthal DW, Eggermont JJ: Electrocochleographic study of Ménière's disease and pontine angle neurinoma, in Ruben RJ, Elberling C, Salomon G (eds): Electrocochleography. Baltimore, Univ Park Pr, 1976

Odenthal DW, Eggermont JJ, Hermans J: Diagnosis by electrocochleography. Rev Laryngol 95:481–488, 1974

Ohlrich ES, Barnet AB: Auditory evoked responses during the first year of life. Electroencephalogr Clin Neurophysiol 32:161–169, 1972

Onishi S, Davis H: Effects of duration and rise time of tone bursts on evoked "V" potentials. J Acoust Soc Am 44:582–591, 1968

Ornitz EM, Ritvo ER, Carr EM, et al: The variability of the auditory averaged evoked response during sleep and dreaming in children and adults. Electroencephalogr Clin Neurophysiol 22:514–524, 1967

Ornitz EM, Walter DO: The effect of sound pressure waveform on human brain stem auditory evoked responses. Brain Res 92:490–498, 1975

Osterhammel PA, Davis H, Wier CC, et al: Adult auditory evoked vertex potentials in sleep. Audiology 12:116–128, 1973

Parmelee AH Jr: Sleep cycles in infants. Dev Med Child Neurol 11:794–795, 1969

Perl ER, Galambos R, Glorig A: The estimation of hearing threshold by electroencephalography. Electroencephalogr Clin Neurophysiol 5:501–512, 1953

Perlman MB, Case TJ: Electrical phenomena of the cochlea in man. Arch Otolaryngol 34:710–718, 1941

Peters JF, Mendel MI: Early components of the averaged electroencephalic response to monaural and binaural stimulation. Audiology 13:195–204, 1974

Picton TW, Goodman WS, Bryce DP: Amplitude of evoked responses to tones of high intensity. Acta Oto-Laryngol (Stockh) 70:77–82, 1970

Picton TW, Hillyard SA: Human auditory evoked potentials: II: Effects of attention. Electroencephalogr Clin Neurophysiol 36:191–199, 1974

Picton TW, Hillyard SA, Krausz HI, et al: Human auditory evoked potentials. I. Evaluation of components. Electroencephalogr Clin Neurophysiol 36:179–190, 1974

Picton T, Woods D, Baribeau-Braun J, et al: Evoked potential audiometry. J Otolaryngol 6:90–119, 1977

Plantz R, Williston JS, Jewett DL: Spatio-temporal distribution of auditory-evoked far-field potentials in rat and cat. Brain Res 68:55–71, 1974

Portmann M, Aran JM: Electro-cochléographie sur le nourrisson et le jeune enfant. Acta Oto-Laryngol (Stockh) 71:253–261, 1971a

Portmann M, Aran JM: Electro-cochleography. Laryngoscope 81:899–910, 1971b

Portmann M, Aran JM: Relations entre "pattern" electrocochleographique et pathologie retrolabyrinthique. Acta Oto-Laryngol 73:190–196, 1972

Portmann M, Aran JM, LeBert G: Potentiels cochléaires obtenues chez l'homme en dehors de toute intervention chirurgicale. Note preliminaire. Rev Laryngol 88:157–164, 1967

Portmann M, Portmann C, Negrevergne M: Four years of clinical use of electrocochleography. Rev Laryngol Otol Rhinol 95:537–539, 1974

Price LL: Evoked response audiometry, in Fulton R, Lloyd LL, (eds): Auditory Assessment of the Difficult-to-Test. Baltimore, Williams and Wilkins, 1975

Price LL, Goldstein R: Averaged evoked responses for measuring auditory sensitivity in children. J Speech Hear Dis 31:248–256, 1966

Price LL, Rosenblut B, Goldstein R, et al: The averaged evoked response to auditory stimulation. J Speech Hear Res 9:361–370, 1966

Rapin I, Bergman M: Auditory evoked responses in uncertain diagnoses. Arch Otolaryngol 90:307–314, 1969

Rapin I, Graziani LJ: Auditory-evoked responses in normal, brain damaged, and deaf infants. Neurology 17:881–894, 1967

Rapin I, Ruben RJ, Lyttle M: Diagnosis of hearing loss in infants using auditory evoked responses. Laryngoscope 80:712–722, 1970

Rapin I, Schimmel H, Cohen MM: Reliability in detecting the auditory evoked response (AER) for audiometry in sleeping subjects. Electroencephalogr Clin Neurophysiol 32:521–528, 1972

Regan D: Evoked Potentials in Psychology, Sensory Physiology and Clinical Medicine. New York, Wiley-Interscience, 1972

Reneau J, Hnatiow GZ: Evoked Response Audiometry: A Topical and Historical Review. Baltimore, Univ Park Pr, 1975

Ritvo ER, Ornitz EM, Walter RD: Clinical application of the auditory averaged evoked response at sleep onset in the diagnosis of deafness. Pediatrics 40:1003–1008, 1967

Roeser R, Price LL, Hnatiow GZ: Evoked response audiometry: Psychiatric patients. Arch Otolaryngol 94:208–213, 1971

Ronis BJ: Cochlear potentials in otosclerosis. Laryngoscope 73:212–231, 1966

Rose DE, Keating LW, Hedgecock LD, et al: A comparison of evoked response audiometry and routine clinical audiometry. Audiology 11:238–243, 1972

Rose DE, Keating LW, Hedgecock LD, et al: Aspects of acoustically evoked responses: Interjudge and intra-judge reliability. Arch Otolaryngol 94:347–350, 1971

Rothman HH: Effects of high frequencies and intersubject variability on the auditory-evoked cortical response. J Acoust Soc Am 47:569–573, 1970

Ruben RJ: Cochlear potentials as a diagnostic test in deafness, in Graham AB (ed.): Sensorineural Hearing Processes and Disorders. Boston, Little, Brown, 1967

Ruben RJ, Bordley JE, Lieberman AT: Cochlear potentials in man. Laryngoscope 71:1141–1164, 1961

Ruben RJ, Elberling C, Salomon G (eds): Electrocochleography. Baltimore, Univ Park Pr, 1976

Ruben RJ, Knickerbocker GG, Sekula J, et al: Cochlear microphonics in man: A preliminary report. Laryngoscope 69:665–671, 1959

Ruben RJ, Lieberman AT, Bordley JE: Some observations on cochlear potentials and nerve action potentials in children. Laryngoscope 72:545–554, 1962

Ruben RJ, Sekula J, Bordley JE, et al: Human cochlear responses to sound stimuli. Ann Otol Rhinol Laryngol 69:459–479, 1960

Ruben RJ, Walker AE: The VIIIth nerve action potential in Ménière's disease. Laryngoscope 73:1456–1461, 1963

Ruhm HB, Jansen JW: Rate of stimulus change and the evoked response: I. Signal rise-time. J Auditory Res 3:211–216, 1969

Ruhm H, Walker E, Flanigin H: Acoustically-evoked potentials in man: Mediation of early components. Laryngoscope 77:806–822, 1967

Salamy A, McKean CM: Postnatal development of human brainstem potentials during the first year of life. Electroencephalogr Clin Neurophysiol 40:418–426, 1976

Salamy A, McKean CM: Habituation and dishabituation of cortical and brainstem evoked potentials. Int J Neuroscience (in press)

Salamy A, McKean CM, Buda FB: Maturational changes in auditory transmission as reflected in human brain stem potentials. Brain Res 96:361–366, 1975

Salomon G, Elberling C: Cochlear nerve potentials recorded from the ear canal in man. Acta Oto-Laryngol (Stockh) 71:319–325, 1971

Saul LJ, Davis H: Action currents in the central nervous system: I. Action currents of the auditory tracts. Arch Neurol Psychiatry 28:1104–1116, 1932

Schimmel H, Rapin I, Cohen MM: Improving evoked response audiometry. Results of normative studies for machine scoring. Audiology 14:466–479, 1975

Schoenberg BS: Richard Caton and the electrical activity of the brain. Mayo Clin Proc 49:474–481, 1974

Schulman-Galambos CA, Galambos R: Brain stem auditory-evoked responses in premature infants. J Speech Hear Res 18:456–465, 1975

Scott TD: A psychophysiological investigation of cortical audiometry during human sleep. Unpublished doctoral dissertation, Univ California, Santa Cruz, 1973

Shagass C: Evoked Brain Potentials in Psychiatry. New York, Plenum, 1972

Simmons FB: Electrocochleography. Ann Otol Rhinol Laryngol 83:312–313, 1974

Simmons FB: Human auditory nerve responses: A comparison of three commonly used recording sites. Laryngoscope 85:1564–1581, 1975

Simmons FB, Glattke T: Electrocochleography, in Bradford LJ (ed): Physiological Measures of the Audio-Vestibular System. New York, Academic, 1975

Skinner PH, Glattke T: Electrophysiologic response audiometry: State of the art. J Speech Hear Dis 42:179–198, 1977

Skinner PH, Antinoro F: The effect of signal rise time and duration on the early components of the auditory evoked cortical response. J Speech Hear Res 14:552–558, 1971

Skinner PH, Jones HC: Effects of signal duration and rise time on the auditory evoked potential. J Speech Hear Res 11:301–306, 1968

Skinner PH, Shimota J: A comparison of the effects of sedatives on the auditory evoked cortical response. J Am Audio Soc 1:71–78, 1975

Smith JC, Marsh JT, Brown WS: Far-field recorded frequency-following responses: Evidence for the locus of brainstem sources. Electroencephalogr Clin Neurophysiol 39:465–472, 1975

Sohmer H, Feinmesser M: Cochlear and cortical audiometry: Conveniently recorded in the same subject. Isr J Med Sci 6:219–223, 1970

Sohmer H, Feinmesser M: Routine use of electrocochleography (cochlear audiometry) in human subjects. Audiology 12:167–173, 1973

Sohmer H, Feinmesser M: Electrocochleography in clinical-audiological diagnosis. Arch Otorhinolaryngol 206:91–102, 1974

Sohmer H, Feinmesser M, Bauberger-Tell L, et al: Routine use of cochlear audiometry in infants with uncertain diagnosis. Ann Otol Rhinol Laryngol 81:72–75, 1972

Sohmer H, Pratt H: Recording of the cochlear microphonic potential with surface electrodes. Electroencephalogr Clin Neurophysiol 40:253–260, 1976

Sohmer H, Pratt H, Feinmesser M: Electrocochleography or evoked cortical responses: Which is preferable in diagnosis of hearing loss? Rev Laryngol 95:515–522, 1974

Starr A: Auditory brainstem responses in brain death. Brain 99:543–554, 1976

Starr A, Achor J: Auditory brainstem responses in neurological disease. Arch Neurol 32:761–768, 1975

Starr A, Amlie R, Martin WH, et al: Development of auditory function in newborn infants revealed by auditory brainstem potentials. Pediatrics, in press

Starr A, Hamilton A: Brain regions generating auditory brainstem responses: Correlating between site of pathology and response abnormalities. Neurology 25:385, 1975

Starr A, Hamilton A: Correlations between confirmed sites of neurological lesions and abnormalities of far-field auditory brainstem responses. EEG J 41:595–608, 1976

Stein L: Clinical study of brainstem evoked response (BER) with untestable and high risk children. Paper presented to the American Speech and Hearing Association Annual Convention, Washington, D.C., 1975

Stillman RD, Moushegian G, Rupert AL: Early tone-evoked responses in normal and hearing impaired subjects. Audiology 15:10–22, 1976

Sudaka J, Chaperon C: Notre experience d'electrocochléographie dans le service d'O.-R.-L. des infants malades. Ann Oto-Laryngol 89:699–706, 1972

Suter CM, Glaser EM, Goldberg A, et al: Auditory brainstem electric response to click trains and continuous tones. J Acoust Soc Am 60 (Suppl 1):516, 1976

Suzuki T, Asawa I: Evoked potential of waking human brain to acoustic stimuli. Acta Oto-Laryngol (Stockh) 48:508–515, 1957

Suzuki T, Origuchi K: Averaged evoked response audiometry in young children during sleep. Acta Oto-Laryngol (Stockh) Suppl 252:19–28, 1969

Suzuki T, Taguchi K: Cerebral evoked response to auditory stimuli in young children during sleep. Ann Otol Rhinol Laryngol 77:102–110, 1968

Taguchi K, Goodman WS, Brummitt WM: Evoked response audiometry in mentally retarded children. Acta Oto-Laryngol (Stockh) 70:190–196, 1970

Taguchi K, Picton T, Orpin J, et al: Evoked response audiometry in newborn infants. Acta Oto-Laryngol (Stockh) Suppl 252:5–17, 1969

Tanguay PE, Lee JCM, Ornitz EM: A detailed analysis of the audiotry evoked response waveform in children during REM and stage 2 sleep. Electroencephalogr Clin Neurophysiol 35:241–248, 1973

Tanguay PE, Ornitz EM, Forsythe AB, et al: Basic rest-activity cycle rhythms in the human auditory evoked response. Electroencephalogr Clin Neurophysiol 34:593–603, 1973

Teas DC, Eldredge DH, Davis H: Cochlear responses to acoustic transients: An interpretation of whole-nerve action potentials. J Acoust Soc Am 34:1438–1459, 1962

Terkildsen K, Osterhammel P, Huis in't Veld F: Electrocochleography with a far field technique. Scand Audiol 2:141–148, 1973

Terkildsen K, Osterhammel P, Huis in't Veld F: Far field electrocochleography, electrode positions. Scand Audiol 3:123–129, 1974

Terkildsen K, Osterhammel P, Huis in't Veld F: Far-field Electrocochleography. Adaptation. Scand Audiol 4:215–220, 1975a

Terkildsen K, Osterhammel P, Huis in't Veld F: Far field electrocochleography. Frequency specificity of the response. Scand Audiol 4:167–172, 1975b

Thompson, D: Influence of selective attention on the averaged electroencephalic response. Unpublished doctoral dissertation, Univ. Wisconsin, Madison, 1972

Thornton A: The effects of stimulus frequency and intensity on the middle components of the auditory averaged electroencephalic response. Unpublished doctoral dissertation, Univ. Iowa, Iowa City, 1975

Thornton A, Mendel MI, Anderson C: Effects of stimulus frequency and intensity on the middle components of the averaged auditory electroencephalic response. J Speech Hear Res 20:81–94, 1977

Thornton ARD: The diagnostic potential of surface recorded electrocochleography. Br J Audiol 9:7–13, 1975a

Thornton ARD: The measurement of surface-recorded electrocochleographic responses. Scand Audiol 4:51–58, 1975b

Thornton ARD: Statistical properties of surface-recorded electrocochleographic responses. Scand Audiol 4:91–102, 1975c

Thornton ARD: Electrophysiological studies of the auditory system. Audiology 15:23–38, 1976

Thornton ARD, Coleman MJ: The adaptation of cochlear and brainstem auditory evoked potentials in humans. Electroencephalogr Clin Neurophysiol 39:399–406, 1975

Tyberghein J, Forrez G: Objective (ERA) and subjective (COR) audiometry in the infant. Acta Oto-Laryngol (Stockh) 71:249–252, 1971

Vaughn HG, Ritter W: The sources of auditory evoked responses recorded from the human scalp. Electroencephalogr Clin Neurophysiol 28:360–367, 1970

Vivion M, Goldstein R, Wolf KE, et al: Middle components of human auditory AER: Waveform variation during averaging. Audiology 16:21–37, 1977

Weitzman E, Fishbein W, Graziani LJ: Auditory evoked responses obtained from the scalp electroencephalogram of the full-term human neonate during sleep. Pediatrics 35:458–562, 1965

Weitzman E, Graziani L: Maturation and topography of the auditory evoked response of the prematurely born infant. Dev Psychobiol 1:79–89, 1968

Weitzman E, Kremen H: Auditory evoked responses during different stages of sleep in man. Electroencephalogr Clin Neurophysiol 18:65–70, 1965

Wever EG, Bray CW: Auditory nerve impulses. Science 71:215, 1930

Williams HL, Tepas DI, Morlock HC: Evoked responses to clicks and electroencephalographic stages of sleep in man. Science 138:685–686, 1962

Withrow FB Jr, Goldstein R: An electrophysiologic procedure for determination of auditory threshold in children. Laryngoscope 68:1674–1699, 1958

Yamada O, Yagi T, Yamane H, Suzuki J-I: Clinical evaluation of the auditory evoked brainstem response. Auris-Nasus-Larynx 2:92–105, 1975

Yanz JL: Frequency specificity of the auditory compound action potential. Unpublished master's thesis, Univ. Iowa, Iowa City, 1976

Yoshie N: Auditory nerve action potential responses to clicks in man. Laryngoscope 78:198–215, 1968

Yoshie, N: Clinical cochlear response audiometry by means of an average response computer: Nonsurgical technique and clinical use. Rev Laryngol Suppl 92:646–672, 1971

Yoshie N: Diagnostic significance of the electrocochleogram in clinical audiometry. Audiology 12:504–539, 1973

Yoshie N, Ohashi T: Clinical use of cochlear nerve action potential responses in man for differential diagnosis of hearing losses. Acta Oto-Laryngol (Stockh) Suppl 252:71–87, 1969

Yoshie N, Ohashi T: Abnormal adaptation of human cochlear nerve action potential responses—clinical observations by nonsurgical recording. Rev Laryngol 92:673–690, 1971

Yoshie N, Ohashi T, Suzuki T: Nonsurgical recording of auditory nerve action potentials in man. Laryngoscope 77:76–85, 1967

Yoshie N, Okudaira T: Myogenic evoked potential responses to clicks in man. Acta Oto-Laryngol (Stockh) Suppl 252:89–103, 1969

Zerlin S, Naunton RF: Early and late averaged electroencephalic responses at low sensation levels. Audiology 13:366–378, 1974

Zerlin S, Mowry HJ, Naunton RF: Effect of frequency and intensity on early components of the evoked cortical response. Paper presented to the American Speech and Hearing Association Annual Convention, Chicago, 1971

Zerlin S, Naunton RF, Mowry HJ: The early evoked cortical response to third octave clicks and tones. Audiology 12:242–249, 1973

Zöllner C, Karnahl T, Stange G: Input-output function and adaptation behavior of the five early potentials registered with the earlobe-vertex pick-up. Arch Otorhinolaryngol 212:23–33, 1976

Zvonar M, Zvonar-Kuhndl B, Odenthal DW: Anesthesia and sedation for electrocochleography, in Eggermont JJ, Odenthal DW, Schmidt PH, Spoor A (eds): Electrocochleography, Basic Principles and Clinical Application. Acta Oto-Laryngol (Stockh) Suppl 316:37–38, 1974

III

The Consequences

Robert L. Koegel
and Susan Felsenfeld

12
Sensory Deprivation

With good cause, there has been considerable concern about the multitude of learning, language, social, and neurologic handicaps imposed on hearing-impaired individuals. Although it is obvious that those with a hearing loss suffer from varying degress of auditory deprivation, what is not so apparent is the number of secondary deprivations which a hearing impairment might produce. While the normal-hearing child (or adult) is continually interacting with his environment and receiving an abundance of novel sensory input, the hearing handicapped individual is very often left in a state of relative social isolation, which, in turn, has the potential of further interrupting his reception of sensory information.

Although there has been very little research conducted directly on the effects of sensory deprivation resulting from a hearing loss, there is a considerable amount of research on sensory deprivation per se. The results of this research, taken as a whole, suggest very strongly that additional damage to hearing-impaired individuals may result from the sensory deprivation imposed by a hearing deficit. Consequently, in this chapter, we present research on the effects of sensory deprivation, and discuss its implications for early detection of auditory impairment.

The writing of this manuscript was facilitated in part by United States Public Health Service Research Grant No. MH28210 from the National Institute of Mental Health.

SENSORY DEPRIVATION DEFINED

Sensory deprivation is defined as a period of time when an organism experiences absence of sensory stimulation. Functionally, stimulus novelty (including such things as variations in intensity, complexity, contrast, pitch, texture, movement, hue, etc.), appears to be the major variable influencing whether or not an individual will experience sensory stimulation, and, if so, what the total impact of the stimulation will be (Fiske and Maddi, 1961). Therefore, an individual who suffers from a hearing loss can be said to experience sensory deprivation as a consequence of: (1) experiencing less total stimulation than a hearing person, and/or (2) experiencing less variety of stimulation, since certain sound intensities and/or frequencies are unavailable to the individual as a source of novelty. This latter effect becomes particularly concerning when one considers that a hearing handicap can produce many secondary absences of stimulus novelty through the aforemented social isolation frequently encountered by such individuals.

SENSORY DEPRIVATION AND NEUROLOGIC DEVELOPMENT

There is a considerable body of literature showing that animals deprived of sensory input at a young age often suffer from permanent neurological damage. In a classic study by Wiesel and Hubel (1965), for example, one eye of a newborn kitten was sutured shut for the first 3 months of its life. When the eye was opened examination of the visual cortex revealed structural damage to cells in the striate cortex, as well as functional blindness in the deprived eye. Most importantly, however, when the animal was reexamined 5 years later, only limited recovery in cortical physiology and only a slight return of vision were observed.

Deprivation-induced deficits in sensory function, in some cases, have been even more directly linked to neurological impairment resulting from such deprivation. For instance, Krech, Rosenzweig, and Bennett (1966) have discovered differences in brain anatomy and chemistry between rats raised in experimentally enriched environments, and their litter mates raised in isolation in experimentally impoverished environments. In addition to quantitative differences, the investigators noted qualitative differences as well; that is, the more impoverished the environment, the more the experimental rats differed from their enriched litter mates in brain anatomy and chemistry. Further, Rosenzweig (1976) has demonstrated that, while certain portions of the cortex of the brain actually become thicker and heavier with exposure to stimulating environments, the converse also holds true. That is, lack of exposure to complex environments can actually lead to failure of neuron formation.

Greenough (1975) has reviewed a number of studies on this topic, and has provided data showing that the formation of synaptic connections may not occur unless environmental stimulation is provided. In a design similar to that of Krech, Rosenzweig, and Bennett (1966), Greenough looked at rats raised in experimentally rich versus impoverished environments, and found that the neurons of rats from the complex environment had more higher-order dendritic branches, and more dendritic synapses per neuron, than did the impoverished animals. In addition, he noted that, in certain areas of the brain, a greater number of dendritic synapses was formed during post-natal maturation when the rats were kept in a complex environment.

Results such as these raise several interesting questions pertaining to the specificity of deprivational effects. Several studies have been conducted in an effort to determine whether specific deprivational experiences generally influence the entire cortex, or if only those cortical areas directly related to the deprivational situation are involved. Addressing this question, Greenough et al. (1973) studied dendritic branching in rapid Golgi-stained neurons in occipital, frontolateral, and temporal regions of the cortex of rats who were exposed to differentially complex types of environmental stimulation. The experimental paradigm involved introducing the rats to environments differing relatively greatly in visual stimulation, differing moderately in auditory stimulation, and differing very little in motor stimulation. The results showed a qualitative difference in dendritic branching as a function of the degree of stimulation. Thus, relatively large differences were found in dendritic branching in the occipital cortex (associated primarily with visual stimulation). That is, greater complexity in visual stimulation produced larger degrees of dendritic branching. Similarly, there were moderate differences in a region of the temporal cortex that receives input from the auditory system. Thus, moderate differences in auditory stimulation produced directly correlated moderate differences in dendritic branching. Finally, the absence of any differences in motor activity between the environments produced no differences in the effects of complexity in the frontolateral cortex (an area associated primarily with body sensation and motor activity). These results have important implications with respect to individuals suffering from a hearing loss. Since the hearing-impaired person experiences a state of constant auditory sensory deprivation, it would seem likely that he would have a relatively low level of dendritic formation in the temporal cortex associated with the auditory system. Further, these results suggest that no amount of compensation in other areas (e.g., visual or motor stimulation) would reduce the loss of neural formation in the auditory cortex.

THE EFFECT OF AGE

Although stimulus deprivation may be harmful at any age, its effects appear to be particularly devastating when the organism is youngest. For example, Wiesel and Hubel (1965) have demonstrated severely reduced visual ability as a result of visual stimulus deprivation during maturation of the visual system in cats. In a subsequent study (1970), Hubel and Wiesel further refined these data by demonstrating that there seemed to be an age-dependent period of high susceptibility for cellular damage due to monocular deprivation in kittens. In short, they found that the period of approximately four to five weeks of age was the time during which the visual system was most susceptible to damage, so much so, in fact, that a closure for as little as six days during this time span would reduce the number of functional cells in the deprived eye to a fraction of what was normal. However, if the eye was not sutured until after the sensitive period—approximately four months—virtually no permanent damaging effects to the visual system occurred. Therefore, it does appear that, in certain cases, if animals are given some exposure to normal stimulation prior to the introduction of the deprivation, the adverse effects of the deprivation are greatly reduced. Some (e.g., Valverde 1967, 1971; Coleman and Riesen, 1968) have formulated a possible explanation to account for such results. Briefly, they have suggested that deprivation at an early age might inhibit the development of certain neural formations which serve as necessary antecedents for future neural developments. If, however, early neurons are allowed to form through exposure to normal stimulation, any later deprivation would not effect subsequent developments relating to those neurons.

In certain instances, it also appears that if a previously sensory-deprived animal is exposed to subsequent normal stimulation, the severity of the effect of the original deprivation can be offset somewhat (Baxter, 1966; Hubel, 1967; Hubel and Wiesel, 1970; Riesen 1966; Walk and Gibson, 1961). Valverde has also studied the spine growth on the dendrites of nerve cells in the visual cortex of dark-reared mice, and has concluded that, if these visually deprived animals were exposed to light later in life, some new spines would eventually form although the number would never reach that of the normal light-reared mouse. The implications of these findings to early detection of hearing-impairments should be readily apparent. First of all, it appears that the age of greatest susceptibility to at least certain kinds of permanent damage due to sensory deprivation is quite young; and, secondly, if a hearing loss is discovered and subsequently treated relatively early, some of the detrimental effects of the auditory deprivation may be alleviated.

When one discusses the importance of early deprivation effects, it is also important to consider the consequent influence that early deprivation might impose on later sensory stimulation. For example, in the case of a hearing impairment that is to be corrected, it would be useful to predict how an individual would be likely to adjust to his newly-acquired auditory acuity. Baldwin and Baldwin (1976) indirectly address this issue when they theorize that the effects of a given type of sensory input may vary with age, and an organism's need for sensory stimulation also changes over time as a function of its experience with sensory input. In other words, Baldwin and Baldwin hypothesize that, through a process of gradual habituation, the sensory input that an organism will seek will proceed toward greater complexity. In short, an activity that may be overstimulating to a young infant may well be understimulating to an older infant who has already habituated to that input level. To illustrate, a child of three months might be perfectly content to merely touch her mother or observe her surroundings passively, while a 12-month-old child would probably require a good deal more sensory input (through climbing, running, manipulating toys, etc.) to keep amused. Additionally, Baldwin and Baldwin claim that the same sensory stimulus (a nursery rhyme, for example) might have an entirely different effect on two individuals dependent on whether or not that stimulus input was reinforcing.

If we accept this idea, then a prolonged period of sensory deprivation would be expected to change entire areas of the developmental sequence. To clarify this, imagine that a child who has had a hearing loss for the first several years of life has just had his hearing corrected surgically. Such a child, of course, would be exposed immediately to amounts of auditory input for which there had been no time to habituate. In all likelihood, this input would prove too complex to be assimilated easily. At any rate, it is fairly safe to assume that this sudden exposure to sound would have a completely different effect than it would have had had the child experienced gradual change in auditory input throughout these years as normal children do. Indeed, we must be aware of not only how sensory deprivation adversely affects an organism, but also how the removal of deprivation can cause problems as well. It would appear that more research is needed on this subject so that we might be better equipped to understand the aurally deprived.

SENSORY DEPRIVATION AND LEARNING

Several studies have indicated that differences in learning abilities and performance levels may be attributable to stimulus deprivation. Greenough et al. (1972) performed an experiment in which mice were raised in complex (versus impoverished) environments and subsequently tested on a Lashley type III maze. The results demonstrated that the mice from the complex environment tended to make fewer errors on the maze than those from the isolated environments, and also tended to learn the mazes and visual discrimination for food rewards much more readily than their isolated counterparts.

The characteristics of an organism's performance level may also be affected by his level of stimulus deprivation. Numerous studies have shown that an organism will work to receive stimulus input (Kish, 1966). Furthermore, the time of stimulation the organism will work to provide appears to be influenced by the type of prior deprivation it has experienced. For example, Odom (1964) found that a group of children deprived of visual stimulation developed a subsequent preference for visual stimuli, whereas another group of children deprived of auditory stimulation developed a subsequent preference for auditory stimuli. Thus, as Reese and Lipsett (1970) point out, it would be expected that stimulus deprivation could facilitate performance in certain situations and impede performance in other situations, depending on the organism's current state of deprivation and functioning.

EMOTIONAL DEVELOPMENT

When one considers the implications of an inability to receive a specific type of sensory input, as is the case with hearing-impaired individuals, it seems quite likely that such a deficit would directly influence a person's emotional development. In fact, there are several accounts which report that the hearing-impaired often do lag behind in emotional maturity and adaptibility, and frequently score as highly anxious, hypersensitive, and irritable on psychologic batteries (Toscher and Rupp, 1974). However, it is interesting to note that, when awake, normal human infants are generally active and irritable under conditions of relative auditory stimulus deprivation (in an extremely quiet environment) as well (e.g., Bartoshuk, 1962; Birns et al., 1965; Brackbill et al., 1966; Irwin, 1941; Irwin and Weiss, 1934a–c). Presentation of a particular kind of auditory stimulus (such as a metronome, lullaby, monotone, heartbeat, etc.), however, will almost certainly quiet a restless child (Brackbill et al., 1966; Salk, 1960, 1961, 1962). Brackbill et al., for instance, studied 102 newborns in the hospital nursery over several consecutive days, and observed 60% more crying during the no-sound condition than during the sound (heartbeat) condition.

It is crucial to note that only certain sounds within a rather limited frequency and intensity range have been effective in calming the neonates. For example, Bench (1969) has found an inverse relationship between the effectiveness of the sound stimulation in quieting the infant and the frequency of the tone presented; that is, tones of middle or low frequencies were shown to be best at this task, while tones in the higher frequencies merely aroused the infants more. These data, as well as those of Eisenberg (1965), point out that it is not only the loss of hearing per se, but the loss of hearing at certain frequencies, which can produce the greatest effects of sensory deprivation. In the previous example, for instance, if a child had a low-frequency hearing loss, presentation of a low-frequency lullaby would probably not have the same effect on him as it would on a normal hearing child, for instead of calming him, the noise might confuse or irritate him. This indicates that compensation across frequencies is unlikely even if the above child had perfect high-tone hearing, this would not make-up for his deficit in the lower frequencies, and vice versa.

Although it is not clear if auditory deprivation will influence personality disturbance, such effects have been frequently reported in individuals deprived of visual stimulation (Freedman, 1971). Massive sensory deprivation, usually accomplished under experimental conditions, is known frequently to result in reports of a loss of touch with reality, and in many cases, hallucinations, deprivation-induced images, and dreams. These images range from merely seeing flashing lights or geometric forms and hearing bits of conversations and music to full-blown sagas involving "a procession of squirrels with sacks over their shoulders marching purposefully" across the visual field. It should be pointed out that nearly everyone who has served as a subject in a sensory deprivation experiment reports the experience to be highly aversive, even for relatively short periods of time, and many subjects actually suffered from a good deal of anxiety during the procedure (Zubek, 1969).

SENSORY DEPRIVATION AND INFANTILE AUTISM

Prolonged periods of extreme sensory deprivation may have severe effects on an organism's psychologic development, sometimes to the point where the organism will develop deficiencies in many areas, and begin to engage in numerous stereotyped mannerisms which appear to be performed primarily for the purpose of providing sensory input (Harlow and Harlow, 1966; Harlow and Zimmermann, 1959). It also has been noted that the behaviors occurring under such conditions frequently bear many similarities to the behaviors of autistic children.

While no direct evidence exists to connect the behavior of autistic children to extreme sensory deprivation, there are findings in the study of autism that relate to research on stimulus deprivation. Taken as a whole, these studies show that, first of all, autistic children appear very withdrawn, and often respond only to very restricted portions of their stimulus environment perhaps resulting in their receiving reduced sensory input (Anthony, 1958; Hermelin and O'Connor, 1971; Kanner, 1943; Koegel and Schreibman, 1976; Lovaas et al., 1971; Ornitz and Ritvo, 1968; Rimland, 1964; Schopler,

1965). Koegel and Schreibman, for example, discovered that a functionally deaf autistic child named Robert was not suffering from an organic hearing impairment at all, but was responding differentially to certain auditory stimuli to his environment and ignoring all else. Although Robert did not respond to white noise unless it was presented at an intensity level over 86 dB, he would consistently respond to the noise of a candy machine which was producing a 53-dB output. Thus, although Robert did not suffer from a peripheral sensory impairment, he most certainly could be considered auditively deprived for, in responding to only select environmental inputs, he was excluding a great deal of relevant sensory information, and, as such, his detection and remediation are no less crucial than that of a child with a peripheral involvement.

In addition, several studies have also shown that autistic children work very hard to provide themselves with sensory input. In fact, these children often engage in numerous stereotyped mannerisms which appear to be performed primarily for the purpose of providing sensory input, such as head banging, rocking, twirling objects in front of the eyes, etc. (Hutt et al., 1965; Lovaas, 1967). Since these behaviors, frequently called self-stimulation or self-stimulatory behaviors, appear very similar to behaviors performed by children with sensory losses it is worth considering the research on self-stimulation in more detail. This is particularly true since certain investigators (e.g., Ornitz, 1976) have theorized that a dysfunction in the circuitry connecting the vestibular system (located within the ear) with the cerebellum and the brain stem may be responsible for the bizarre sensorimotor behavior observed in autistic children.

Rincover et al. (1974) and Ferris and Newsom (1974) have reported that, in the absence of any external reinforcement, autistic children will engage in fairly high levels of self-stimulatory behavior for indefinitely long periods of time with no evidence of extinction. It appears as if the sensory input itself may serve to reinforce the behavior. Further, Ferris and Newsom reported that if one type of self-stimulation (e.g., arm flapping) is suppressed, then another form (e.g., finger twiddling) appears to replace the suppressed form. That is, it appears as if the children are striving to maintain a particular level of sensory input and will replace suppressed behaviors in a manner permitting maintenance of that level. Further evidence to support this contention has been provided by Koegel and Covert (1972) and Koegel et al. (1974). In these studies, all forms of autistic self-stimulation were suppressed. Instead of sitting and doing nothing, the children appeared to replace the self-stimulation with more normal attempts to gain sensory input. For example, the children in the Koegel et al. study began to engage in high levels of appropriate toy play. Figure 12-1 shows the results of suppressing large amounts of self-stimulatory behavior in two autistic children. That figure's ordinate shows the percent occurrence of both self-stimulation and approp-

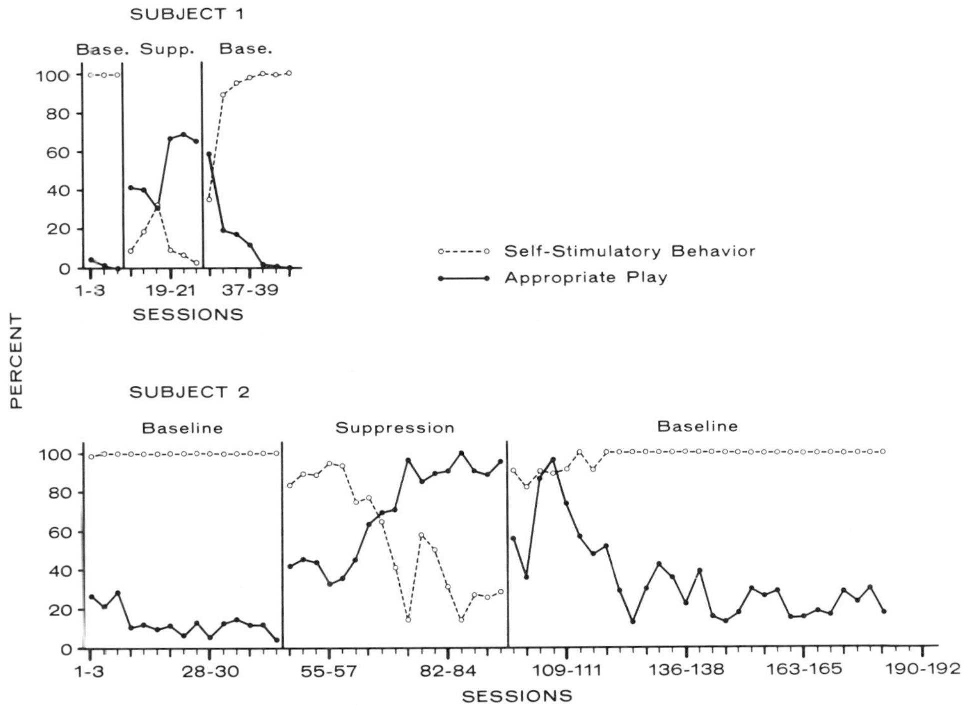

Fig. 12-1. Percent of time-sample intervals in which self-stimulatory and appropriate play behaviors occurred during baseline, suppression of self-stimulation conditions, and reversal. (From Koegel et al: J Appl Behav Anal 1974.)

riate play. Sessions are plotted in groups of three along the abscissa. Both children showed extensive amounts of self-stimulatory behavior during the baseline condition. Also, during the self-stimulation suppressive condition, both children seemed to compensate for the loss of self-stimulatory behavior by beginning to engage in large amounts of appropriate play. During the second baseline condition, the children were again permitted to engage in self-stimulation, and their levels of appropriate play again decreased. The importance of this result is that it suggests that large portions of an individual's behavioral repertoire may be influenced by changes in the amount of stimulation the individual receives. Table 12-1 shows the complete list of self-stimulatory behaviors and Table 12-2 shows the complete list of covary-

Table 12-1.
Complete List of Self-Stimulatory Responses for Subject 1 and Subject 2.

Subject 1

1. Eye crossing
2. Finger manipulations (moving the hands with continuous flexion and extension)
3. Repetitive vocalizations (excluding recognizable words)
4. Feet contortions (tight sustained flexions)
5. Leg contortions (tight sustained flexions)
6. Rhythmic manipulation of objects (repeatedly rubbing, rotating, or tapping objects with fingers)
7. Grimacing (corners of mouth drawn out and down, revealing the upper set of teeth)
8. Staring or gazing (a fixed glassy-eyed look lasting more than 3 sec)
9. Hands repetitively rubbing mouth
10. Hands repetitively rubbing face
11. Mouthing of objects (holding nonedible objects in contact with the mouth)
12. Locking hands behind head
13. Hands pressing on or twisting ears

Subject 2

1. Staring or gazing (a fixed glassy-eyed look lasting more than 3 sec)
2. Grimacing (corners of mouth drawn out and down, revealing the upper set of teeth)
3. Hand waving vertically or horizontally with fingers outstretched in front of eyes
4. Hands vigorously and repetitively rubbing eyes
5. Hands vigorously and repetitively rubbing nose
6. Hands vigorously and repetitively rubbing mouth
7. Hands vigorously and repetitively rubbing ears
8. Hands vigorously and repetitively rubbing hair
9. Hands vigorously and repetitively rubbing clothes
10. Hands vigorously and repetitively rubbing objects

11. Hand flapping in air
12. Hand wringing (hands alternately rubbing and clutching each other)
13. Finger contortions (tight sustained flexions)
14. Tapping fingers against part of body or an object
15. Tapping whole hand against part of body or object
16. Mouthing of objects (holding nonedible objects in contact with mouth)
17. Rocking (moving the trunk at the hips rhythmically back and forth or from side to side)
18. Head weaving (moving head from side to side in a figure-eight pattern)
19. Body contortions (sustained flexions or extensions of the torso)
20. Repetitive vocalizations (excluding recognizable words)
21. Teeth clicking (audibly and rapidly closing teeth together)
22. Tongue rolling and clicking
23. Audible saliva swishing in mouth
24. Repetitive tapping feet on floor
25. Repetitive tapping toes inside shoes (visible through canvas tennis shoes)
26. Leg contortions (tight sustained flexions)
27. Repetitive knocking knees against each other
28. Repetitive knocking ankles against each other
29. Tensing legs and suspending feet off the ground
30. Head shaking (rapid small movements from side to side)
31. Tensing whole body and shaking

From Koegel R et al. J App Behav Anal, 1974

Table 12-2.
Complete List of Appropriate Play Responses for Child 1 and Child 2.

Child 1

1. Making a distinct line or curve on the paper with a crayon
2. Placing a tile in the pegboard
3. Matching a block to its printed representation, with at least 50% of the block overlapping the picture

Child 2

1. Making a distinct line or curve on the paper with a crayon
2. Placing a plastic object into the appropriately shaped slot in the mailbox or retrieving it from the compartment in the bottom of the mailbox
3. Manipulating the appropriate mechanism (lever, button, dial, switch, handle) to make one of five animal heads pop up, or pushing the head piece back down to reset the toy

From Koegel R et al. J App Behav Anal 7:521–528, 1974

ing appropriate play behaviors. The implication of such covariations for the area of hearing losses is that the imposed loss of auditory input could produce behavioral covariations in seemingly different areas of an individual's behavioral repertoire, influencing even areas not typically associated directly with auditory stimulation. Similar results in the covariation of other behaviors in other environments have been reported by Brethower and Reynolds (1962), Buell et al., (1968), Lovaas and Simmons (1969), Sajwaj, Twardosz, and Burke (1972), and Wahler et al. (1970). Such results are consistent with Berlyne's (1960) theory that organisms will seek out an optimal level of stimulation, and thus attempt to compensate for losses in one area by increasing their input in another area. The overall effects of such altered behavioral repertoire are in need of further research.

As a whole, the literature on self-stimulation suggests that this behavior appears to be performed primarily for its sensory consequences, and that if an organism is deprived of the opportunity to engage in one type of self-stimulatory behavior, then that organism will work very hard to engage in other behaviors (presumably to regain the previous level of sensory input).

CONCLUSION

The literature on sensory deprivation suggests that fairly high levels of sensory input appear to be necessary for normal neurological development. Any deprivation imposed on the organism seems to result in the organism's attempt to replace that input with another form of sensory input, generally resulting in alterations in normal patterns of behavior. Continued deprivation appears not only to be highly aversive, resulting in emotional upset, irritability, and changes in learning strategies, but in some cases to result in actual neurological impairment. When this impairment occurs at a young age, it is frequently permanent with far reaching effects resulting in subsequent additional abnormal sensory functioning and learning ability as the organism matures. Although there has been relatively little research on the consequences of auditory sensory deprivation occurring specifically as a function of a hearing impairment, the results of the related research discussed in this chapter suggest that it may be very important to learn more in this area.

In summary, we can say that pediatric audiometry has several important values. First, there is the potential of detecting hearing impairments at an early age. Thus, through remediation of the impairment, or through amplification, severe permanent deprivation consequences can be prevented. Secondly, pediatric audiometry has the potential to detect children who, for any reason, are receiving low levels of auditory input (as in the case of withdrawn or autistic children). Functionally, this may be just as important as detecting a peripheral hearing loss. For example, Griffiths (1967) has pointed out that children with normal hearing, deprived of adequate listening opportunities early in life, will subsequently fail to respond to sound and perform as if they were deaf, showing both lack of response to sound and failure to develop speech. Early detection offers the possibility (perhaps the only possibility) for early remediation of such deficits. The research suggests that if sensory abnormalities are detected early enough, most, if not all, permanent impairment may be avoided. Thus, when one considers the extreme differences between prevention of severe often permanent consequences through the early detection of a hearing loss, and the development of severe handicaps through the sensory deprivation imposed by a failure to detect such a loss (for even a period of 1–2 years), research in the area of pediatric audiometry seems as if it may hold considerable potential.

REFERENCES

Anthony J: An experimental approach to the psychopathology of childhood: Autism. Br J Med Psych 31:211–225, 1958

Baldwin J, Baldwin J: The role of learning phenomena in the ontogeny of exploration and play, in Chevalier-Skolnikoff S, Poirier F (eds): Bio-Social Development Among Primates. New York, Garland, 1976

Bartoshuk AK: Response decrement with repeated elicitation of human neonatal cardiac acceleration to sound. J Comp Physiol Psychol 55:9–13, 1962

Baxter BL: Effect of visual deprivation during postnatal maturation on the electroencephalogram of the cat. Exp Neurol 14:224–237, 1966

Bench J: Some effects of audio-frequency stimulation of the crying baby. J Audit Res 9:122–128, 1969

Berlyne DE: Conflict, Arousal and Curiosity. New York, McGraw-Hill, 1960

Birns B, Blank M, Bridger WH, et al: Behavioral inhibition in neonates produced by auditory stimuli. Child Dev 36:639–645, 1965

Brackbill Y, Adams G, Crowell DH, et al: Arousal level in neonates and preschool children under continuous auditory stimulation. J Exp Child Psychol 4:178–188, 1966

Brethower DM, Reynolds GS: A facilitative effect of punishment on unpunished behavior. 5:191–199, 1962

Buell J, Stoddard P, Harris F, et al: Collateral social development accompanying reinforcement of outdoor play in a preschool child. J Appl Behav Anal 1:167–173, 1968

Coleman PD, Riesen AH: Environmental effects on cortical dendritic fields: I. Rearing in the dark. J Anat 102:363–374, 1968

Eisenberg RB: Auditory behavior in the human neonate. Paper presented at the biennial meeting of the Society for Research in Child Development, Minneapolis, 1965

Ferris C, Newsom C: An experimental analysis of symptom substitution. Paper presented at the Western Psychological Association Annual Convention, San Francisco, 1974

Fiske DW, Maddi SR: Functions of Varied Experience. Homewood, Il., Dorsey, 1961

Freedman DA: Congenital and perinatal sensory deprivation: Some studies in early development. Am J Psychiatry 127:115–121, 1971

Greenough WT, Experiential modification of the developing brain. Am Sci 63:37–46, 1975

Greenough WT, Volkmar FR, Juraska JM: Effects of rearing complexity on dendritic branching in frontolateral and temporal cortex of the rat. Exp Neurol 41:371–378, 1973

Greenough WT, Wood WE, Madden TC: Possible memory storage differences among mice reared in environments varying in complexity. Behav Biol 7:712–722, 1972

Griffiths C: Auditory training in the first year of life. Paper presented to the International Conference on Oral Education of the Deaf, Northampton, Mass., 1967

Harlow HF, Zimmerman RR: Affectional responses in the infant monkey. Science 130:421–432, 1959

Harlow MK, Harlow HF: Affection in primates. Discovery 27:11–17, 1966

Hermelin B, O'Connor N: Psychological Experiments With Autistic Children. Oxford, Pergamon, 1971.

Hubel DH: Effects of distortion of sensory input on the visual system of kittens. Physiologist 10:17–45, 1967

Hubel DH, Wiesel TN: The period of susceptibility to the physiological effects of unilateral eye closure in kittens. J Physiol 206:419–436, 1970

Hutt SJ, Hutt C, Lee D, et al: A behavioral and encephalographic study of autistic children. J Psychiatr Res 3:181–197, 1965

Irwin OC: Effect of strong light on the body activity of newborns. J Comp Psychol 32:233–236, 1941

Irwin OC, Weiss LA: Differential variations in the activity and crying of the newborn infant under different intensities of light: a comparison of observational with polygraph findings. Univ Iowa Studies Child Welfare 9:139–147, 1934a

Irwin OC, Weiss LA: The effect of clothing on the general vocal activity of the newborn infant. Univ Iowa Studies Child Welfare 9:151–162, 1934b

Irwin OC, Weiss LA: The effect of darkness on the activity of newborn infants. Univ Iowa Studies Child Welfare 9:163–175, 1934c

Kanner L: Autistic disturbances of affective contact. Nerv Child 2:217–250, 1943

Kish GB: Studies of sensory reinforcement, in Honig WK (ed): Operant Behavior: Areas of Research and Application. New York, Appleton, 1966

Koegel RL, Covert A: The relationship of self-stimulation to learning in autistic children. J Appl Behav Anal 5:381–387, 1972

Koegel RL, Firestone PB, Kramme KW, et al: Increasing spontaneous play by suppressing self-stimulation in autistic children. J Appl Behav Anal 7:521–528, 1974

Koegel RL, Schreibman L: Identification of consistent responding to auditory stimuli by a functionally "deaf" autistic child. J Autism Child Schizo 6:147–156, 1976

Krech D, Rosenzweig MR, Bennett E: Environmental impoverishment, social isolation and changes in brain chemistry and anatomy. Physiol Behav 1:99–104, 1966

Lovaas OI: Behavior therapy approach to the treatment of childhood schizophrenia, in Hill JP (ed): Minnesota Symposia on Child Development. Minneapolis, Univ Minnesota, 1967

Lovaas OI, Schreibman L, Koegel RL, et al: Selective responding by autistic children to multiple sensory impact. J Abn Psychol 77:211–222, 1971

Lovaas OI, Simmons JQ: Manipulation of self-destruction in three retarded children. J Appl Behav Anal 2:143–157, 1969

Odom RD: Effects of auditory and visual stimulus deprivation and satiation on children's performance in an operant task. J Exp Child Psych 1:16–25, 1964

Ornitz EM: The modulation of sensory input and motor output in autistic children, in Schopler E, Reichler RJ (eds): Psychopathology and Child Development. New York, Plenum 1976

Ornitz EM, Ritvo ER: Perceptual inconstance in early infantile autism. Arch Gen Psych 18:76–98, 1968

Reese HW, Lipsitt LP: Experimental Child Psychology. New York, Academic, 1970

Riesen AH: Sensory deprivation, in Stellar E, Sprague JM (eds): Progress in Physiological Psychology. New York, Academic, 1966

Rimland B: Infantile Autism. New York, Appleton, 1964

Rincover A, Newsom C, Carr T: Studies in motivation: Sensory stimulation as reinforcement. Paper presented at Western Psychological Association Annual Convention, San Francisco, 1974

Rosenzweig MR: Effects of environment on brain and behavior in animals, in Schopler E, Reichler RJ (eds): Psychopathology and Child Development. New York, Plenum, 1976

Sajwaj T, Twardosz S, Burke M: Side effects of extinction procedures in a remedial preschool. J Appl Behav Anal 5:163–176, 1972

Salk L: The effects of the normal heartbeat sound on the behavior of the newborn infant: Implications for mental health. World Mental Health 12:168–175, 1960

Salk L: The importance of heartbeat rhythm to human nature: Theoretical, clinical, and experimental observations. Proceedings of the Third World Congress of Psychiatry. Montreal, McGill Univ Pr, 1961

Salk L: Mother's heartbeat as an imprinting stimulus. Trans NY Acad Sci 24:753–763, 1962

Schopler E: Early infantile autism and the receptor processes. Arch Gen Psychiatry 13:327–335, 1965

Toscher M, Rupp R: The psychological implications of deafness; the human factor. Michigan Speech Hearing Assoc J 10:60–67, 1974

Valverde F: Apical dendritic spines of the visual cortex and light deprivation in the mouse. Exp Brain Res 3:337–352, 1967

Valverde F: Rate and extent of recovery from dark rearing in the visual cortex of the mouse. Brain Res 33:1–11, 1971

Wahler RG, Sperling KA, Thomas MR, et al: The modification of childhood stuttering: some response-response relationships. J Exp Child Psych 9:411–428, 1970

Walk RD, Gibson EJ: A comparative and analytical study of visual depth perception. Psych Monogr 75:1–44, 1961

Wiesel TN, Hubel DH: Comparison of the effects of unilateral and bilateral eye closure on cortical unit responses in kittens. J Neurophysiol 28:1029–1040, 1965

Zubek JP: Sensory Deprivation: Fifteen Years of Research. New York, Appleton, 1969

Carol A. Prutting
and Elizabeth A. Skarakis

13
Communication Development

Aristotle was one of the first to suggest that the instinct of language and speech did not exist in the hearing-impaired individual; a notion that has prevailed through the centuries. The traditional position concerning language has been that the hearing-impaired child is linguistically deficient. Hearing-impaired children have been described as language deprived, seriously retarded in language, and as essentially alinguistic (Schmitt, 1966; Moores, 1970; Dale, 1976).

It is possible to follow the reasons for this belief based on the following quotes from past years:

> . . . The deaf child is almost entirely dependent upon formal education in acquiring language. Unlike hearing children he does not live in a language environment . . . (Pinter and Paterson, 1916).

> Deaf child misses all sound experience . . . He misses words and sentences which are symbols for ideas and consequently is unable to form associations in his mind between an incident, a person, or thing, and its language symbol (Fitzgerald, 1961).

> Language acquisition is particularly difficult for the deaf because it is an auditory vocal process . . . Deaf children can't learn language because they can't hear it (Blanton, 1968).

It is interesting that these investigators refer only to the hearing-impaired child developing oral language. No reference is made to the hearing-impaired child's native language, the language of signs (Cicourel and Boese, 1972).

In this chapter, the language and cognitive development of the hearing-impaired are discussed. Specific recommendations for communication and the hearing-impaired are presented.

LANGUAGE DEVELOPMENT

Experimental Research Using an Oral Language Model

Several different approaches have been utilized to investigate the language of the hearing-impaired individual. One group of studies focused on the secondary language skills of reading and writing; another focused on word association skills; and a third group of studies dealt with the hearing-impaired individual's use of word classes and syntax.

Cooper and Rosenstein (1966) reviewed language acquisition studies which were based on the secondary language skills, reading and writing. Subjects in these studies were between seven and 21 years of age. Language performance was measured using standardized reading achievement tests (Pinter and Paterson, 1916; Pugh, 1946; Goetzinger and Rousey, 1959; Myklebust, 1960) or by evaluation of written compositions according to parts of speech used, sentence complexity, and quantity of language used (Heider and Heider, 1940; Myklebust, 1960; Simmons, 1962). Results were obtained through comparison of hearing-impaired and normal hearing subjects' linguistic performances. The results of these studies indicated that hearing-impaired subjects were markedly retarded in all areas of language achievement as measured by standardized achievement tests. In addition, it was noted that the hearing-impaired subjects' written language performance was similar to that of a younger hearing child in terms of sentence complexity, use of certain parts of speech, and in quantity of language used. Schulze (1965), using a longitudinal design, found hearing-impaired children to have a four-year lag from hearing children in their written vocabulary.

Other investigators have approached the language acquisition of the hearing-impaired individual by studying word association abilities. Hearing-impaired adolescents and young adults served as subjects in these studies. The Kent and Rosanoff (1910) word association lists and controlled continuous word association tasks (Johnson, Johnson, and Mark, 1951) were used to investigate word association ability in hearing-impaired persons. Subjects were presented words from the Kent-Rosanoff list and required to write the first word they associated with the stimulus (Schein, 1961; Blanton and Nunnally, 1964; Nunnally and Blanton, 1966; Koplin et al., 1967; Restaino, 1969; McGettigen and Rosenstein, 1969). In controlled continuous word association tasks, subjects were given five word categories (fruit, clothing, tools, animals, and jobs) and were asked to write down as many examples of each category as possible (Fremer and MacGinitie, 1969). Tweney and Holmann (1973) investigated syntagmatic-paradigmatic shift in word associations of hearing-impaired subjects compared to hearing subjects. Both groups, aged

7–13 years, demonstrated clear syntagmatic-paradigmatic shift, though the level of paradigmatic responding was lower for the deaf subjects.

All investigators conducting word association studies consistently found that, when compared to hearing controls, the hearing-impaired subjects exhibited: (1) general language immaturity; (2) a greater tendency to give category and subordinate responses; (3) a restricted repertoire of responses; (4) a tendency to give detail or attributive responses; (5) a lesser ability to identify synonyms and associations correctly; and (6) a weakness in the ability to give affective or evaluative responses.

A third approach to language acquisition in the hearing-impaired individual has been to investigate the use of word classes and syntax. One type of such study focused on the written language of hearing-impaired subjects 7–18 years of age. Odom, Blanton, and Nunnally (1967) used a Cloze procedure, in which systematic omissions in written material are completed by subjects, to investigate grammatical and syntactic processes of hearing-impaired children. They found that hearing-impaired subjects exhibited a weakness in the use of function words and confusion in their use of words within a syntactic class. MacGinitie (1964) used a sentence completion task to investigate the hearing-impaired child's ability to supply missing words. He found, as did Odom, Blanton, and Nunnally, uniform retardation in the hearing-impaired child's ability to supply content and function words.

A second type of study investigating word classes and syntax dealt with the comprehension and production of the language of hearing-impaired subjects 8–18 years of age. In such studies, spontaneous sentences are elicited through the use of pictures and recorded orthographically by the investigators. Goda (1964) analyzed hearing-impaired subjects' spontaneous responses according to Fries' (1952) description of word classes in the English sentence. Goda found hearing-impaired subjects used fewer auxiliary and expansion words and fewer different types of words than normal hearing subjects. Brannon (1968) evaluated spontaneous responses according to a system designed by Jones et al. (1963). The system provided a classification of words into 14 grammatical classes for comparison of aphasic and normal subjects. He found, as did Goda, hearing-impaired subjects produced fewer total words and fewer different types of words than hearing subjects. Brannon and Murray (1966) evaluated spoken sentences according to an error classification system devised by Myklebust (1954). Categories in this classification included word additions, word omissions, word substitutions, and word order errors. These investigators found a general retardation in the spoken language of the hearing-impaired subjects, and identified word substitution as the most common syntactic error made. The comprehension and production of the passive sentence was investigated by Schmitt (1968). He indicated that hearing-impaired children up to 14 years of age were able to comprehend and produce sentences in the passive voice, but, by 17 years of age, about 60% could comprehend passive sentences, however only 30% could produce such sentences. Powers and Quigley (1973) also investigated hearing-impaired adolescents' comprehension and production of the passive voice. The comprehension task consisted of moving objects or picture selection while the production task consisted of writing in the passive marker using a closure technique. It was found that, in the oldest age group, fewer than half understood the passive form correctly. Normal children in the preschool years are able to perform comprehension tasks which demonstrate their understanding of the passive voice. In another study, Quigley et al. (1974) studied question formation and conjoined sentences (Wilbur, Quigley and Montanelli, 1975) in the language of students who were ten to nineteen years of age. They were asked to judge grammaticality of question form and conjunctions. The results were compared to hearing children's ability, ages 8–10 years. Results indicated that even the youngest hearing subject consistently obtained higher scores than the majority of hearing-impaired subjects. These authors also analyzed specific aspects of performance and concluded that there is a coexistence of normal and deviant rules in the hearing-impaired subjects.

The experimental research on the language acquisition of the hearing-impaired child is summarized according to methodology and results. The general methodology used in these studies was: (1) utilization of hearing-impaired subjects 7–21 years of age; (2) written language as the primary linguistic behavior measured; and (3) comparison of hearing-impaired to normal hearing subjects to determine the linguistic performance of the hearing-impaired persons. The results across all studies indicated an immaturity or retardation in the linguistic performance of the hearing-impaired subjects in relation to normal hearing subjects; supporting the position which claims linguistic deficiency in hearing impaired individuals.

Descriptive Research Using a Sign Language Model

The study of natural language acquisition has developed rapidly in the past 20 years. Study of the pragmatic level of language has provided researchers with procedures for describing nonverbal communication, and these procedures have been employed to study the young hearing-impaired child.

Present knowledge about language acquisition can be summarized as follows: the child is an active participant in the process of language acquisition (Brown and Bellugi, 1964); the progression of syntactic development is similar for all children (Brown et al., 1968; Slobin, 1966); child language is systematic and rule governed, not an incomplete copy of adult language (Klima and Bellugi, 1966); a small set of semantic relations, possibly universal, exists, accounting for a majority of the meaning expressed in two-word utterances (Bloom, 1970; Schlesinger, 1971; Brown, 1973); language development occurs as part of the child's general cognitive development (Bloom, 1970; Sinclair-de-Zwart, 1973; Edwards, 1973; Brown, 1973); the child has knowledge and expresses semantic and pragmatic functions nonverbally and in conjunction with situational cues before he can express grammatical relations verbally (Greenfield and Smith, 1976; Dore, 1974; Bates, 1976; Halliday, 1975); language development exists as a continuum from early communication with intention conveyed through gesture, facial expression, joint action with an adult, and vocalization, to language proper with full symbolic representational power (Dore, 1974; Bates, 1976; Bruner, 1975a, b; Halliday, 1975; Greenfield and Smith, 1976).

The research in the area of natural language acquisition has provided two very important contributions to the study of the hearing-impaired child's acquisition. First, descriptive methodology has been developed to study the young hearing-impaired child's nonverbal communication. Second, the fact that normal children's nonverbal communication (semantic-pragmatic development) was found to provide the basis upon which later verbal language development (phonologic–syntactic development) was formed added credibility to the study of the hearing-impaired child's nonverbal language.

Bellugi and Klima (1972) studied a hearing-impaired child of hearing-impaired parents who was acquiring American Sign Language. Their preliminary results indicated: the child's sign vocabulary covered the full range of concepts expressed by hearing children of comparable age; early sign combinations expressed all the semantic relations expressed by normal hearing children; signed sequences steadily increased in length paralleling the increase found in normal hearing children's language. They concluded that stages of language development appeared to be the same regardless of modality.

Schlesinger and Meadow (1972) studied the acquisition of sign language in four hearing-impaired children, two with hearing-impaired parents and two with normal hearing parents. The first child (of hearing-impaired parents) was studied between the ages of 8 and 22 months. Schlesinger and Meadow reported the first formal sign appeared at 12 months, after which a rapid vocabulary growth took place. They also reported single signs were used with a range of meaning; first produced with the referent present and later spontaneously without a referent. Results indicated parallel development of sign language and verbal language. The second child was also of hearing-impaired parents. She was observed between the ages of two years-ten months and three years-six months, during the period of two-sign combinations. Results indicated that the same semantic relations observed in the normal hearing child were present in the hearing-impaired child's language. The third child, of normal hearing parents, had been receiving formal sign language input from age one year-six months. Schlesinger and Meadow reported that by three years of age the child had a sign vocabulary of 384 signs, which doubled four months later. The last child, also of hearing parents, was observed from age three years-nine months to five years-three months. Fingerspelling and Signed English served as linguistic input for the child. Results demonstrated that by age three years-six months the child consistently used the past tense, plural, and present progressive morphemes appropriately. Schlesinger and Meadow concluded, as did Bellugi and Klima (1972), that stages in the development of sign language paralleled those in the acquisition of verbal language.

Nash (1975) studied the language acquisition of a profoundly hearing-impaired child whose linguistic input was first Cued Speech and later Signed English. Parents provided consistent linguistic input of Cued Speech from the time the child was 1 year old, until three years of age. Preliminary results indicated that during this period the child's receptive vocabulary developed similarly to normal hearing children of comparable age reported in the natural acquisition studies (Brown, 1973; Slobin, 1971; McNeill, 1966). Nash reported the child's expressive verbal vocabulary consisted of 13 intelligible words, and concluded that cued speech was not capable of being a basis for a separate linguistic community as evidenced by the lack of expressive behavior compared to that found in normal language acquisition literature. At three years of age, linguistic input to the child was changed to Signed English. Preliminary results revealed that: two months after the onset of signing, the child produced two-sign combinations and progressed into more complete phrases; within one year, techniques for indicating negation and verb tense had developed; nine months after the onset of signing, the child produced well-formed English sequences of up to eight signs.

Goldin-Meadow and Feldman (1975) studied the ontogenesis of symbolic communication in four hearing-impaired children of normal hearing parents. The subjects were between one year-six months and four years of age. None had any formal language input: oral, manual, or total communication. Spontaneous communication samples were analyzed for meaning and semantic relations based on Bloom's (1970) work. Gestural combinations were assigned semantic roles or cases (Fillmore, 1968). Results indicated hearing-impaired subjects developed gestural communication systems despite the lack of formal linguistic input. Goldin-Meadow and Feldman identified three stages in the development of a gestural system. The first stage was characterized by the use of few different gestures. During the second stage, specific lexical items were created for objects and actions, and relations between objects and actions were expressed in two-unit sequences according to the child's own order rule. Both action and objects were expressed through action gestures. The third phase marked the expression of multiple semantic relations in phrases of more than two gestures. The investigators hypothesized that the hearing-impaired child generalizes and abstracts from actions in his environment in order to generate names for objects and actions. Goldin-Meadow and Feldman concluded that symbolic communication could be developed by children with auditory impairment even with the lack of any obvious linguistic models.

Skarakis (1976) studied four preschool deaf children between the ages of 2.1 and 4.2 years. She used a natural language acquisition approach (Greenfield and Smith, 1976; Dore, 1974) to describe the early semantic-pragmatic behavior in the spontaneous communication of these children in four different communicative settings. Results revealed that the hearing-impaired subjects exhibited the same semantic functions and pragmatic communicative intentions in spontaneous communication as those identified in the young normal hearing child's linguistic repertoire. It is of interest to note that all four subjects were receiving oral language training at the John Tracy Clinic summer session and previously had no formal sign language instruction. Three of the children were profoundly deaf (80-dB loss or more) and were predominantly using esoteric gestures or signs for purposes of communication. The other child was classified as hard of hearing (50-dB loss or less) and was using verbal communication as the dominant style of interaction. This finding supports the premise that the hearing-impaired child's native language, regardless of educational training, is the language of signs.

The descriptive research using a sign language model and natural language acquisition procedures has yielded two major findings. First, investigators demonstrated that the hearing-impaired child could generate language spontaneously (Schlesinger and Meadow, 1972; Nash, 1975; Goldin-Meadow and Feldman, 1975). Second, the development of the hearing-impaired child's language has been described as paralleling that of normal hearing children (Bellugi and Klima, 1972; Schlesinger and Meadow, 1972; Nash, 1975; Skarakis, 1976). These findings demonstrate that the hearing-impaired child is capable of learning language just as a normally hearing child. The position claiming linguistic deficiency in the young hearing-impaired is not substantiated when the young child's native language, the language of gestures and signs, is described.

COGNITIVE DEVELOPMENT

Researchers have emphasized the intimate relationship between cognitive and language development (Bloom, 1970; Brown, 1973; Edwards, 1973; Sinclair-de-Zwart, 1973). Bloom maintained that linguistic expression was interrelated with the child's cognitive-perceptual development and with the child's interaction in a world of objects, events, and relations. The others (cf. supra) utilized the cognitive developmental theory of Piaget (1926) to account for the relationship between the set of semantic functions which first emerge in a child's language and the child's cognitive development. They proposed that the early semantic relations expressed by a child parallel his sensori-motor stage of cognitive development.

The following section summarizes the literature regarding the conceptual abilities of the hearing-impaired. The most prevalent emphasis is to compare the hearing-impaired to what the hearing are capable of doing on verbal experimental conceptual tasks. Another group of researchers has been concerned with the question: What conceptual tasks are the deaf capable of performing using nonverbal tasks? Lastly, is the question of whether the hearing-impaired perceive, organize, or categorize their experiences differently from the hearing individual.

Conceptual Abilities as Measured by Verbal Tasks

When hearing-impaired children are compared to hearing children on abstract reasoning tasks (Getz, 1953; Farrant, 1964; Myklebust, 1964, 1967), they are found to be retarded in tasks that involve any sort of verbal comprehension. Eight concepts from the Stanford Achievement Test were used by Austin (1975) to study both hearing-impaired and hearing subjects. On some concepts, the hearing-impaired subjects lagged behind the hearing; however, on concepts relevant to everyday experiences, the hearing-impaired demonstrated a normal pattern of growth. The apparent lag in development of the other concepts may reflect social and educational experiences.

In various learning skill experiments examining writing skills, an apparent learning plateau has been reported that is reached by the hearing-impaired in certain areas of conceptual thought (Neyhus and Myklebust, 1967; Furth, 1967; Fremer and MacGinitie, 1969; Vandenberg, 1971). This plateau begins to emerge at approximately nine to eleven years of age. The hearing-impaired and hearing are often of equal conceptual ability until this time. The major finding among these researchers is that without sufficient language abilities, social or educational experience, the deaf cannot compete with the conceptual abilities of the hearing. None of these studies dealt with subjects taught using a manual means of communication. In addition, age of onset of hearing loss, early language intervention, the opportunity to learn concepts, differences in school emphasis, and the deaf child raised by deaf parents were not considered in the experimental designs.

Ross and Hormann (1975) provided hearing-impaired subjects with classroom training on probability problems which they had been unable to perform. The hearing-impaired subjects made significant progress which led these investigators to conclude that experience and teaching procedures could account for differences usually found on probability task performances.

Conceptual Abilities as Measured by Nonverbal Tasks

One group of investigators has concentrated on devising nonverbal conceptual tasks to determine the hearing-impaired child's conceptual abilities (Rosenstein, 1960; Kates, Yudin, and Tiffany, 1962; Furth and Youniss, 1971; Furth, 1970). These studies demonstrate no differences between hearing-impaired children and hearing children in organizing and categorizing as measured by nonverbal conceptual tasks. Hearing-impaired children's performance varies as a function of the modality tested. Tasks that are verbal demonstrate a deficit, while tasks presented nonverbally demonstrate parallel cognitive performance when compared to hearing subjects. The testing modality has been demonstrated as having a pervasive impact on the findings.

Recently investigators have addressed themselves to whether cognitive processing differences exist for the hearing-impaired individual in contrast to the hearing individual (Bellugi et al., 1974). A short-term memory task was administered to a group of hearing and deaf college students, the hearing-impaired being children of hearing-impaired parents. A list of words was presented to each group according to its mode of communication. The hearing-impaired were given the list in American Sign Language; and the hearing, orally. Both groups were then asked to write those words they remembered. The researchers reported results according to the error types made by the subjects. For the hearing, phonetic, or sound, confusions were made; but, for the hearing-impaired, the errors were visual confusions. After translating the written errors of the hearing-impaired back to sign language, it was found that the errors were specific and systematic. All but one of the parameters of the original sign were preserved in the errors. The basic form of the original sign (e.g., one hand, two hands, active or passive role of hand, etc.) did not change the errors. It appeared that the signs were actually coded by the hearing-impaired in terms of such parameters as movement, orientation with respect to the body, handshape, and location. Signs seemed to be processed with systematic and internal analysis and not as unitary holistic patterns. In other words, this study suggests that the hearing-impaired, because of using a different modality for communication than the hearing, actually may process the world differently.

COMMUNICATION AND THE DEAF

The hearing-impaired are found to be less competent than their hearing counterparts in both language and cognitive abilities when measured using verbal tasks. On the other hand, the hearing-impaired have been found to be equal to the hearing in language and cognitive performance when measured using nonverbal tasks. This finding simply suggests that, when the hearing-impaired are tested in their native language, visual-gestural, they perform better than when tested in their second language, auditory-verbal. One would expect these findings. Hearing-impaired children appear to operate in a bi-modal manner regardless of educational training. They are most proficient, however, using signs which capitalize on the visual-gestural modality rather than the auditory-verbal approach which utilizes the hearing and speech mechanisms. Since the hearing-impaired have an intact visual mechanism, and have a pathological hearing mechanism, this finding is not surprising.

Some hearing-impaired children are taught to communicate using an oral approach. The oral approach focuses on auditory training procedures combined with lipreading procedures. A recent study by Farwell (1976) has shown that the ability to learn the skill of lipreading is not related to IQ or amount of educational training. If this is the case, an important question is: Is lipreading a learned skill which can be taught? Also 40 to 60 percent of the phonemes in English are not discriminable through speech reading. Johnson (1976) conducted a study in which he investigated the communicative characteristics of students entering the National Technical Institute for the Deaf. He found that 56% of the students were rated as having unintelligible speech and 34% could not speech read well enough to comprehend the content of conversations. There are some hearing-impaired people who become proficient using the oral mode of communication. These individuals seem to be exceptions, while the majority of hearing-impaired individuals has great difficulty communicating orally.

Others are taught using a variety of nonverbal communication methods: American Sign Language (Ameslan) Signing Exact English$_1$ (SEE$_1$), Signing Exact English$_2$ (SEE$_2$), Linguistics of Visual English (LOVE), the Rochester Method, and total communication. There is much disagreement as to which sign language mode should be taught. Gustason and Rosen (1975) stated "Now that we've got many people to accept signs, we have to confuse them with this battle over which kind of signs."

There is no doubt that some educational system must be chosen as soon as possible for the young child identified as hearing-impaired. The dispute goes on: oral vs manual, and now a new focus—if manual, which procedure? Scherer (1971) stated: "For decades, we have polarized ourselves into opposing philosophical positions while we have spent undue energy defending our positions, deaf children have continued to grow to adulthood with limited language and communication, and severe educational retardation.'' Vernon (1975–76) summarized the literature regarding the hearing-impaired child of hearing-impaired parents taught manual communication compared to hearing-impaired children of hearing parents taught orally. In all studies, the hearing-impaired child using manual communication performed better than the oral group on these dimensions: general educational achievement, reading, vocabulary, and written language (Quigley and Frisina, 1961; Stuckless and Birch, 1966; Meadow, 1968; Quigley, 1969; Moores, 1970; Vernon and Koh, 1970). There were no differences found in speech intelligibility and speech reading (Meadow, 1968; Montgomery, 1966; Quigley, 1968; Vernon and Koh, 1970). It appears that hearing-impaired children of hearing-impaired parents taught manual communication at an early age are at a distinct advantage educationally over hearing-impaired children of hearing parents taught orally. It has been documented that hearing parents of hearing-impaired children rarely use sign language (Schlesinger and Meadow, 1972; Freeman et al., 1975; Dagleish, 1975). In a survey of 243 hearing parents of hearing-impaired children, 216 parents said they did not use sign language (Brill, 1960). If parents of hearing-impaired children do learn sign language, it is usually not until their child reaches adolescence (Bellugi and Klima, 1972). However, it is important that language input begins during the first days of life, especially since there are critical periods for language acquisition (Lenneberg, 1967; Lewis and Freedle, 1972; Schlesinger and Meadow, 1972). Hearing-impaired children who do not know signs have neither adequate auditory nor visual feedback. For the development of cognition, there must be a symbol system which is attached to ideas in order to communicate. Reliance on an impaired sensory system has been demonstrated as a hindrance to the cognitive system (Tomlinson-Keasey and Kelly, 1974). The first few years of life are crucial for cognitive and language development. Early mother-child reciprocal interactions constitute an important step toward communicative development (Bruner, 1975a,b; Seitz and Marcus, 1976).

Bragg (1973), a renowned member of the National Theater of the Deaf, describes Ameslish (derived from a combination of Ameslan and English) as the language that most deaf individuals use. Ameslish is defined as ''speaking, mouthing, fingerspelling, gesture, Ameslan grammer, pantomine, initialized signs of SEE_2, body and facial expression, acting and whatever else you have to communicate with.'' What he is really describing is the deaf adult's use of any available method to convey meaning. Bragg presents the idea that what matters most is communication itself, not which language modality. The high verbal hearing-impaired can communicate orally, while the low verbal will depend more on various forms of signs. Both high verbal and low verbal hearing-impaired individuals will find themselves in various communicative settings which will predict which code they will use regardless of proficiency. In other words, the hearing-impaired communicator will be a code switcher and will need to know the language of the hearing as well as the language of the deaf. The sociolinguistic literature documents that a hearing person switches codes as a function of the nature of the communicative interaction (Labov, 1969).

It is also well documented that the deaf population exists in a well-integrated social group which is separate, however, from the larger society (Lunde, 1960; Stokoe, 1960; Boese, 1964; Vernon, 1969; Cicourel and Boese, 1972; Markowicz, 1972). Generally, this subculture, the hearing-impaired living among the hearing-impaired, is a result of the difficulty they have in communicating with the hearing society around them as opposed to the ease with which they interact among themselves. Markowicz reported Brill as stating:

> Even when they are fairly good speakers and lipreaders which is true of only a small percentage, there is a difficulty in the means of ordinary communication and the result is that they will isolate themselves.

It seems to be that, socially, most deaf people prefer other hearing-impaired people, and this seems to be a healthy adjustment to this physical handicap. Why would anyone seek the company of others with whom it is difficult to communicate?

RECOMMENDATIONS

It is highly recommended that the deaf child be given every opportunity to learn both a system of signs or systems of signs as well as by an oral approach. The deaf individual's prime language appears to be a combination of signs, speech, and various other means called Ameslish. In addition, the deaf may encounter situations in which they will have to be more verbal or less verbal depending on the communicative setting. Therefore, it seems appropriate to recommend that parents, educators, audiologists, and others encourage the deaf child to become a bimodal communicator. Based on the information we now have, this seems to be the most beneficial approach for providing the deaf child with a flexible communicative system, flexible enough to communicate with both the hearing and hearing-impaired. In this manner, the deaf child will be able to switch codes, and presumably utilize and choose the most effective system for any given communicative setting. It is often only through contact with the hearing-impaired adult population that the hearing professional can understand their needs. In addition, joint efforts of both hearing and deaf professionals is needed to insure the upgrading of the quality of the education of the hearing-impaired.

REFERENCES

Austin G: Knowledge of selected concepts obtained by an adolescent deaf population. Am Ann Deaf 120:360–370, 1975

Bates E: Language and Context: The Acquisition of Pragmatics. New York, Academic, 1976

Bellugi U, Klima E: The roots of language in the sign talk of the deaf. Psych Today 6:60–76, 1972

Bellugi U, Klima E, Siple P: Remembering in signs. Cognition 3:93–125, 1974–75

Blanton RL: Language learning and performance in the deaf, in Rosenberg S, Koplin J (eds): Developments in Applied Psycholinguistic Research. New York, Macmillan, 1968

Blanton RL, Nunnally J: Evaluation of language in the deaf. Psychol Rep 15:891–894, 1964

Bloom L: Language Development: Form and Function in Emerging Grammars. Cambridge, MIT Pr, 1970

Boese R: Differentiations in the deaf community; a paper presented to the Department of Sociology, University of British Columbia, 1964

Bragg B: Ameslish—our American heritage. Am Ann Deaf 118:672–674, 1973

Brannon J: Linguistic word classes in spoken language of normal, hard of hearing, and deaf children. J Speech Hear Res 11:279–287, 1968

Brannon J, Murray T: The spoken syntax of normal, hard of hearing, and deaf children. J Speech Hear Res 9:604–610, 1966

Brill RG: A study in the adjustment of three groups of deaf children. Except Child 26:464–466, 1960

Brown R: A First Language. Cambridge, Harvard Univ Pr, 1973

Brown R, Bellugi U: Three processes in the child's acquisition of syntax. Harvard Educa Rev 34:133–151, 1964

Brown R, Cazden C, Bellugi U: The child's grammer from 1 to 3, in Hill J (ed): Minnesota Symposium on Child Psychology. Minneapolis, Univ Minnesota Pr, 1968

Bruner J: The ontogenesis of speech acts. Child Lang 2:1–19, 1975a

Bruner J: From communication to language. A psychological perspective. Cognition 3:255–287, 1975b

Cicourel AV, Boese R. Sign language acquisition and the teaching of deaf children, in Cazden C, John V, Hymes D (eds): Functions of Language in the Classroom. New York, Teachers College Pr, 1972

Cooper R, Rosenstein J: Language acquisition of deaf children. Volta Rev 68:46–56, 1966

Dagleish B: Communication preference and the social conditions of language learning in the deaf. Am Ann Deaf 120:70–77, 1975

Dale PS: Language Development. New York, Holt Rinehart, 1976

Dore J: A pragmatic description of early language development. J Psycholinguist Res 3:343–350, 1974

Edwards D: Sensory-motor intelligence and semantic relations in early child grammar. Cognition 2/4:395–434, 1973

Farrant R: The intellectual abilities of deaf and hearing children. Am Ann Deaf 109:306–325, 1964

Farwell R: Speech reading: A research review. Volta Rev 78:19–30, 1976

Fillmore C: The case for case, in Bach E, Horms R (eds): Universals in Linguistic Theory. New York, Holt Rinehart, 1968

Fitzgerald M: Workshop in Language for the Deaf. Philadelphia School for the Deaf, 1961

Freeman R, Malkin S, Hasting J: Psychosocial problems of deaf children and their family: A comparative study. Am Ann Deaf 120:391–405, 1975

Fremer J, MacGinitie W: The content of controlled continuous word association, in Rosenstein J, MacGinitie W (eds): Verbal Behavior of the Deaf Child. New York, Teachers College Pr, 1969

Fries CC: The Structure of English. New York, Harcourt, Brace, 1952

Furth H: A review and perspective on the thinking of deaf people, in Hellmuth J (ed): Cognitive Studies. New York, Brunner/Mazel, 1967

Furth H: A review and perspective on the thinking of deaf people, in Hellmuth J (ed): Cognitive Studies. New York, Brunner/Mazel, 1970

Furth H, Youniss J: Formal operations and language: A comparison of deaf and hearing adolescents. Int J Psych 6:49–64, 1971

Getz S: Environment and the Deaf Child. Springfield, IL, Thomas, 1953

Goda S: Spoken syntax of normal, deaf and retarded adolescents. J Verbal Learn Verbal Behav 3:401–405, 1964

Goetzinger C, Rousey CL: Educational achievement of deaf children. Am Ann Deaf 104:221–231, 1959

Goldin-Meadow S, Feldman H: The creation of a communication system: A study of deaf children of hearing parents. Sign Lang Stud 8:225–236, 1975

Greenfield P, Smith H: The Structure of Communication in Early Language Development. New York, Academic, 1976

Gustason G, Rosen R: Effective Sign Communication for Instructional Purposes: Manual English and American Sign Language. North Carolina: paper delivered at the Convention of American Instructors of the Deaf, 1975

Halliday M: Learning How to Mean. London, Edward Arnold, 1975

Heider F, Heider G: A comparison of sentence structure of deaf and hearing children. Psychol Monogr 52:42–103, 1940

Johnson D: Communication characteristics of a young deaf adult population: Technique for evaluating their communication skills. Am Ann Deaf 121:409–424, 1976

Johnson DM, Johnson RG, Mark AL: A mathematical analysis of verbal fluency. J Gen Psych 44:121–128, 1951

Jones C, Goodman M, Wepman J: The classification of parts of speech for the characterization of aphasics. Lang Speech 6:94–104, 1963

Kates S, Yudin L, Tiffany R: Concept attainment by deaf and hearing adolescents. J Education Psych 53:119–126, 1962

Kent G, Rosanoff A: A study of association in insanity. Am J Insanity 67:37–96, 317–390, 1910

Klima E, Bellugi U: Syntactic regularities in the speech of children, in Lyons J, Wales R (eds): Psycholinguistic Papers. Edinburgh, Edinburgh Univ Pr, 1966

Koplin J, Odom P, Blanton R, et al: Word association test performance of deaf subjects. J Speech Hear Res 10:126–132, 1967

Labov W: The Study of Nonstandard English. Washington, D.C., Center for Applied Linguistics, 1969

Lenneberg EH: Biological Foundations of Language. New York, Wiley, 1967

Lewis M, Freedle R: Mother-Infant Dyad: The Cradle of Meaning. Bethesda, MD: ERIC Document Reproduction Service, ED 067 149, 1972

Lunde A: The sociology of the deaf, in Stokoe W (ed): Studies in Linguistics. Buffalo, Univ Buffalo, 1960

MacGinitie W: Ability of deaf children to use different word classes. J Speech Hear Res 7:141–150, 1964

Markowicz H: Some sociological considerations of American sign language. Sign Lang Stud 2:15–37, 1972

McGettigen J, Rosenstein J: The influence of associative strength on identification of word meanings, in Rosenstein J, MacGinitie W (eds): Verbal Behavior of the Deaf Child. New York, Teachers College Pr, 1969

McNeill D: The creation of language by children, in Lyons J, Wales R (eds): Psycholinguistic Papers, Edinburgh, Edinburgh Univ Pr, 1966

Meadow K: Early manual communication in relation to the deaf child's intellectual, social and communicative functioning. Am Ann Deaf 113:29–41, 1968

Montgomery G: The relationship of oral skills to manual communication in profoundly deaf students. Am Ann Deaf 111:557–565, 1966

Moores D: Psycholinguistics and deafness. Am Ann Deaf 115:37–48, 1970

Myklebust H: Auditory Disorders in Children. New York, Grune and Stratton, 1954

Myklebust H: Psychological effects of deafness. Am Ann Deaf 105:372–385, 1960

Myklebust H: The Psychology of Deafness (2nd ed.). New York, Grune and Stratton, 1964

Myklebust H: Development and Disorders of Written Language. New York, Grune and Stratton, 1967

Nash J: Cues or signs: A case study in language acquisition. Sign Lang Stud 8:79–91, 1975

Neyhus A, Myklebust H: Early-life deafness and mental development, in McConnell F, Ward P (eds): Deafness in Childhood. Nashville, Vanderbilt Univ Pr, 1967

Nunnally J, Blanton R: Patterns of word association in the deaf. Psychol Rep 18:86–92, 1966

Odom P, Blanton R, Nunnally J: Some "Cloze" technique studies of language capability in the deaf. J Speech Hear Res 10:816–827, 1967

Piaget J: The Language and Thought of the Child. New York, Harcourt, Brace, 1926

Pinter R, Paterson D: A measurement of the language ability of deaf children. Psychol Rev 23:413–426, 1916

Powers D, Quigley S: Deaf children's acquisition of the passive voice. J Speech Hear Res 16:5–11, 1973

Pugh G: Summaries from appraisal of the silent reading abilities of acoustically handicapped children. Am Ann Deaf 91:331–349, 1946

Quigley S: The influence of fingerspelling on the development of language, communication, and educational achievement in deaf children, report of research grant RD

12996. Washington: Rehabilitation Services Administration, Department of Health, Education and Welfare, 1969

Quigley S, Frisina R: Institutionalized and psychoeducational development of deaf children. Council for Exceptional Children Research Monograph, Series A, No. 3, 1961

Quigley S, Smith N, Wilbur R: Comprehension of relativized sentences by deaf students. J Speech Hear Res 17:325–341, 1974

Quigley S, Wilbur R, Montanelli D: Question-formation in the language of deaf students. J Speech Hear Res 17:699–713, 1974

Restaino L: Word association of deaf and hearing child, in Rosenstein J, MacGinitie W (eds): Verbal Behavior of the Deaf Child. New York, Teachers College Pr, 1969

Rosenstein J: Cognitive abilities of deaf children. J Speech Hear Res 3:108–119, 1960

Ross B, Hormann H: The attainment of formal operations. Genet Psychol Monogr 91:61–119, 1975

Schein J: Word association conformity on deaf and hearing college students. Paper presented at the meeting of the American Psychological Association, New York, 1961

Scherer P: An open letter to educators of the deaf. Am Ann Deaf 116:404–407, 1971

Schlesinger H: Language in four deaf children, in Schlesinger H, Meadow K (eds): Deafness and Mental Health: A Developmental Approach. San Francisco, Langley Porter Inst., 1971

Schlesinger H, Meadow K: Sound and Sign: Childhood Deafness and Mental Health. Berkeley: Univ California Pr, 1972

Schmitt P: Language instruction for the deaf. Volta Rev 68:85–108, 1966

Schmitt P: Deaf Children's Comprehension and Production of Sentence Transformations and Verb Tenses. Unpublished doctoral dissertation, University of Illinois, Champaign-Urbana, 1968

Schulze G: An evaluation of vocabulary development by thirty-two deaf children over a three year period. Am Ann Deaf 110:424–435, 1965

Seitz S, Marcus S: Mother-child interactions: A foundation for language development. Excep Child 42:445–449, 1976

Simmons A: A comparison of the type-token ratio of spoken and written language of deaf and hearing children. Volta Rev 64:417–421, 1962

Sinclair-de-Zwart H: Language acquisition and cognitive development, in Moore T (ed): Cognitive Development and the Acquisition of Language. New York, Academic, 1973

Skarakis E: Early Communication: Semantic Functions and Communicative Intentions in the Communication of the Preschool Child with Impaired Hearing. Unpublished master's thesis, University of California, Santa Barbara, 1976

Slobin D: Grammatical transformations in childhood and adulthood. J Verbal Learn Verbal Behav 5:219–227, 1966

Slobin D: Developmental psycholinguistics, in Dingwall W (ed): A Survey of Linguistic Science. College Park, Md, College Park Pr, 1971

Stokoe W: Sign language structure, in Stokoe W (ed): Studies in Linguistics. Buffalo, Univ Buffalo, 1960

Stuckless E, Birch J: The influence of early manual communication on the linguistic development of deaf children. Am Ann Deaf 111:452–460, 499–504, 1966

Tomlinson-Keasey O, Kelly R: The development of thought processes in deaf children. Am Ann Deaf 119:693–699, 1974

Tweney R, Holmann H: The development of semantic associations in profoundly deaf children. J Speech Hear Res 16:309–318, 1973

Vandenberg D: The Written Language of Deaf Children. New York, Whitcombe and Tombs, 1971

Vernon M: Sociological and psychological factors associated with hearing loss. J Speech Hear Res 12:541–563, 1969

Vernon M: Total communication. Talk, No. 78:10–15, 1975–76

Vernon M, Koh S: Effects of manual communication on deaf children's educational achievement, linguistic competence, oral skills and psychological development. Am Ann Deaf 115:527–536, 1970

Wilbur R, Quigley S, Montanelli D: Conjoined structures in the language of deaf students. J Speech Hear Res 18:319–335, 1975

Robert J. Hanson, Jr.

14 Articulatory Development

The consequences of a hearing loss that remains uncorrected throughout a child's preschool years are drastic and easily heard in the speech of most hearing-impaired children. In order to provide effective and efficient help for these children, one must not only detect hearing losses early, but, equally importantly, one must be able to provide hearing aids and training which maximize the child's use of any residual hearing for learning during those crucial first years of life. Unfortunately, our knowledge of articulatory development in hearing-impaired children is not sufficient to permit definite answers to all questions which must be addressed concerning optimization of programs of therapy and the efficacy of different amplification systems. One reason for this lack of information is that so few infants have losses diagnosed before their first vocalizations. Therefore, researchers have worked of necessity with older hearing-impaired children. Moreover, the development of speech skills in normal infants during the first year of life has not been studied in enough detail to permit comparisons between deaf and normal articulation from the onset of development.

However, there is sufficient information to address three topics of major importance for our understanding of articulatory development in the hearing-impaired child: (1) What is the importance of the first years of a child's life for articulatory development? (2) What is the prognosis for approaching normal articulatory development if hearing aids can be fitted and programs of therapy initiated early? (3) What are some of the characteristics of articulation of the hearing-impaired that must be corrected or possibly avoided if the loss is detected early? This chapter attempts to answer these questions by describing some important ways in which vocalizations of deaf and hearing children differ, as well as ways in which the sequence of articulatory development differs.

THE FIRST YEARS

Normal articulatory development progresses very rapidly in the first years of a child's life. The child's ability to control speech passes from the rudimentary babbling stage to recognizable utterances in about 24 months. Babbling begins around three to six months for both normal and hearing-impaired infants (Lenneberg, 1966). At onset, babbling is a spontaneous activity, independent of the amount of human speech in the infant's environment (Lenneberg et al., 1965). Within two or three months, the normal infant will begin to respond to a familiar voice by babbling (Fry, 1975). This communicative act, albeit primitive, marks the beginning of language acquisition. This is also the point where the sequence of articulatory development for the hearing and the deaf infant will diverge. For the hearing-impaired infant this point will either be significantly delayed or, as often happens with profound losses, the child may simply stop babbling. Symptoms such as these could alert clinicians and parents to the possibility of a hearing loss. Other aspects of the infant's vocalizations may also signal a hearing problem. Stark (1972) reported that deaf infants produce fewer noncrying sounds than normal infants, and that of the consonants produced by the deaf infant there is a predominance of bilabials as opposed to the alveolar stops which are expected to predominate in the vocalizations of hearing infants.

Even a relatively small hearing loss will have an effect on the child's speech and language development. Goetzinger (1962) found that a loss of 20–35 dB was sufficient to have a marked effect on auditory discrimination, and thus on speech development. He further hypothesized that a loss of 30–35 dB would cause approximately a 1 year delay in development. However, from what little evidence is available, it appears that if the loss is detected within 6–8 months after birth, and corrective measures are taken, the prognosis for nearly normal articulatory development is excellent. The basis for this prediction lies in the fact that the child's later ability to produce intelligible speech is not determined as much by the severity of the hearing loss as it is by the amount of language to which the child is exposed aurally (Whetnall and Fry, 1971). For reasons to be discussed, the sooner a child receives some corrective measures for hearing loss, the higher our expectations will be for nearly normal speech development due to the increase in information about the speech signal received by the child.

The importance of the first years of a child's life for articulatory development can hardly be overstated. From about the age of six months until about six years is the period of most rapid development for all aspects of language. It is during this period that the brain is most receptive to organizing acoustic cues and articulatory gestures into the phonetic and phonologic system of the language in the child's environment (Lenneberg, 1967). Physiologic development is also very rapid during this period, with the most rapid growth of the vocal tract occurring between three and five years of age (Eguchi and Hirsh, 1969). While the tract is changing so quickly, it is necessary, of course, for the child to receive high quality auditory feedback to be able to compensate for changes in the size and relationship of articulators.

By the time the hearing child is five or six years old, he has mastered the phonetic and phonologic systems of his native language (Fry, 1975), although there still remains much for him to learn about other aspects of the language. The first years of a child's life are so important for language development that children deprived of hearing any speech at all during this period may never be able to acquire oral language. For this reason, this initial rapid development period has been termed the critical learning period for language. If we compare the speech abilities of children whose hearing loss developed after the critical learning period, or who received the benefits of aids and training during the period, with the abilities of children who had neither advantage, we can easily understand the importance of this difference for the speech production abilities of the hearing-impaired.

SPEECH INTELLIGIBILITY

In the discussion so far, we have established the importance of the first few years of life for articulatory development, and for providing the hearing-impaired child with as much information about the speech signal as possible. Providing information about the full complexity of the speech signal, however, entails that we already know: (1) which features of the speech signal are necessary and sufficient for comprehension and normal speech development; (2) how to extract these features from the speech signal; and (3) to transform this information into the residual hearing range or into other sensory modalities for training the hearing-impaired child. In point of fact, we do not have a complete enough understanding of the speech signal or of sensory integration to allow a complete solution to this problem. One avenue that is open to us is to explore those aspects of articulation which usually cause the most difficulty for the hearing-impaired speaker and then to infer which acoustic cues might be crucial for a complete understanding of the phonetic and phonologic systems underlying the speech signal.

Severity of Hearing Loss

There is an obvious relationship between severity of hearing loss and amount of acoustic information that will be available to the child. However, the relationship between audiometric findings and speech production ability is not so straightforward. That is, there is no simple way to predict from the amount of hearing loss at any particular frequency how well—or how poorly—a hearing-impaired person will be able to produce particular sounds or particular phonetic features. Such simple metrics do not control for many factors, including the amount of training a person may have had or the amount of time he has worn a hearing aid. More importantly, however, they fail to capture the fact that phonetic features are not signaled exclusively by the presence or absence of energy at one frequency. Thus, even if a feature's primary acoustic cue is inaudible to the person, there are often secondary cues of that feature which can reliably signal the presence or absence of the feature. On the other hand, when too many cues are inaudible, the hearing-impaired learner will either use the feature inappropriately, or not use it at all because he failed to recognize its relevance for the production of intelligible speech.

Phonetics

One basic question which must be answered before comparing the speech of normals with that of the hearing-impaired is whether the hearing-impaired use the same phonetic feature framework as hearing speakers. Pickett et al. (1972) reported that the deaf do use the same features. We might wonder, though, whether the lack of acoustic information in certain frequencies (usually the higher frequencies) would lead hearing-impaired speakers to rank the features in a different order of importance than normals. In a study of phonemic responses from hard-of-hearing and deaf subjects. Danhauer and Singh (1975) found differences in feature usage which were presumably linked to the severity of the hearing loss. Based on these findings, it seems reasonable to assume that hearing-impaired speakers do ascribe different degrees of importance to certain phonetic features than normals; but that they do use the same features.

Another related question concerns the features of articulation which cause the most difficulty for hearing-impaired speakers. This question may be phrased in a way which reflects the experimental methodology used; that is, which features of hearing-impaired speech do normal listeners find most disturbing? We might suppose—with a number of researchers in this area (Fry, 1975; Pickett et al., 1972)—that, since the majority of hearing-impaired persons have residual hearing in the low-frequency range, they should have a good command over features whose primary cues lie within that range or over features which are temporal rather than spectral in nature. Unfortunately, as the data in the following paragraphs demonstrate, no such simple relationship exists.

An example of a temporal feature of speech is vowel duration. There are both phonetic and phonological regularities affecting vowel duration (Lehiste, 1976). Despite severe attenuation of the higher frequencies, we would still expect deaf speakers to be able to judge fairly accurately the onset and offset of the vocalic portions of an utterance and thus be able to perceive and produce vowel length differences. However, Monsen (1974) found that deaf speakers adopted a fixed difference between tense and lax vowels which did not take into account environmentally conditioned length changes. In the speech of his subjects, /i/ was always longer than /ɪ/ by about the same amount; whereas, in the speech of normals, there will be considerable overlap in the durations of instances of /i/ and /ɪ/. One cause of this variability is the influence of the consonant succeeding the vowel. In English, a vowel may be as much as fifty percent longer before a voiced consonant than before a voiceless one. It is well known, however, that hearing-impaired speakers make many voiced/voiceless errors in consonant production (Hudgins and Numbers, 1942). Thus, it is not surprising that they would not produce a vowel length difference which is conditioned by a consonant voicing contrast which they also do not maintain.

Interestingly enough, the voiced/voiceless contrast for stop consonants can be reliably signaled by durational features. In normal speech, the period of closure for voiceless stops is significantly longer than that for voiced stops. Calvert (1962), however, found that not only were the closure periods of stop consonants produced by deaf speakers four to five times longer than normal, but the voiced/voiceless closure duration difference was often reversed. Another durational feature which has been shown to reliably signal the voiced/voiceless contrast is voicing onset time (the time from release of the stop to the onset of voicing). Stark (1972) reported that, while both deaf and hearing infants started out producing voicing onset times which would characterize the stops as voiced, hearing children went on to master the longer voicing onset times of voiceless stops much sooner than did deaf infants, who never produced the distinction consistently.

Other temporal features of speech are distorted in the speech of the hearing-impaired. John and Howarth (1965) found that temporal distortions contributed significantly to the poor intelligibility of deaf children, and that removal of some of these abnormalities greatly improved their performance. One of the ways in which temporal distortion seemed to affect these speakers was their slower rate of articulation. Not only were many sounds much longer than in the speech of normals, but transitions from sound to sound were much slower. A perceptual correlate of these lengthened transitions is the introduction of extraneous sounds, especially preceding and succeeding stop consonants. These slow, deliberate transitions do not show as much coarticulatory effect as do transitions in the speech of the hearing (Rothman, 1972).

An example of a spectrally based feature with at least primary cues in the lower frequencies is nasality. Here again expectations are not met with regard to the hypothesized control deaf speakers should have over such features. In fact, one of the most widely reported abnormalities of deaf speech is its hypernasality. Not all of this hypernasality can be attributed to improper control of the velopharyngeal port. Colton and Cooker (1968) found that much of the perceived nasality might be due to the slower rate of articulation and longer duration of sounds. They found that normal speakers were also rated as being more nasal when they reduced the tempo of their speaking. Even when reduced tempo is taken into consideration, their remains considerable abnormality in the use of nasalization in the speech of the deaf. Stevens et al. (1976) have demonstrated that an objective measure of nasality can be tied to a subjective rating of velar control. Their measure of nasality, based on a measurement of nasal energy, has proved useful in helping hearing-impaired speakers improve control over nasalization. In this application, an index of nasality curve produced by an instructor is presented visually to the students who attempt to match it. This study indicates that deaf subjects are able to integrate information obtained visually with their speech production abilities.

Since the primary nasal resonance is fixed in the lower frequency range, we must assume that other cues for nasality are inaudible or severely distorted for the hearing-impaired person. One possible candidate is the nasal antiresonances that lie in the higher frequencies and affect formant energy. Another possible reason why nasality is incorrectly perceived may be due to misperception of the coarticulatory effect that nasals have on adjacent sounds. If nasality is not perceived consistently in all types of sounds by deaf speakers, then it may appear to them to be a random variable with little linguistic import especially since it would not be obvious that the source of the nasalization (when it was perceived correctly) was the nasal in the utterance. One observation in support of such a hypothesis is that the deaf sometimes inappropriately denasalize nasal consonants as well as nasalizing nonnasalized sounds (Stevens et al., 1976).

Another area of difficulty for deaf speakers is vowel intelligibility. Since vowel identity is signaled primarily by the relative frequency of the first three formants, it is not surprising that hearing-impaired speakers would have problems especially with the higher frequency formants. In a study of the speech of deaf adolescents, Angelocci, Kopp, and Holbrook (1964) found that the higher the formant frequency was, the more restricted its range. In other words, the higher frequency formants did not vary nearly enough to adequately signal vowel identity. The collapsing of distinctions between vowels in the speech of the hearing-impaired has been termed a reduced phonologic space (Monsen, 1976a).

Problems with higher frequency formants are carried over to other aspects of articulation where formant dynamics are also important. As noted previously in this discussion, transitions from consonants to vowels are very important for signaling both place of articulation and voicing. Changes in frequency of the second formant are especially important in this regard. Monsen (1976b) has demonstrated that deaf children have second formant transitions which are much slower and not as wide ranging in frequency as those of hearing children of the same age.

Vowel intelligibility may be further degraded by differences in the manner of vocal fold vibration. Monsen, Engebertson, and Fisher (1974) studied the glottal waveform of deaf children and found several differences. One acoustic result of these differences was greater attenuation of high frequencies than would be seen in the glottal waveform spectrum of normal children. This means that the speech of deaf children will have even less energy at higher frequencies where their hearing deficit is greatest. This will render the higher frequency formants less audible in their own speech, and more than likely contribute to their inability to correctly discriminate and produce vowel formants at higher frequencies.

REMEDIATION

The discussion so far has highlighted only a few of the more prominent features of the speech of the hearing-impaired, and yet the effects of misusing these features are drastic. A basic problem, therefore, is to bring these features into range of perception in a way which is meaningful for learning correct articulation. Other than the future possibility of prosthetic devices to circumvent the impairment, we are left with two approaches which have produced some successful results. The first approach is to increase the capacity of what residual hearing there is by high gain amplification and possibly frequency recoding of the higher frequencies into a lower range (Velmans, 1975). A second approach is to transform particular features of speech into some type of sensory stimulation other than auditory.

The technical details of these approaches are beyond the scope of the present discussion. What is of interest here is that hearing-impaired learners have shown some improvement using recoded and transformed information. While they may be receiving more acoustic information about the speech signal, they still are not hearing speech as the normal listener would. Apparently what is necessary for these learners is that the important cues for speech perception and production be presented in a manner which maintains a simple correspondence between articulatory position and acoustic result. Either method relies on neural plasticities, that is, the ability of the subject to detect regularities in a signal received through one modality, and to reproduce those regularities in another modality. Although the vast majority of language learners use the auditory channel for receiving and analyzing the signal, there is no reason to believe that this is the only modality that can be used.

Initial efforts to visually present a complete spectral analysis of the speech signal for training the hearing-impaired (Potter, Kopp, and Green, 1947) did not live up to expectations. The lack of success with this technique is presumably due to the fact that features of importance for the learner were "embedded" along with less important features in the display, making it very difficult for the learners to interpret. More recently, efforts in this area have been aimed at presenting only selected features of the speech signal, and giving the subjects very rapid feedback on their performance. One such technique was mentioned previously in the discussion of nasalization (Stevens et al., 1976). Other examples include visual displays of fundamental frequency (Abberton and Fourcin, 1976) and vibrotactile displays of selected frequency components (Goldstein and Stark, 1976). Of course, there are many others, but these exemplify the direction this research has taken.

All of these techniques have been demonstrated to improve to some extent the speech of children trained with them. Continued success in improving these and developing future techniques will depend, in large part, on an improved understanding of articulatory development of the hearing-impaired.

REFERENCES

Abberton E, Fourcin AJ: Visual feedback and the acquisition of intonation, in Lenneberg EH, Lenneberg E (eds): Foundations of Language Development. New York, Academic, 1975

Angelocci A, Kopp G, Holbrook A: The vowel formants of deaf and normal-hearing eleven to fourteen-year-old boys. J Speech Hear Dis 29:156–170, 1964

Calvert DR: Speech sound duration and the surd-sonant error. Volta Rev 64:401–402, 1962

Colton RH, Cooker HS: Perceived nasality in the speech of the deaf. J Speech Hear Res 11:553–559, 1968

Danhauer JL, Singh S: A multidimensional scaling analysis of phonemic responses from hard-of-hearing and deaf subjects of three languages. Language Speech 18:42–64, 1975

Eguchi S, Hirsh IJ: Development of speech sounds in children. Acta Oto-laryngol (Stockh) Suppl 257, 1969

Fry DB: Phonological aspects of language acquisition in the hearing and the deaf, in Lenneberg EH, Lenneberg E (eds): Foundations of Language Development. New York, Academic, 1975

Goetzinger CP: Effects of small perceptive losses on language and on speech discrimination. Volta Rev 64:408–414, 1962

Goldstein MH, Jr, Stark RE: Modification of vocalizations of preschool deaf children by vibrotactile and visual displays. J Acoust Soc Am 59:1477–1481, 1976

Hudgins CV, Numbers FT: An investigation of the intelligibility of the speech of deaf and normal subjects. Genet Psychol Monogr 25:289–392, 1942

John GEG, Howarth GN: The effect of time distortions on the intelligibility of deaf children's speech. Language Speech 8:127–134, 1965

Lehiste I: Suprasegmental features of speech, in Lass N (ed): Contemporary Issues in Experimental Phonetics. New York, Academic, 1976

Lenneberg EH: The natural history of language, in Smith F, Miller GA (eds): The Genesis of Language. Cambridge, MIT Pr, 1966

Lenneberg EH: Biological Foundations of Language, New York, Wiley, 1967

Lenneberg EH, Rebelsky FG, Nichols IA: The vocalizations of infants born to deaf and hearing parents. Human Dev 8:23–27, 1965

Monsen RB: Durational aspects of selected consonant-vowel combinations in the speech of deaf and normally hearing children. J Speech Hear Res 17:386–398, 1974

Monsen RB: Normal and reduced phonological space: The production of English vowels by deaf adolescents. J Phonet 4:189–198, 1976a

Monsen RB: Second formant transitions of selected consonant-vowel combinations in the speech of deaf and normal-hearing children. J Speech Hear Res 19:279–289, 1976b

Monsen RB, Engebertson AM, Fisher WM: Some characteristics of the glottal sound source of deaf children. J Acoust Soc Am 56:561(A), 1974

Pickett JM, Martin ES, Johnson D, et al: On patterns of speech feature reception by deaf listeners, in Fant G (ed): Proceedings of the International Symposium on Communication Ability in Profound Deafness, Stockholm, 1970. Washington, D.C., A. G. Bell Association for the Deaf, 1972

Potter RK, Kopp GA, Green HC: Visible Speech, New York, Van Nostrand, 1947

Rothman HB: An acoustic and electromyographic investigation of consonant-vowel transitions in the speech of deaf adults. J Acoust Soc Am 52:159(A), 1972

Stark RE: Some features of the vocalizations of young deaf children, in Bosma JE (ed): Third Symposium on Oral Sensation and Perception: The Mouth of the Infant. Springfield, IL, Thomas, 1972

Stevens KN, Nickerson RS, Boothroyd A, et al: Assessment of nasalization in the speech of deaf children. J Speech Hear Res 19:393–416, 1976

Velmans M: Effects of frequency recoding on the articulation learning of perceptively deaf children. Language Speech 18:180–193, 1975

Whetnall E, Fry DB: The Deaf Child. London, Heinemans, 1971

Roberta A. Jackson

15
Social and Educational Development

The scope of this book centers around infancy and the detection, prevention, and management of hearing impairment. When considering social and educational development, one necessarily looks at the period from birth to 3 years of age as the relevant time for the transmission of language, culture, and social values. The precursors to cognition center around the experiential backgrounds of children (Schlesinger and Meadow, 1972).

When considering social and educational development of children with hearing losses, it is necessary to distinguish those etiologies of deafness which lead to handicaps in addition to hearing impairment. Genetic factors, viral infections during pregnancy, blood incompatabilities, and low birth weight all are known to be associated with other neurologic and physiologic handicaps. Brain damage, mental retardation, and various learning handicaps are evidenced in the deaf population. Because the presence of deafness or severe hearing loss sometimes is evidence in itself of brain damage—as for example in cases of meningitis or severe perinatal hypoxia—it is likely that secondary handicaps will be manifested among many deaf children. The knowledge of a confounding secondary handicap places the social and educational development of a hearing-impaired child in another light. On the other hand, as noted by Brill (1970), genetically deaf children are the least likely to be multiply handicapped and have a mean I.Q. higher than the general population. Furthermore, hereditary factors constitute the largest single category of congenital deafness.

SOCIAL AND COGNITIVE DEVELOPMENT

Human intelligence is a kind of biologic achievement which allows an individual to interact effectively with the environment. If one examines such social interaction in a child, an overlap of communicative, cognitive, and emotional development appears to occur. The mode in which the social values of a society are presented indicates that the family and peer group are major providers (Blumer, 1966) and that the development of the self requires the manipulation of symbols—the use of language. Communication skills are learned as a product of a child's interaction with his environment.

Piaget's Observations

Piaget (1971) defined intelligence as "a particular instance of biological adaptation." He believes that knowledge of the world, reality, is discovered and constructed by the activity of the child. Hence, the Piagetian view of intellectual development suggests that physical interaction of a child with his environment is what leads to the emergence of cognitive skills or of intelligence. It is essential to note (as in Chap. 13) that cognitive skills which emerge as a child physically interacts with his environment do not require verbal language. All humans inherently possess the ability to interact with the environment, and the emergence of the intellect unfolds throughout childhood.

The first 2 years of life correspond roughly with what Piaget calls the sensorimotor period. It is during this period that the interaction with the environment through direct manipulation by the child sets up ever-changing schema which help the child to organize and adapt to the sensory information he experiences. Regardless of his hereditary and neurophysiological constitution, each human is capable of interacting with the environment in a sensory way. Support for intense environmental stimulation should encourage the development of any child's cognitive and social skills.

Early intervention programs foster attitudes of caretakers of hearing-impaired children which help support the child's opportunity for interaction with the world. This direct interaction with the physical world creates an organized pattern of behavior which Piaget (1955) called scheme. During the sensorimotor period, a child develops schemes which allow immediate experience of the world. Toward the end of the sensorimotor period (from about 18 months to two years of age), a child develops the ability to use mental symbols and words to refer to absent objects. The emergence of language allows the child to be able to experience the world without a concrete here and now experience.

Furth's Observations

Although Piaget observed hearing children and noted that the emergence of verbal language signaled the beginning of thought, Furth (1966) recognized that verbal labels were not prerequisites for thought. Any symbol structure which represents concrete objects can be said to be language. It is this manipulation of symbols which provides for the escalation of schemes and the environmental interactions of the children.

This observation underlies the necessity of having the goal of parent education to encourage the hearing-impaired child's participation in the world. Comments such as the following one of Elkin (1960) are simply not true: ". . . a child born deaf cannot, since he does not hear his own voice, learn to use language without special training." Encouragement of participation in the world on the part of a deaf child will establish language in the sense in which Furth demonstrated it.

Furth has noted that hearing children and deaf children behave quite similarly as infants. Smiling, laughing, crying, the child expresses curiosity in the environment around him. The deaf infant achieves the same developmental milestones as the hearing infant. He will sit up, crawl, handle things, and place objects in his mouth. Until the diagnosis of hearing impairment is made, parents treat deaf children just as they would hearing children. And, in fact, deaf infants coo, cry, and babble very much like hearing children.

It needs to be emphasized that deaf children develop into normal, healthy individuals; their only handicap is one of oral communication. This, in itself, is not a serious obstacle for healthy development of intelligence and personality. Although a child may not have verbal language, he does develop an internalized system of language. The individual's use of language depends upon his own adaptation (Furth, 1973).

PSYCHOSOCIAL DEVELOPMENT

After a diagnosis of severe hearing impairment has been confirmed in an infant, parents begin to doubt the overall capabilities of their child. Unfounded concerns develop about mental retardation and/or brain damage. Parents may enter into a period of mourning and experience the same stages of mourning that Kubler-Ross (1969) has described in her work with the terminally ill. Undoubtedly this parental reaction has its effects on the development of an otherwise healthy and normal child.

Schlesinger and Meadow (1972)—in their study of the interactions between hearing mothers and their deaf children—found that the behavior of mothers appeared to be inflexible, controlling, didactic, intrusive, and disapproving. They observed:

> The deaf children with fewer communicative skills appeared to be less happy, to enjoy interaction with their mothers less, to be less compliant and creative . . .

Schlesinger and Meadow also noted child-rearing practices which reflected constant supervision of the child to protect him from accident, a narrowed range of disciplinary techniques, and feelings of frustration regarding mother–child communication. They hypothesized that the differing form of mother–child interaction may have been due to shifts in style arising from the frustration of trying to deal with a reduced communication system. Also, this style may be due to conflicting philosophies on how to raise a deaf child. These hearing mothers may have felt inadequate in their knowledge of proper parenting skills and which ways are seen to be correct. Undoubtedly the historic conflicts which have arisen over the method of communication training—that is, oralism versus manualism versus total—have added still more pressures on the interactions of hearing mothers with their deaf children. Perhaps most significantly, Schlesinger and Meadow found none of these difficulties in deaf mothers of deaf children.

EDUCATIONAL CONSIDERATIONS

Of course, social development of a very young child cannot be separated from educational development. With a hearing-impaired child, the social-educational process begins when the child is an infant. From the time of identification of hearing impairment, the infant and his parents are very likely to be involved in some type of language stimulation program. Schlesinger (1971) noted that parental over-concern was characteristic of deaf children. The parents in her study tended to protect and avoid just those social interactive situations which would have helped stimulate the cognitive and linguistic abilities of their children. It is apparent, then, that parenting skills for caretakers of hearing-impaired infants should constitute a primary goal of early intervention programs. Early intervention programmed goals are directed at helping parents to cope with their child's hearing difference while encouraging the parents to provide maximal stimulation in all areas of growth and development. For example, the Santa Barbara County Schools' Family Infant Support Program (FISP) provides home activities for hearing-impaired children under 3 years of age in which the parents are primary stimulators of language and social development. A similar program is the infant deaf education program of the Santa Clara County Schools. The goal of such programs is to help parents feel confident about their child's overall abilities; to involve the parents physically and emotionally with their child. Other early intervention programs (e.g., the South Carolina project) take parent education and support as their primary goals.

It is important, also, to be reminded of the findings reported in Chapter 12 on sensory deprivation. First, we now have solid neuroanatomical evidence that early release from deprivation results in cortical development. On the other hand, release which comes too late may be useless; we don't know. But no competent audiologist, otologist, pediatrician, or educator of the deaf would ever adopt the old wait-and-see attitude. Similarly, those who teach the hearing-impaired are virtually unanimous in their opinion that children who receive amplification in the first year of life somehow do better later on in school.

Social and educational development begin at birth. They need some encouraging when that birth results in a child with a severe hearing impairment.

REFERENCES

Blumer M: Sociological implication of the thought of George Herbert Mead. Am J Sociol 71:535–544, 1966

Brill RG: The superior I.Q.'s of deaf children of deaf parents. J Rehabil Deaf 4:45–53, 1970

Elkin F: The Child and Society. New York, Random House, 1960

Furth H: Thinking Without Language. New York, Free Pr, 1966

Furth H: Deafness and Learning. Belmont, CA, Wadsworth, 1973

Kubler-Ross E: On Death and Dying. New York, Macmillan, 1969

Piaget J: The Language and Thought of the Child. New York, Meridian, 1955

Piaget J: Biology and Knowledge. Chicago, Univ Chicago Pr, 1971

Schlesinger H: Language acquisition in four deaf children, in Schlesinger H, Meadow K (eds): Deafness and Mental Health: A Developmental Approach. San Francisco, Langley Porter Institute, 1971

Schlesinger H, Meadow K: Sound and Sign. Berkeley, Univ California Pr, 1972

Sanford E. Gerber

16
Public Health Considerations

All of the preceding text is without force unless public health agencies act on these recommendations. There is some question, however, about whether the outlined procedures and techniques should be mandated at all; and, if they should, whether by state or by federal agencies. A few states have acted, and so have some countries. In this country, it is rather likely that at least some of the recommendations may be covered by a form of national health insurance. If that becomes the case, then, the states probably should not act. The fact is that one or two states have acted quite responsibly, while others have acted rather irresponsibly; and most have not acted at all. The purpose of this final brief chapter is to explore what has been done and to consider some other possibilities.

The first resolution of the Nova Scotia Conference on the Early Identification of Hearing Loss (Mencher, 1976) includes the statement: "We recommend that the World Health Organization, national and local governments, and health agencies adopt this program by legal mandate." What legal mandates, in fact, have been adopted?

THE UNITED STATES

Few states have addressed this question; and some which have, have done so irresponsibly. In this writer's opinion, the state which has acted most intelligently is Texas. According to Glorig and Curtis (1976), the instructions of the legislature given to that state's education agency imply a provision for "establishing identification and evaluation programs." The Director of Education for the Deaf has appointed an Early Detection and Diagnosis Advisory

Council which has recommended that education for the deaf should start at as early an age as possible. Glorig and Curtis estimate that "there will be about fifteen thousand high risk children, including 150 deaf children, born per year in Texas." Their estimation of the number of deaf children to be included among those who are at risk may be rather conservative. Their estimate is that one in one hundred high risk children will prove to be deaf; however, the estimates of Downs (1976) and Stewart (1974) in Colorado suggest that the figure will be closer to one in fifty. Using those figures, 300 deaf children should be expected to be born each year in Texas; hence, we should expect approximately 300 deaf children per year to become of school age in that state.

Glorig and Curtis have recommended to the state of Texas that it employ the five-item questionnaire contained in the 1973 Statement of the Joint Committee on Newborn Hearing. In addition, they have recommended the use of the rest of that statement, that is, the part dealing with follow-up testing. It was their recommendation that all those who failed the high-risk questionnaire should be reported to the state Director of Eduation for the Deaf. They then directed that the regional school superintendents would be responsible for initiating procedures for follow-up evaluations on all those neonates who are suspected of being deaf within a given region of the state. They further propose a number of "approved evaluation teams" to be located at 30 places throughout the state, making maximum use of existing facilities. Of primary importance in the Texas plan is its insistence on the agreed position that there is no age at which one is too young to begin habilitation. Furthermore, any delay of habilitation after the time of detection is inexcuseable. The proposed "Texas plan" should be a model for all states, and one that ought to be followed by all states.

The Commonwealth of Massachusetts, in 1971, passed a law which should serve as a model for no one to emulate. Sections F67G and 67H of Chapter 111 of the General Laws of that state specify certain high risk conditions which merit further examination. The Massachusetts law defines the high-risk conditions: "(1) Before birth (a) family history of deafness as indicated by one or more deaf or hard of hearing children in family; (b) maternal thyroid abnormality; (c) maternal German measles in the first three months of pregnancy; (d) maternal influenza or chicken pox in the first three months of pregnancy, and (2) newborn difficulty (a) Mycin drugs administered to infant; (b) multiple abnormalities of infant from whatever cause." Of course, it is apparent that this high-risk register differs from the one recommended by the Joint Committee on Newborn Hearing. It differs in two significant ways: what it includes and what it excludes. Including the family history of deafness is consistent with the Joint Committee's Statement; however, item 1 pertaining to maternal thyroid abnormality, while important, is statistically rather insignificant. While maternal thyroid disease does lead to deafness, one's concern really is limited to Pendred's Syndrome which, according to Fraser (1964), accounts for 7½% of all deaf children. In fact, according to Brown (1967), Pendred's is the most common syndrome which includes deafness; but other enzyme defects are also associated with deafness. Regarding that state's item about rubella, one can have no serious argument except for the fact that the first trimester of pregnancy is not the only time period that is hazardous (Bordley et al., 1967). With regard to other viral diseases during pregnancy, there are those that lead to congenital deafness; but there is no reason to limit the law to the study of influenza and chicken pox, and then only in the first trimester. Kapur (1977) reported the incidence of small pox, chicken pox, and measles in his deaf patients. The attack on mycin drugs is certainly unwarranted; only a few of those drugs have been shown to be ototoxic. One would not want to follow up an infant for neurosensory deafness because he had received, for example, terramycin. On the other hand it would have been useful for that law to specify, above all, kanamycin and gentamycin.

The principal difficulty with the Massachusetts law, however, is not the conditions which are specified as constituting high risk. The main difficulty lies in how the high-risk register is to be employed. Nowhere does the law require that the infants be examined, either physically or by a study of the records. The law instead requires that "the parent or legal guardian of the child" will be provided with literature which describes these conditions. This literature then asks the parents to discuss these high risk factors with their physicians to make the determination. If, then, such a determination is made, they are to be referred to one of four centers in that state where diagnostic work may be done. This handing out of literature is reminiscent of the maxim of leading horses to water. What is commendable in the act is that this diagnostic work may be done at no cost to the family, but it is curious that one of the four centers doing follow-up evaluations is a department of orthopedics. In the five years since that act has been passed by the legislature of the Commonwealth of Massachusetts, there have been no reports that it works.

The states of Indiana and Minnesota have instituted comprehensive service for the hearing-impaired; however, as far as we know, no data have been published. There are eleven states which have legislative mandate to provide services for the handicapped beginning at birth, but many of them have not produced the regulations which would be necessary to implement such legislation. In California, some really strange legislative proposals have been made. These included, for example, a bill that would require the detection of deafness in the newborn nursery. This bill did not describe how deafness was to be detected, by whom it was to be detected, or what ought to be done with the infants who were detected in this mysterious manner. Fortunately, that bill never arrived on the floor of the legislature. Following the failure of that bill the health committee of the state assembly decided to hold hearings on the subject and some experts were called to testify. A year later, the assembly passed a resolution directing the Department of Health to determine the feasibility and cost of detecting deafness in the newborn. To date, no action has been taken, although the report (Gerber, 1976) required by that resolution has been submitted to the assembly. The report recommended the high risk questionnaire of the 1973 Statement by the Joint Committee on Newborn Hearing, and further recommended that it be implemented in a manner similar to that of the Texas plan.

As of this writing, at least to my knowledge, only the state of Utah has a program in force and operating. The Utah program began in 1967 as a Maternal and Child Health demonstration project. From that time until 1972, a mass screening program was conducted in seven hospitals. At that time, and in response to the Joint Committee's statement, a pilot questionnaire was introduced. As of January, 1977 they had processed over 26,000 questionnaires and are now working in all but three of the hospitals in the state (Mahoney, 1977). In essence, the Utah program adheres to the recommendations of the Joint Committee's 1973 statement. They employ a seven item questionnaire, which is shown as Fig. 16-1. The questionnaire is enclosed in a packet of materials given to the parents at the time of preparing the birth certificate information. Hospitals collect the questionnaires and send them to the state Division of Health, Speech Pathology/Audiology section, and the personnel of this section make the high risk decision. To date about 19% of births have been considered to be high risk; this probably reflects a high false positive rate but also reflects a low false negative rate. The follow-up program is also interesting. The first contact is made by telephone when the child is 6–8 months of age; only about 2% are considered at risk after this step. Utah is planning to increase its contacts to 25,000 this year alone, so the reduction in number becomes important. If, at the time of the telephone call, the infant is still thought to be at risk, then referral is made to an audiology center or to one of seven itinerant clinics. Sometimes additional data are provided to the parents. After confirmation of the hearing loss, appropriate otolaryngologic, pediatric, and educational steps are taken. Although the data have not yet been published, Mahoney (1977) reports "a number of children with moderate or greater sensorineural losses" have been found.

As of this time, most states have not dealt with this matter at all. There has been activity in some states which have not been active in the past, for example, Oklahoma and New Jersey. On the other hand, the prospect of federal legislation becomes greater all the time. The uniformity of procedure which may be realizable under federal legislation is desirable regardless of

NEWBORN HEARING SCREENING QUESTIONNAIRE

Please PRINT

Baby's Name ______ Birthdate ______ Sex ______

Parent's Name ______ Home Phone ______ Date ______

Address ______ City ______ Zip ______

Hospital ______ Baby's Doctor ______

Dear Parent: Please fill out this information by circling YES or NO. ANSWER ALL QUESTIONS. If you need assistance, please contact the hospital nurse.

1.	Has a close relative of the baby had a hearing loss SINCE CHILDHOOD?	YES	NO
2.	During the pregnancy, was the mother exposed to RUBELLA (3 day, German, or "soft" measles)?	YES	NO
3.	At birth, did the baby weigh LESS THAN 3½ pounds (1500 grams)?	YES	NO
4.	Was there an RH (blood incompatibility) problem that required blood transfusion?	YES	NO
5.	At birth, were there any defects involving the baby's head, ears, nose, or throat?	YES	NO
6.	Has the baby been SERIOUSLY ill since birth?	YES	NO
7.	Do you have reason to be concerned about this child's hearing?	YES	NO

IF additional information is required, you may expect to receive a telephone call from a professional staff member within approximately six months. Should you have any questions, call 533-6175, Salt Lake City, Utah.

HOSPITAL STAFF: Please mail the original to this address and place the carbon in the baby's file, if desired.

Speech Pathology/Audiology Section
Utah State Division of Health
44 Medical Drive
Salt Lake City, Utah 84113

SDH–BSHS–10–3/76

Fig. 16-1. The Utah high-risk register. (Mahoney, 1977)

how one may feel about centralization. As the prospect of national health insurance becomes more likely, it is hoped that the detection of deafness and other congenital neurosensory deficits will be included.

In the fall of 1975, the president signed into law the Education of All Handicapped Children Act (PL94-142). This law requires each state to provide educational opportunities for all handicapped children, including hearing-impaired, to the youngest age. Early detection is thereby explicit in this law.

OTHER COUNTRIES

Some countries have done so well that they merit our attention and perhaps our emulation. In Sweden, where virtually all births occur in hospitals, they have essentially universal detection programs (Barr, 1965). The Swedish government has a Committee on Care and Education of Preschool Children. According to Stensland-Junker (1976), this committee has stressed the importance of early recognition of children "with special needs for stimulation." She describes special needs children as those who require medical, educational, and/or social intervention. She adopts the bias which is evident throughout this book that "their cooperation is not a question for future consideration. It concerns the present day . . ." Using a universal mass screening procedure, Barr (1965) reported successful correct detection of one deaf infant in 2000 births. Such a mass screening procedure works very well in a country such as Sweden because of its massive public welfare programs. That is to say, in a place where virtually all births occur in hospitals and virtually all children are seen thereafter in well baby clinics, mass screening is possible. Whether it is desirable, however, is another question.

Such mass screening has been tried, for example, in Israel. The Department of Otolaryngology at Hadassah University Hospital in Jerusalem embarked upon such a large scale program. Over a period of about 3 years, nearly 18,000 newborns were screened using a behavioral method. In addition to the behavioral screen, they introduced a high-risk register. In total, they examined 17,731 infants of whom 23 were identified as suffering severe bilateral sensory-neural deafness. Only six of the 23 failed the behavioral screen; conversely, 17 deaf children would have been cleared by the behavioral test. As a consequence, Feinmesser and Tell (1976) concluded that only children who have profound losses may be detected by a behavioral method, and that such a test is "not sensitive enough for detection of deafness in newborns and, therefore, is not valid for screening purposes." On the other hand, the Israelis have excellent health care delivery, and children are characteristically brought to well-baby clinics. This makes it possible for screening to be done at later ages: 85% of children are seen in baby clinics at the age of five or six months, and at that time the screening did turn out to be practical. Some two percent of these children failed at that age. Children were available to be seen again later: 65% at 18–24 months of age, and 44% at three years. Even with this excellent follow-up, Feinmesser and Tell conclude that a restricted high risk register should be applied in the newborn nursery.

At the Research Institute for Mother and Child in Warsaw, Poland, they have the objective of testing hearing in every child three times before the age of seven years (Borkowska-Gaertig et al., 1976). It has been their assumption that the program developed at that institute would be available for testing throughout the country, and, in fact, field experiments have been carried out in Warsaw, in Cracow, and in Szczecin, with more than 12,000 children having been tested. These children are aged between eight and twelve months, but we have been unable to determine if the Poles are doing nursery screening. Apparently they don't test before the age of 8 months (Borkowska-Gaertig, 1975). Their data have revealed thirteen hearing-impaired children per every thousand examined, an extremely high figure indeed; however, it includes all levels of hearing impairment, not only those which are severe or profound. Examining the data of children under the age of one year, the Polish figures agree essentially with those from other parts of the world, that is, about $^{1}/_{10}$ of 1%. It appears, as of this writing, that the programs conducted in Poland have been mostly for research purposes rather than for public health purposes although that is a primary goal.

It has been the attitude of Italian researchers (Rossi and Guidotti, 1976) that the early detection of deafness must come from programs in "all childhood health care structures." The Italian data are similar to the Polish in that they have detected five deaf children of somewhat more than 5000 newborns examined. In addition to the five detected early, there were two false negatives detected later. While Rossi and Guidotti did not report the nature of any legislative mandate in their country, they did state an opinion that the limitation of screening to the high risk population would be unwise. They feel that hospitals "are not ready to select babies reliably enough." Their program was conducted by volunteer help, however, and specially trained volunteers or, preferably, paraprofessionals might solve that problem for them. They recommend encouraging frequent use of a high risk questionnaire in pediatricians' offices for the purpose of referral to audiological centers.

Infant screening and follow-up can be done by service organizations, and apparently quite successfully. In Canada, the Elks have implemented a project called the Deaf Detection and Development Program for Early Identification of the Hearing Impaired. The clinical division of this program has been examining infants in three age groups: 48 hours to 1 week, 3 months to one year, and nine months to one year. They employ a high risk questionnaire for the newborns and see the older children in public health facilities or in cooperating audiologic facilities (Alexander, Coulling, and Coulling, 1976). For the neonates, they use both the high-risk register and a pure tone screen. Similar procedures are applied for the older infants but the screening is done at 60 dB rather than at 90 dB. By the end of 1974, they had examined nearly 10,000 infants in newborn nurseries; of the 10,000, nearly 600 were not cleared. This figure, again, is consistent with that reported in other countries. Among those children referred to public health agencies, 15 of 383 were not cleared. The province of British Columbia has recommended that all children should be screened by using a neonatal high risk register with follow-up implementation between the ages of 6 months and 18 months (Zink, 1976). The program of this province has stressed the significance of follow-up procedures, an important matter which has been insufficiently stressed elsewhere.

In at least four centers in Yugoslavia, successful programs of research on the causes of deafness are being carried out. Mencher (1972) reported on visits he made to two centers in Ljubljana, one in Zagreb, and one in Belgrad. At the time of that writing, they had examined about 4000 babies, but were reporting an extraordinarily high incidence of false positives. One hopes that their methods improve before programs are adopted on a broader scale.

CONCLUSIONS

It is difficult to draw any general or very meaningful conclusions from the preceding discussion. In general, it appears that most of the responsible public health agencies have not addressed the question of hearing impairment at all. Among those which have, the variations are equal in number to the institutions doing the considering. Models range from nonexistent (as in most places) to useless (as in Massachusetts) to purely research oriented (as in Poland and Yugoslavia) to very good detection and follow-up (as in Texas, British Columbia, and Sweden). It is to be hoped that uniformity can be attained. This uniformity was proposed in the resolutions of the Nova Scotia Conference on Early Identification of Hearing Loss (Mencher, 1976). As we stated at the beginning of this chapter, those resolutions requested that agencies which have the authority to do so must act responsibly. There is yet no evidence that many are doing so.

REFERENCES

Alexander PT, Coulling L, Coulling RK: The Elks deaf detection and development program for early identification of the hearing impaired, in Mencher GT (ed): Early Identification of Hearing Loss. Basel, Karger, 1976

Barr B: Early primary screening, in Davis H (ed): The Young Deaf Child. Acta Otolaryngol (Suppl) (Stockh) 206:45–47, 1965

Bordley JE, Brookhouser PE, Hardy J, et al: Observations on the effect of prenatal rubella in hearing, in McConnell F, Ward PH (eds): Deafness in Childhood.

Nashville, Vanderbilt Univ Pr, 1967
Borkowska-Gaertig D: Study of Hearing Impairments in Children in Poland. Warsaw, Research Institute of Mother and Child, 1975
Borkowska-Gaertig D, Urbanska I, Sobieszczanska-Radoszewska L, et al: Evaluation of the three-stage hearing testing programme for children in Poland, in Mencher GT (ed): Early Identification of Hearing Loss. Basel, Karger, 1976.
Brown KS: The genetics of childhood deafness, in McConnell F, Ward PH (eds): Deafness in Childhood. Nashville, Vanderbilt Univ Pr, 1967
Downs MP: Early identification of hearing loss: Where are we? Where do we go from here? in Mencher GT (ed): Early Identification of Hearing Loss. Basel, Karger, 1976
Feinmesser M, Tell L: Evaluation of methods for detecting hearing impairment in infancy and early childhood, in Mencher GT (ed): Early Identification of Hearing Loss. Basel, Karger, 1976
Fraser GR: Profound childhood deafness. J Med Genet 1:118–150, 1964
Gerber SE: Unpublished report on behalf of California Department of Health, Bureau of Maternal and Child Health, 1976
Glorig A, Curtis GA: Considerations in implementing program of identification and evaluation of deaf persons (birth-Twenty-one) in Texas, in Mencher GT (ed): Early Identification of Hearing Loss. Basel, Karger, 1976
Kapur YP: Viral otitis media in children, in Jazbi B (ed): Pediatric Otorhinolaryngology, Otolaryngologic Clinics of North America. Philadelphia, Saunders, 1977, Vol. 10, No. 1, p. 251
Mahoney T: (personal communication, 1977)
Mencher GT: Report of a Visit to Israel and Yugoslavia. Lincoln, University of Nebraska, 1972
Mencher GT (ed): Early Identification of Hearing Loss. Basel, Karger, 1976
Rossi P, Guidotti E: Problems associated with the early diagnosis of deafness in newborn babies, in Mencher GT (ed): Early Identification of Hearing Loss. Basel, Karger, 1976
Stensland-Junker K: BOEL-A child welfare program for early screening of communication abilities, in Mencher GT (ed): Early Identification of Hearing Loss. Basel, Karger, 1976
Stewart J: High risk screening. Meeting of the Western Society for Pediatric Research, Carmel, CA, 1974
Zink GD: Comprehensive programming for early detection and management of communication disorders, in Mencher GT (ed): Early Identification of Hearing Loss. Basel, Karger, 1976

Bibliography

Abberton E, Fourcin AJ: Visual feedback and the acquisition of intonation. *In* Lenneberg EH, Lenneberg E (eds): Foundations of Language Development. New York, Academic, 1975

Abe M: Electrical responses of the human brain to acoustic stimulus. Tohoku J Exp Med 60:47–58, 1954

Ackner B: A simple method for recording respiration. J Psychosom Res 1:144–146, 1956

Adrian E: The microphonic action of the cochlea in relation to theories of hearing. *In* Report of a Discussion of Audition of the Physical Society of London, 1931

Akiyama Y, Schulte FJ, Schultz MA, et al: Acoustically evoked responses in premature and full term newborn infants. Electroencephalogr Clin Neurophysiol 26:371–380, 1969

Alberti P: Stapedial reflex estimation and the loudness recruitment phenomenon. *In* Rose D, Keating L (eds): Impedance Symposium. Chicago, Zenith Hearing Inst. Corp., 1972

Alexander PT, Coulling L, Coulling RK: The Elks deaf detection and development program for early identification of the hearing impaired. *In* Mencher GT (ed): Early Identification of Hearing Loss. Basel, Karger, 1976

Altenau MM: Histopathology of sensorineural hearing loss. *In* Glasscock ME (ed): Sensorineural hearing loss in children: Early detection and intervention. Otolaryngol Clin North Am 8:49–58, 1975

Amadeo M, Shagass C: Brief latency click-evoked potentials during waking and sleeping in man. Psychophysiology 10:244–250, 1973

Anch AM: The auditory evoked brain response during adult human sleep. Unpublished doctoral dissertation, Saint Louis University, 1971

Anders T, Emde R, Parmelee AH Jr: A Manual of Standardized Terminology, Techniques and Criteria for Scoring of States of Sleep and Wakefulness in Newborn Infants. Los Angeles, UCLA Brain Information Service/BRI Publ Office, 1971

Anderson H, Jepsen O, Ratjen E: Ossicular chain defects—diagnosis and treatment. Acta Oto-Laryngol (Stockh) 54:393–402, 1962

Anderson H, Wedenberg E: Audiometric identification of normal hearing carriers of genes for deafness. Acta Oto-Laryngol (Stockh) 65:535–554, 1968

Andreev AM, Arapova AA, Gersuni GV: On electrical potentials in the human cochlea. J Physiol 26:205–212, 1939

Angelocci A, Kopp G, Holbrook AJ: The vowel formants of deaf and normal-hearing eleven to fourteen-year-old boys. J Speech Hear Dis 29:156–170, 1964

Anson BJ: Developmental anatomy of the ear. *In* Paparella MM, Shumrick DA (eds): Otolaryngology. Philadelphia, Saunders, 1973

Anthony J: An experimental approach to the psychopathology of childhood: Autism. Br J Med Psychol 31:211–225, 1958

Antinoro F, Skinner PH, Jones JJ: Relation between sound intensity and amplitude of the AER at different stimulus frequencies. J Acoust Soc Am 46:1433–1436, 1969

Appleby SV: The slow vertex maximal sound evoked response in infants. *In* Davis H (ed): The Young Deaf Child: Identification and Management. Acta Oto-Laryngol (Stockh) Suppl 206:146–152, 1965

Aran JM: The electro-cochleogram: recent results in children and in some pathological cases. Archiv Klin Exp Ohren–Nasen Kehlkopfh 198:128–141, 1971

Aran JM: Clinical measures of VIIIth nerve functions. Adv Otol Rhinol Laryngol 20:374–394, 1973

Aran JM, Delaunay J: Étude électrophysiologique de l'audition humaine. Rev Acoust 14:91–94, 1971

Aran JM, LeBert G: Les réponses nerveuses cochleaires chez l'homme image du fonctionnement de l'orielle et nouveau test d'audiométrie objective. Rev Laryngol 89:361–378, 1968

Aran JM, Negrevergne M: Clinical study of some particular pathological patterns of eighth nerve responses in the human being. Audiology 12:488–503, 1973

Aran JM, Pèlerin J, Lenoir J, et al: Aspects théoriques et pratiques des enregistrements électro-cochléographique selon la méthode établie à Bordeaux. Rev Laryngol (Suppl):601–644, 1971

Aran JM, Portmann C, Delaunay J, et al: L'électrocochléogramme: Méthodes et premiers résultats chez l'enfant. Rev Laryngol 90:615–634, 1969

Aran JM, Portmann M: L'électrocochléogramme. J Fran Otol Rhinol Laryngol 21:211–221, 1972

Aran JM, Portmann M, Portmann C, et al: Electro-cochleography in adults and children: electrophysiological study of the peripheral receptor. Audiology 11:77–89, 1972

Ashton R: The state variable in neonatal research; a review. Merrill–Palmer Q Beh Dev 19:1–9, 1973

Austin G: Knowledge of selected concepts obtained by an adolescent deaf population. Am Ann Deaf 120:360–370, 1975

Baldwin JL: Dysostosis craniofacialis of Crouzon. Laryngoscope 78:1660–1676, 1968

Baldwin J, Baldwin J: The role of learning phenomena in the ontogeny of exploration and play. *In* Chevalier-Skolnikoff S, Poirier F (eds): Bio-Social Development among Primates. New York, Garland, 1976

Bancaud J, Bloch V, Paillard J: Contribution EEG a l'étude des potentiels evoques chez l'homme au niveau du vertex. Rev Neurol 89:399–418, 1953

Barlow J: An electronic method for detecting evoked responses of the brain and for reproducing their average waveforms. Electroencephalogr Clin Neurophysiol 9:340–343, 1957

Barnet AB: Averaged evoked electroencephalographic responses to clicks in the infant. *In* Davis H (ed): The Young Deaf Child: Identification and Management. Acta Oto-Laryngol (Stockh) Suppl 206:134–146, 1965

Barnet AB: Evoked response audiometry in 241 normal and hearing impaired children under three years. Arch Klin Exp Ohren Nasen Kehlkopfh 198:154–157, 1971

Barnet AB: EEG and evoked response correlates of mental retardation. Clin Proc

Child Hosp 94:250–260, 1971

Barnet AB, Goodwin RS: Averaged evoked electroencephalographic responses to clicks in the human newborn. Electroencephalogr Clin Neurophysiol 18:441–450, 1965

Barnet AB, Goodwin RS: Averaged evoked electroencephalographic responses to clicks in the human newborn. *In* Brackbill Y (ed): Behavior in Infancy and Early Childhood: A Book of Readings. New York, Free Press, 1967

Barnet AB, Lodge A: Diagnosis of deafness in infants with the use of computer-averaged electroencephalographic responses to sound. J Pediatr 69:753–758, 1966

Barr B: Early primary screening. *In* Davis H (ed): The Young Deaf Child: Identification and Management. Acta Oto-Laryngol (Stockh) Suppl 206:45–47, 1965

Barr B, Junker KS: Functional Contact Test for Babies as a Screening Method. Stockholm, Lekateket Pa Blockhusudden, 1969

Bartoshuk AK: Response decrement with repeated elicitation of human neonatal cardiac acceleration to sound. J Comp Physiol Psychol 55:9–13, 1962

Bartoshuk AK: Human neonatal cardiac acceleration to sound; habituation and dishabituation. Percept Motor Skills 15:15–27, 1962

Bartoshuk AK: Human neonatal cardiac response to sound; a power function. Psychon Sci 1:151–152, 1964

Bates E: Language and Context: The Acquisition of Pragmatics. New York, Academic, 1976

Baxter BL: Effect of visual deprivation during postnatal maturation on the electroencephalogram of the cat. Exp Neurol 14:224–237, 1966

Beagley HA, Kellogg SE: A comparison of evoked response and subjective auditory thresholds. Int Audiol 8:345–353; 1969

Beagley HA, Kellogg SE: Amplitude of the auditory evoked response at high intensities. Sound 4:86–90, 1970

Beagley HA, Knight JJ: Changes in auditory evoked response with intensity. J Laryngol Otol 81:861–873, 1967

Beck A: Oznaczenie lokalizacyi w mozgu i rdzeniu za pomoca zjawisk elektry czynch. Krakow, University Jagiellonski, 1890

Beiter RC, Hogan DD: Effects of variations in stimulus rise–decay time upon the early components of the auditory evoked response. Electroencephalogr Clin Neurophysiol 34:203–206, 1973

Bellugi U, Klima E: The roots of language in the sign talk of the deaf. Psychol Today 6(June):60–76, 1972

Bellugi U, Klima E, Siple P: Remembering in signs. Cognition 3:93–125, 1974–5

Bench J: Some effects of audio-frequency stimulation of the crying baby. J Aud Res 9:122–128, 1969

Bench J: Audio-frequency and audio-intensity discrimination in the human neonate. Int Audiol 8:615–625, 1969

Bench J: The law of initial value: A neglected source of variance in infant audiometry. Int Audiol 9:314–322, 1970

Bench J, Collyer Y, Mentz L, et al: Studies in infant behavioural audiometry: I.

Neonate. Audiology 15:85–105, 1976

Bench J, Collyer Y, Mentz L, et al: Studies in infant behavioural audiometry: II. Six-week-old infants. Audiology 15:302–314, 197

Bench J, Collyer Y, Mentz L, et al: Studies in infant behavioural audiometry: II. Six-month-old infants. Audiology 15:384–394, 1976

Bench J, Parker A: Hyper-responsivity to sounds in the short-gestation baby. Dev Med Child Neurol 13:15–19, 1971

Benjamin L: Statistical treatment of the law of initial values in autonomic research: A review and recommendation. Psychosom Med 25:556–566, 1963

Berger H: Über das Elektrenkephalogramm des Menschen. Arch Psychiatr Nervenkrankh 87:527–570, 1929

Bergstrom L: Congenital deafness. *In* Northern JL (ed): Hearing Disorders. Boston, Little Brown, 1976

Berlin CI: New developments in evaluating central auditory mechanisms. Ann Otol Rhinol Laryngol 85:833–841, 1976

Berlin CI, Gondra MI: Extratympanic clinical electrocochleography with clicks. *In* Ruben RJ, Elberling C, Salomon G (eds): Electrocochleography. Baltimore, University Park, 1976

Berlyne DE: Conflict, Arousal and Curiosity. New York, McGraw–Hill, 1960

Berry H, Briant TD, Winchester BT: Electrophysiologic assessment of the lower portion of the auditory pathway in the human subject. J Otolaryngol 5:3–11, 1976

Bickford RG: Physiological and clinical studies of microreflexes. Recent Cont Neurophysiol, EEG 31(Suppl):93–108, 1972

Bickford RG, Jacobson J, Cody D: Nature of average evoked potentials to sound and other stimuli in man. Ann NY Acad Sci 112:204–223, 1964

Birns B, Blank M, Bridger WH, et al: Behavioral inhibition in neonates produced by auditory stimuli. Child Dev 36:639–645, 1965

Black FO, Bergstrom L, Downs MP, et al: Congenital Deafness. Boulder, Colorado Associated Univ Press, 1971

Blanton RL: Language learning and performance in the deaf. *In* Rosenberg S, Koplin J (eds): Developments in Applied Psycholinguistic Research. New York, Macmillan, 1968

Blanton RL, Nunnally J: Evaluation of language in the deaf. Psychol Rep 15:891–894, 1964

Blegvad B: Binaural summation of surface-recorded electro-cochleographic responses. Normal hearing subjects. Scand Audiol 4:233–238, 1975

Bloom L: Language Development: Form and Function in Emerging Grammars. Cambridge, MIT, 1970

Blumer M: Sociological implication of the thought of George Herbert Mead. Am J Sociol 71:535–544, 1966

Bochenek Z, Bochenek W: Early (12–16 ms) responses evoked by tones and clicks. Rev Laryngol 96:114–120, 1975

Boese R: Differentiations in the deaf community. Dept Sociol, Univ Br Columbia, 1964 (unpublished)

Bordley JE, Brookhouser PE, Hardy JW, et al: Observations on the effect of prenatal rubella in hearing. *In* McConnell F, Ward PH (eds): Deafness in Childhood.

Nashville, Vanderbilt Univ Press, 1967

Borkowska-Gaertig D: Study of Hearing Impairments in Children in Poland. Warsaw, Research Institute of Mother and Child, 1975

Borkowska-Gaertig D, Urbanska I, Sobieszczanska-Radoszewska L, et al: Evaluation of the three-stage hearing testing programme for children in Poland. *In* Mencher GT (ed): Early Identification of Hearing Loss, Basel, Karger, 1976

Borsanyi SI: Some aspects of auditory evoked potentials in man. Ann Otol Rhinol Laryngol 73:61–71, 1964

Brackbill Y, Adams G, Crowell DH, et al: Arousal level in neonates and preschool children under continuous auditory stimulation. J Exp Child Psychol 4:178–188, 1966

Brackmann DE, Selters WA: Electrocochleography in Ménière's disease and acoustic neuromas. *In* Ruben RJ, Elberling C, Salomon G (eds): Electrocochleography. Baltimore, Univ Park, 1976

Bradford LJ: Respiration audiometry. *In* Bradford LJ (ed): Physiological Measures of the Audio-Vestibular System. New York, Academic, 1975

Bradford LJ, Rousey CL, Bradford MA: Respiration audiometry with the preschool child. The Menninger Foundation, Topeka, 1968

Bragg B: Ameslish—our American heritage. Am Ann Deaf 118:672–674, 1973

Brannon J: Linguistic word classes in spoken language of normal, hard of hearing, and deaf children. J Speech Hear Res 11:279–287, 1968

Brannon J, Murray T: The spoken syntax of normal, hard of hearing, and deaf children. J Speech Hear Res 9:604–610, 1966

Brazier M: The historical development of neurophysiology. *In* Field J, Magoun H, Hall V (eds): Handbook of Physiology. Section 1, Neurophysiology, Vol. 1. Baltimore, Williams and Wilkins, 1959

Brazier M, Barlow J: Some applications of correlation analysis to clinical problems in electroencephalography. Electroencephalogr Clin Neurophysiol 8:325–331, 1956

Brethower DM, Reynolds GS: A facilitative effect of punishment on unpunished behavior. J Exp Anal Behav 5:191–199, 1962

Bridger WH, Reiser MF: Psychophysiologic studies of the neonate: An approach toward the methodological and theoretical problems involved. Psychosom Med 21:265–276, 1959

Brill RG: A study in the adjustment of three groups of deaf children. Excep Child 26:464–466, 1960

Brill RG: The superior I.Q.'s of deaf children of deaf parents. J Rehab Deaf 4:45–53, 1970

Brooks D: Electro-acoustic impedance bridge studies on normal ears of children. J Speech Hear Res 14:247–253, 1971

Brown JL: States in newborn infants. Merrill–Palmer Q Behav Dev 10:313–327, 1964

Brown KS: The genetics of childhood deafness. *In* McConnell F, Ward PH (eds): Deafness in Childhood. Nashville, Vanderbilt Univ Press, 1967

Brown R: A First Language. Cambridge, Harvard Univ Press, 1973

Brown R, Bellugi U: Three processes in the child's acquisition of syntax. Harvard Educ Rev 34:133–151, 1964

Brown R, Cazden C, Bellugi U: The child's grammar from 1 to 3. *In* Hill J (ed): Minnesota Symposium on Child Psychology. Minneapolis, Univ Minn Press, 1968

Bruner J: The ontogenesis of speech acts. Child Language 2:1–19, 1975

Bruner J: From communication to language. A psychological perspective. Cognition 3:255–287, 1975

Buchsbaum M: Average evoked response: Techniques and applications. Schizophr Bull 3:10–18, 1970

Buchwald JS, Huang CM: Far-field acoustic response: Origins in the cat. Science 189:382–384, 1975

Buell J, Stoddard P, Harris F, et al: Collateral social development accompanying reinforcement of outdoor play in a preschool child. J Appl Behav Anal 1:167–173, 1968

Callaway E: Brain Electrical Potentials and Individual Psychological Differences. New York, Grune & Stratton, 1975

Calvert DR: Speech sound duration and the surd-sonant error. Volta Rev 64:401–402, 1962

Caton R: The electric currents of the brain. Br Med J 2:278, 1875

Celesia GC, Puletti F: Auditory cortical areas of man. Neurol 19:211–220, 1969

Cicourel AV, Boese R: Sign language acquisition and the teaching of deaf children. *In* Cazden C, John V. Hymes D (eds): Functions of Language in the Classroom. New York, Teachers Coll Press, 1972

Clark W Jr: Average response computer (ARC-1). Quarterly progress report, MIT Research Lab of Elec, 1958, pp 114–117

Clifton RK, Graham FK, Hatton HM: Newborn heart-rate response and response habituation as a function of stimulus duration. J Exp Child Psychol 6:265–278, 1968

Clifton RK, Meyers WJ: The heart-rate response of four-month-old infants to auditory stimuli. J Exp Child Psychol 7:122–135, 1969

Coats AC: On electrocochleographic electrode design. J Acoust Soc Am 56:708–711, 1974

Coats AC, Dickey JR: Nonsurgical recording of human auditory nerve action potentials and cochlear microphonics. Ann Otol Rhinol Laryngol 79:844–852, 1970

Coats AC, Dickey JR: Postmasking recovery of human click action potentials and click loudness. J Acoust Soc Am 52:1607–1612, 1972

Cody DTR, Klass DW, Bickford RG: Cortical audiometry: An objective method of evaluating auditory acuity in awake and sleeping man. Trans Am Acad Ophthal Otolaryngol 71:81–91, 1967

Cohen L, Peters R: Response behaviors of infants to simulated moving sound stimuli. Eighth International Congress on Acoustics, London, 1974

Cohen MM, Rapin I, Lyttle M, et al: Auditory evoked response (AER)—Consistency of detection in young sleeping children. Arch Otolaryngol 94:214–219, 1971

Coleman PD, Riesen AH: Environmental effects on cortical dendritic fields: I. Rearing in the dark. J Anat 102:363–374, 1968

Colton RH, Cooker HS: Perceived nasality in the speech of the deaf. J Speech Hear

Res 11:553–559, 1968

Cooper R, Rosenstein J: Language acquisition of deaf children. Volta Rev 68:46–56, 1966

Cotes JE: Lung Function: Assessment and Application in Medicine (2nd ed). Oxford, Blackwell, 1968

Crowley DE, Davis H, Beagley HA: Survey of the clinical use of electrocochleography. Ann Otol Rhinol Laryngol 84:297–307, 1975

Cullen JK, Berlin CI, Gondra MI, et al: Electrocochleography in children: A retrospective study. Arch Otolaryngol 102:482–486, 1976

Cullen JK, Ellis MS, Berlin CI, et al: Human acoustic nerve action potential recordings from the tympanic membrane without anesthesia. Acta Oto-Laryngol (Stockh) 74:15–22, 1972

Dagleish B: Communication preference and the social conditions of language learning in the deaf. Am Ann Deaf 120:70–77, 1975

Dahle AJ, McCollister FP, Hamner BA, et al: Subclinical congenital cytomegalovirus infection and hearing impairment. J Speech Hear Dis 39:320–329, 1974

Dale D: Applied Audiometry for Children. Springfield, Thomas, 1962

Dale PS: Language Development. New York, Holt, 1976

Dallos P: The Auditory Periphery, Biophysics and Physiology. New York, Academic, 1973

Daly DM, Roeser RJ, Moushegian G: The frequency-following response in subjects with profound unilateral hearing loss. Electroencephalogr Clin Neurophysiol 40:132–142, 1976

Danhauer JL, Singh S: A multidimensional scaling analysis of phonemic responses from hard-of-hearing and deaf subjects of three languages. Lang Speech 18:42–64, 1975

Davis H: Enhancement of evoked cortical potentials in humans related to a task requiring a decision. Science 145:182–183, 1964

Davis H: Sedation of young children for evoked response audiometry (ERA). Summary of a symposium. Audiology 12:55–57, 1973

Davis H: Brain stem and other responses in electric response audiometry. Ann Otol Rhinol Laryngol 85:3–14, 1976a

Davis H: Principles of electric response audiometry. Ann Otol Rhinol Laryngol 28–85 (Suppl):1–96, 1976b

Davis H, Davis PA, Loomis A, et al: Electrical reactions of the human brain to auditory stimulation during sleep. J Neurophysiol 2:500–514, 1939

Davis H, Derbyshire AJ, Lurie M, et al: The electric response of the cochlea. Am J Physiol 107:311–332, 1934

Davis H, Fernandez C, McAuliffe DP: The excitatory process in the cochlea. Proc Natl Acad Sci 36:580–587, 1950

Davis H, Gernandt BE, Riesco-MacClure JS, et al: Aural microphonics in the cochlea of the guinea pig. J Acoust Soc Am 21:502–510, 1949

Davis H, Hirsh SK: Clinical trial of fast responses of ERA. Third Symposium of the Intl Electric Response Audiometry Study Group, Bordeaux, 1973

Davis H, Hirsh SK: The audiometric utility of brain stem response to low-frequency

sounds. Audiology 15:181–195, 1976
Davis H, Hirsh SK, Shelnutt J, et al: Further validation of evoked response audiometry (ERA). J Speech Hear Res 10:717–732, 1967
Davis H, Mast TE, Yoshie N, et al: The slow response of the human cortex to auditory stimuli: recovery process. Electroencephalogr Clin Neurophysiol 21:105–113, 1966
Davis H, Onishi S: Maturation of auditory evoked potentials. Int Audiol 8:24–33, 1969
Davis H, Zerlin S: Acoustic relations of the human vertex potential. J Acoust Soc Am 39:109–116, 1966
Davis PA: Effects of acoustic stimuli on the waking human brain. J Neurophysiol 2:494–499, 1939
Davis RC, Buchwald AM, Frankmann RW: Autonomic and muscular responses and their relation to simple stimuli. Psychol Mono #405, 1955
Dawson G: Cerebral responses to electrical stimulation of peripheral nerve in man. J Neurol Neurosurg Psychiatry 10:134–140, 1947
Dawson WW, Doddington HW: Phase distortion of biological signals: extraction of signal from noise without phase error. Electroencephalogr Clin Neurophysiol 34:207–211, 1973
Derbyshire AJ, Fraser A, McDermott M, et al: Audiometric measurements by electroencephalography. Electroencephalogr Clin Neurophysiol 8:467–478, 1956
Desmedt JE, Brunko E, Debecker J, et al: The system bandpass required to avoid distortion of early components when averaging somatosensory potentials. Electroencephalogr Clin Neurophysiol 37:407–410, 1974
Desmond MM, Franklin RR, Vallbona C, et al: The clinical behavior of the newlyborn. J Pediatr 62:307–325, 1963
DiBartolomeo JR: The auditory system: Pre- and post-natal development. *In* Anon: Sensory and Perceptual Dysfunctioning in Infants: Identification, Diagnosis and Current Research. Univ So Calif School Med, Post-Grad Div, 1974
DiGeorge A, Olmsted RW, Harley RD: Waardenburg's syndrome. J Pediatr 57:649–669, 1960
Dix MR, Hallpike CS: The peep show: A new technique for pure tone audiometry in children. Br Med J 2:719–732, 1947
Djupesland G: Middle ear muscle reflexes elicited by acoustic and non-acoustic stimuli. Acta Oto-Laryngol (Stockh) Suppl 188:287–292, 1963
Djupesland G: Use of impedance indicator in diagnosis of middle ear pathology. Int Audiol 8:570–578, 1969
Djupesland G, Zwislocki J: The effect of temporal summation on the human stapedial reflex. Acta Oto-Laryngol (Stockh) 71:262–265, 1971
Doerfler LG: Neurophysiological clues to auditory acuity. J Speech Hear Dis 13:227–232, 1948
Dore J: A pragmatic description of early language development. J Psycholinguist Res 3:343–350, 1974
Downs MP: Testing hearing in infancy and early childhood. *In* McConnell F, Ward PH (eds): Deafness in Childhood. Nashville, Vanderbilt Univ Press, 1967
Downs MP: Early identification of hearing loss: Where are we? Where do we go from

here? *In* Mencher GT (ed): Early Identification of Hearing Loss. Basel, Karger, 1976

Downs MP, Sterritt GM: Identification audiometry in neonates: a preliminary report. J Aud Res 4:69–80, 1964

Downs MP, Sterritt GM: A guide to newborn and infant hearing screening programs. Arch Otolaryngol 85:15–22, 1967

duBois-Reymond E: Untersuchungen über thierische Electricität. Berlin, Reimer, 1848

Dublin WJ: Cytoarchitecture of the cochlear nuchlei. Arch Otolaryngol 100:355–359, 1974

Edwards D: Sensory-motor intelligence and semantic relations in early child grammar. Cognition 2:395–434, 1973

Eggermont JJ: Summating potentials in electrocochleography: Relation to hearing disorders. *In* Ruben RJ, Elberling C, Salomon G (eds): Electrocochleography. Baltimore, Univ Park, 1976

Eggermont JJ, Odenthal DW: Electrophysiological investigation of the human cochlea: Recruitment, masking, and adaptation. Audiology 13:1–22, 1974a

Eggermont JJ, Odenthal DW: Frequency selective masking in electrocochleography. Rev Laryngol 95:489–496, 1974b

Eggermont JJ, Odenthal DW: Methods in electrocochleography. *In* Eggermont JJ, Odenthal DW, Schmidt PH, et al (eds): Electrocochleography, Basic Principles and Clinical Application. Acta Oto-Laryngol (Stockh) Suppl 316:17–24, 1974c

Eggermont JJ, Odenthal DW, Schmidt PH, et al (eds): Electrocochleography, Basic Principles and Clinical Application. Acta Oto-Laryngol (Stockh) Suppl 316:5–84, 1974

Eggermont JJ, Spoor A, Odenthal DW: Frequency specificity of tone-burst electrocochleography. *In* Ruben RJ, Elberling C, Salomon G (eds): Electrocochleography. Baltimore, Univ Park, 1976

Eguchi S, Hirsh IJ: Development of speech sounds in children. Acta Oto-Laryngol (Stockh) Suppl 257:5–51, 1969

Eimas P, Siqueland E, Jusczyk P, et al: Speech perception in infants. Science 171:303–306, 1971

Eisenberg RB: Auditory behavior in the human neonate. Biennial meeting, Society for Research in Child Development, Minneapolis, 1965.

Eisenberg RB: Auditory behavior in the human neonate: functional properties of sound and their ontogenetic implications. Annual convention, American Speech and Hearing Association, Washington, 1966

Eisenberg RB: Auditory behavior in the human neonate: Functional properties of sound and their ontogenetic implications. Int Audiol 8:34–45, 1969

Eisenberg RB, Coursin DB, Rupp NR: Habituation to an acoustic pattern as an index of differences among human neonates. J Aud Res 6:239–248, 1966

Eisenberg RB, Marmarou A, Giovachino P: Infant heart rate changes to a synthetic speech sound. J Aud Res 14:21–28, 1974

Elberling C: Action potentials along the cochlear partition recorded from the ear canal in man. Scand Audiol 3:13–19, 1974

Elberling C, Salomon G: Electrical potentials from the inner ear in man in response to transient sounds generated in a closed acoustic system. Rev Laryngol Suppl:691–707, 1971

Elkin F: The Child and Society. New York, Random House, 1960

Ellingson RJ, Danahy I, Nelson B, et al: Variability of auditory evoked potentials in human newborns. Electroencephalogr Clin Neurophysiol 36:155–162, 1974

Engel R: Early waves of the electroencephalic auditory response in neonates. Neuropädiatrie 3:147–154, 1971

Engel R, Young NB: Calibrated pure tone audiograms in normal neonates based on evoked electroencephalographic responses. Neuropädiatrie 1:149–160, 1969

Evans TR, Deatherage BH: The effect of frequency on the auditory evoked response. Psychon Sci 15:95–96, 1969

Farrant R: The intellectual abilities of deaf and hearing children. Am Ann Deaf 109:306–325, 1964

Farwell R: Speech reading: A research review. Volta Rev 78:19–30, 1976

Feinmesser M, Tell L: Evaluation of methods for detecting hearing impairment in infancy and early childhood. *In* Mencher GT (ed): Early Identification of Hearing Loss. Basel, Karger, 1976

Feinmesser M, Tell L: Neonatal screening for detection of deafness. Arch Otolaryngol 102:297–299, 1976

Feldman A: Acoustic impedance measurement as a clinical procedure. Int Audiol 3:156–165, 1964

Ferris C, Newsom C: An experimental analysis of symptom substitution. Annual convention, Western Psychological Assn, San Francisco, 1974

Ferriss GS, Davis GD, Dorsen M, et al: Maturation of the evoked response to auditory stimuli in human infants. Electroencephalogr Clin Neurophysiol 23:83, 1967

Fillmore C: The case for case. *In* Bach E, Horms R (eds): Universals in Linguistic Theory. New York, Holt, 1968

Fisch L: Deafness as part of an hereditary syndrome. J Laryngol 73:355–382, 1959

Fisch L (ed): Research in Deafness in Children. Oxford, Blackwell, 1964

Fiske DW, Maddi SR: Functions of Varied Experience. Homewood IL, Dorsey, 1961

Fitzgerald M: Workshop in language for the deaf. Philadelphia School for the Deaf, 1961

Flottorp G, Djupesland G, Winther F: The acoustic reflex in relation to critical bandwidth. J Acoust Soc Am 49:457–461, 1971

Franceschetti A, Klein D: Wildervanck syndrome. J Genet Hum 3:176, 1954

Fraser GR: Profound childhood deafness. J Med Gen 1:118–150, 1964

Fraser GR: Genetic approaches to the nosology of deafness. *In* Bergsma D (ed): The Clinical Delineation of Birth Defects: Part IX: Ear. Baltimore, Williams and Wilkins for the National Foundation/March of Dimes, 1971

Fraser GR: Heredity, early identification of hearing loss, and the risk register. *In* Mencher GT (ed): Early Identification of Hearing Loss. Basel, Karger, 1976

Freedman DA: Congenital and perinatal sensory deprivation: Some studies in early development. Am J Psychiatry 127:115–121, 1971

Freeman R, Malkin S, Hasting J: Psychosocial problems of deaf children and their family: A comparative study. Am Ann Deaf 120:391–405, 1975

Fremer J, MacGinitie W: The content of controlled continuous word association. *In* Rosenstein J, MacGinitie W (eds): Verbal Behavior of the Deaf Child. New York, Teachers College Press, 1969

Friedlander BZ: Listening, language, and the auditory environment. *In* Hellmuth J (ed): Exceptional Infant. Vol. 2, Studies in Abnormalities. New York, Brunner/Mazel, 1971

Fries CC: The Structure of English. New York, Harcourt, Brace Jovanovich, 1952

Frisina DR: Measurement of hearing in children. *In* Jerger JF (ed): Modern Developments in Audiology. New York, Academic, 1963

Fröding CA: Acoustic investigation of newborn infants. Acta Oto-Laryngol (Stockh) 52:31–40, 1960

Froeschels E, Beebe H: Testing the hearing of newborn infants. Arch Otolaryngol 44:710–714, 1946

Fromm B, Nylen CO, Zotterman Y: Studies in the mechanism of the Wever and Bray effect. Acta Oto-Laryngol (Stockh) 22:477–486, 1935

Fry DB: Phonological aspects of language acquisition in the hearing and the deaf. *In* Lenneberg EH, Lenneberg E (eds): Foundations of Language Development. New York, Academic, 1975

Furth H: Thinking Without Language. New York, Free Press, 1966

Furth H: A review and perspective on the thinking of deaf people. *In* Hellmuth J (ed): Cognitive Studies. New York, Brunner/Mazel, 1967

Furth H: A review and perspective on the thinking of deaf people. *In* Hellmuth J (ed): Cognitive Studies. New York, Brunner/Mazel, 1970

Furth H: Deafness and Learning. Belmont CA, Wadsworth, 1973

Furth H, Youniss J: Formal operations and language: A comparison of deaf and hearing adolescents. Int J Psychol 6:49–64, 1971

Gardi JN, McKean CM, Merzenich M: Origins of brainstem frequency following response. Annual convention, American Speech and Hearing Association, Chicago, 1977

Garrabrint E, Robertson E, Biggers W: Tympanometry and acoustic impedance changes in newborns. Unpublished.

Geisler C, Frishkopf L, Rosenblith W: Extracranial responses to acoustic clicks in man. Science 128:1210–1211, 1958

Gerber SE: Auditory behavioral responses of some hearing infants. Volta Rev 71:340–346, 1969

Gerber SE: Neonatal auditory testing: A review. *In* Cunningham GC (ed): Conference on Newborn Hearing Screening. Berkeley, California Dept of Health, 1971

Gerber SE: Biomedical technology and the detection of birth defects. Rehab Lit 33:322–325, 1972

Gerber SE: Introductory Hearing Science. Philadelphia, Saunders, 1974

Gerber SE: Unpublished report on behalf of California Dept of Health, Bureau of Maternal and Child Health, 1976

Gerber SE, Cone BK: A study of impedance audiometry in infants. Annual convention, Society for Ear, Nose, and Throat Advances in Children, Mexico City, 1975

Gerber SE, Gilchrist DB: Respiratory rate changes of neonates as responses to speech stimuli. Unpublished.

Gerber SE, Mulac A, Kizziah KT: Effects of respiratory phase on the cardiovascular response to sound. In preparation.

Gerber SE, Mulac A, Lamb ME: The cardiovascular response to acoustic stimuli. Audiology 16:1–10, 1977

Gerber SE, Mulac A, Swain BJ: Idiosyncratic cardiovascular response of human neonates to acoustic stimuli. J Am Audiol Soc 1:185–191, 1976

Gerber SE, Mulac A, Swain BJ: Cardiovascular responses to sound in human neonates. *In* Mencher GT (ed): Early Identification of Hearing Loss. Basel, Karger, 1976

Gerken GM, Moushegian G, Stillman RD, et al: Human frequency-following responses to monaural and binaural stimuli. Electroencephalogr Clin Neurophysiol 38:379–386, 1975

Gerull G, Giesen M, Mrowinski D, et al: Properties of an early AER of 5–10 ms latency. Rev Laryngol 95:560–565, 1974

Getz S: Environment and the Deaf Child. Springfield, Thomas, 1953

Gibbs FA, Davis H, Lennox W: The electroencephalogram in epilepsy and in conditions of impaired consciousness. Arch Neurol Psychiatry 3:1133–1148, 1935

Gidoll SH: Quantitative determination of hearing to audiometric frequencies in the electroencephalogram: Preliminary report. Arch Otolaryngol 55:597–601, 1952

Glaser EM, Suter CM, Dashieff R, et al: The human frequency-following response: Its behavior during continuous tone burst stimulation. Electroencephalogr Clin Neurophysiol 40:25–32, 1976

Glorig A, Curtis GA: Considerations in implementing program of identification and evaluation of deaf persons (birth to twenty-one) in Texas. *In* Mencher GT (ed): Early Identification of Hearing Loss. Basel, Karger, 1976

Goda S: Spoken syntax of normal, deaf, and retarded adolescents. J Verbal Learning Verbal Beh 3:401–405, 1964

Goetzinger CP: Effects of small perceptive losses on language and on speech discrimination. Volta Rev 64:408–414, 1962

Goetzinger CP, Rousey CA: Educational achievement of deaf children. Am Ann Deaf 104:221–231, 1959

Goff W: Human average evoked potentials: Procedures for stimulating and recording. *In* Thompson R, Patterson M (eds): Bioelectric Recording Techniques, Part B, Electroencephalography and Human Brain Potentials. New York, Academic, 1974

Goff W, Allison T, Lyons W, et al: Origins of short latency auditory evoked response components in man. *In* Desmedt J (ed): Cerebral Evoked Potentials in Man. In press.

Goldenberg RA, Derbyshire AJ: Averaged evoked potentials in cats with lesions of auditory pathway. J Speech Hear Res 18:420–429, 1975

Goldin-Meadow S, Feldman H: The creation of a communication system: A study of deaf children of hearing parents. Sign Lang Stud 8:225–236, 1975

Goldstein MH: The auditory periphery. *In* Mountcastle V (ed): Medical Physiology (Vol 1). St Louis, Mosby, 1974

Goldstein MH, Stark RE: Modification of vocalizations of preschool deaf children by vibrotactile and visual displays. J Acoust Soc Am 59:1477–1481, 1976

Goldstein MJ: Cardiac rate response to acoustic stimuli in one-, two-, and three-month-old infants. Unpublished master's thesis, University of California, Santa Barbara, 1972

Goldstein R, McRandle CC: Middle components of the averaged electroencephalic response to clicks in neonates. *In* Hirsh SK, Eldredge DH, Hirsh IJ, et al (eds): Hearing and Davis: Essays Honoring Hallowell Davis. St Louis, Washington Univ Press, 1976

Goldstein R, Rodman LB, Karlovich RS: Effects of stimulus rate and number on the early components of the averaged electroencephalic response. J Speech Hear Res 15:559–566, 1972

Goodhill V: Auditory pathway lesions resulting from Rh incompatability. *In* McConnell F, Ward PH (eds): Deafness in Childhood. Nashville, Vanderbilt Univ Press, 1967

Goodhill V, Lowell EL, Lowell MO: Computerized objective auditory testing in infancy. Final report of project DHEW H-181, 1970

Goodman WS, Appleby SV, Scott JW, et al: Audiometry in newborn children by electroencephalography. Laryngoscope 74:1316–1328, 1964

Graham FK, Clifton RK: Heart rate change as a component of the orienting response. Psychol Bull 65:305–320, 1966

Graham FK, Clifton RK, Hatton HM: Habituation of heart rate response to repeated auditory stimulation during the first five days of life. Child Dev 39:35–52, 1968

Graziani LJ, Weitzman ED, Velasco MSA: Neurologic maturation and auditory evoked responses in low birth weight infants. Peds 41:483–494, 1968

Green DS: The pup-show: a simple inexpensive modification of the peep-show. J Speech Hear Dis 23:118–120, 1958

Greenfield P, Smith H: The Structure of Communication in Early Language Development. New York, Academic, 1976

Greenough WT: Experiential modification of the developing brain. Am Sci 63:37–46, 1975

Greenough WT, Volkmar FR, Juraska JM: Effects of rearing complexity on dendritic branching in frontolateral and temporal cortex of the rat. Exp Neurol 41:371–378, 1973

Greenough WT, Wood WE, Madden TC: Possible memory storage differences among mice reared in environments varying in complexity. Behav Biol 7:712–722, 1972

Griffiths C: Auditory training in the first year of life. International Conference on Oral Education of the Deaf, Northampton, MA, 1967

Grisanti G, Restivo S, LaBarbera L: Risultati dell'audiometria comportamentale nei neonati a termine. Il Valsalva 47:161–170, 1971

Gustason G, Rosen R: Effective sign communication for instructional purposes: Manual English and American sign language. Convention of Am Instr Deaf, North Carolina, 1975

Habener S, Snyder J: Stapedius reflex amplitude and decay in normal hearing ears. Arch Otolaryngol 100:294–297, 1974

Haller MW: The reactions of infants to changes in the intensity and pitch of pure tones. J Gen Psychol 40:162–180, 1932

Halliday M: Learning How to Mean. London, Arnold, 1975

Hallpike CS, Rawdon-Smith A: The origin of the Wever–Bray phenomenon. J Physiol 83:243–254, 1934

Hamilton LR, Derbyshire AJ, Joseph ME: Testing variables in infant audiometry. Annual convention of the American Speech and Hearing Association, New York, 1970

Hardy JW: Studies in hearing in neonates. *In* Davis H (ed): The Young Deaf Child: Identification and Management. Acta Oto-Laryngol (Stockh) Suppl 206:34–36, 1965

Hardy WG: Evaluation of hearing in infants and young children. *In* Glorig A (ed): Audiometry: Principles and Practices. Baltimore, Williams and Wilkins, 1965

Harker LA, Hosick EC, Voots RJ, et al: Influence of succinylcholine on middle component auditory evoked potentials. Arch Otolaryngol 103:133–137, 1977

Harlow HF, Zimmerman RR: Affectional responses in the infant monkey. Science 130:421–432, 1959

Harlow MK, Harlow HF: Affection in primates. Discovery 27:11–17, 1966

Hawkins JE Jr: Iatrogenic toxic deafness in children. *In* McConnell F, Ward PH (eds): Deafness in Childhood. Nashville, Vanderbilt Univ Press, 1967

Hecox K: Electrophysiological correlates of human auditory development. *In* Cohen LB, Salapatek P (eds): Infant Perception from Sensation to Cognition, Vol II: Perception of Space, Speech, and Sound. New York, Academic, 1975

Hecox K, Galambos R: Brain stem auditory evoked responses in human infants and adults. Arch Otolaryngol 99:30–33, 1974

Hecox K, Squires N, Galambos R: Brainstem auditory evoked responses in man. I. Effect of stimulus rise–fall time and duration. J Acoust Soc Am 60:1187–1198, 1976

Heider F, Heider G: A comparison of sentence structure of deaf and hearing children. Psychol Monogr 52:42–103, 1940

Hemenway WG, Bergstrom L: The pathology of acquired viral endolabyrinthitis. *In* McConnell F, Ward PH (eds): Deafness in Childhood. Nashville, Vanderbilt Univ Press, 1967

Henderson D: Behavioral and human evoked response thresholds as a function of frequency. J Speech Hear Res 15:390–394, 1972

Herer GR: Evaluation of hearing in infants and young children. Clin Proc Child Hosp Wash 23:18–33, 1967

Hermelin B, O'Connor N: Psychological Experiments with Autistic Children. Oxford, Pergamon, 1971

Heron TG, Jacobs R: A physiological response of the neonate to auditory stimulation. Int Audiol 7:41–47, 1968

Heron TG, Jacobs R: Respiratory curve responses of the neonate to auditory stimulation. Int Audiol 8:71–84, 1969

Hillis JW, Oyer HJ: Success of play audiometry as a function of chronological age. Annual convention, American Speech and Hearing Assn, Los Angeles, 1960

Hood DC: Central effects on the human peripheral auditory system. Unpublished doctoral dissertation, Northwestern Univ, 1971

Hood DC: Evoked cortical response audiometry. *In* Bradford LJ (ed): Physiological Measures of the Audio-Vestibular System. New York, Academic, 1975

Horwitz S, Larson S, Sances A: Evoked potentials as an adjunct to the auditory evaluation of patients. Proc Symp Biomed Eng 1:49–52, 1966

Hosick E, Mendel MI: Effects of secobarbitol on the late components of the auditory evoked potentials. Rev Laryngol 96:185–191, 1975

Hrbek A, Hrbkova M, Lenard H: Somato-sensory, auditory, and visual evoked responses in newborn infants during sleep and wakefulness. Electroencephalogr Clin Neurophysiol 26:597–603, 1969

Hubel DH: Effects of distortion of sensory input on the visual system of kittens. Physiologist 10:17–45, 1967

Hubel DH, Wiesel TN: The period of susceptibility to the physiological effects of unilateral eye closure in kittens. J Physiol 206:419–436, 1970

Hudgins CV, Numbers FT: An investigation of the intelligibility of the speech of deaf and normal subjects. Genet Psychol Monogr 25:289–392, 1942

Hung I, Dallos P: Study of the acoustic reflex in human beings. I: Dynamic characteristics. J Acoust Soc Am 52:1168–1180, 1972

Hutt SJ, Hutt C, Lee D, et al: A behavioral and electroencephalographic study of autistic children. J Psychiatr Res 3:181–197, 1965

Hyde ML, Stephens SDG, Thornton ARD: Stimulus repetition rate and the early brainstem responses. Br J Audiol 10:41–50, 1976

Innitzer J, Schmid E: General anesthesia in children—a modified ketamine hydrochloride application. Bienniel meeting, International Electric Response Audiometry Study Group, London, 1975

Irwin OC: Effect of strong light on the body activity of newborns. J Comp Psychol 32:233–236, 1941

Irwin OC, Weiss LA: Differential variations in the activity and crying of the newborn infant under different intensities of light: a comparison of observational with polygraph findings. Univ Iowa Stud Child Welfare 9:139–147, 1934

Irwin OC, Weiss LA: The effect of clothing on the general vocal activity of the newborn infant. Univ Iowa Stud Child Welfare 9:151–162, 1934

Irwin OC, Weiss LA: The effect of darkness on the activity of newborn infants. Univ Iowa Stud Child Welfare 9:163–175, 1934

Itakura S: Electroencephalography and sound stimulation. Folia Psychiatr Neurol Jpn 9:280–281, 1955

Jaffe BF: Pinna anomalies associated with congenital conductive hearing loss. Pediatrics 57:332–341, 1976

Jasper HH, Carmichael L: Electrical potentials from the intact human brain. Science 81:51–53, 1935

Jazbi B: Audiometry for children. Ninth International Congress on Audiology, London, 1968

Jepsen O: Middle ear muscle reflexes in man. *In* Jerger JF (ed): Modern Developments in Audiology. New York, Academic, 1963

Jerger JF: Clinical experience with impedance audiometry. Arch Otolaryngol 92:311–324, 1970

Jerger JF, Armstrong L, Jerger S, et al: Studies in impedance audiometry. III: Middle ear disorders. Arch Otolaryngol 99:165–191, 1974

Jerger JF, Burney P, Mauldin L, et al: Predicting hearing loss from the acoustic reflex. J Speech Hearing Dis 39:11–22, 1974

Jerger JF, Harford E, Clemis J, et al: The acoustic reflex in eighth nerve disorders. Arch Otolaryngol 99:409–413, 1974

Jerger JF, Jerger S, Mauldin L: Studies in impedance audiometry. I: Normal and sensorineural ears. Arch Otolaryngol 96:513–523, 1972

Jerger S, Jerger JF, Segal P, et al: Studies in impedance audiometry. II: Children less than six years old. Arch Otolaryngol 99:1–9, 1974

Jewett DL: Averaged volume-conducted potentials to auditory stimuli in the cat. Physiologist 12:262, 1969

Jewett DL: Volume-conducted potentials in response to auditory stimuli as detected by averaging in the cat. Electroencephalogr Clin Neurophysiol 28:609–618, 1970

Jewett DL, Romano MN: Neonatal development of auditory system potentials averaged from the scalp of rat and cat. Brain Res 36:101–115, 1972

Jewett DL, Romano MN, Williston JS: Human auditory evoked potentials: Possible brain stem components detected on the scalp. Science 167:1517–1518, 1970

Jewett DL, Williston JS: Auditory-evoked far fields averaged from the scalp of humans. Brain 94:681–696, 1971

Johansson B, Wedenberg E, Westin B: Measurement of tone response by the human foetus. Acta Oto-Laryngol (Stockh) 57:188–192, 1964

John GEG, Howarth GN: The effect of time distortions on the intelligibility of deaf children's speech. Lang Speech 8:127–134, 1965

Johnson D: Communication characteristics of a young deaf adult population: Technique for evaluating their communication skills. Am Ann Deaf 121:409–424, 1976

Johnson DM, Johnson RG, Mark AL: A mathematical analysis of verbal fluency. J Gen Psychol 44:121–128, 1951

Jones C, Goodman M, Wepman J: The classification of parts of speech for the characterization of aphasics. Lang Speech 6:94–104, 1963

Jordan RE: Symposium: Conservation of hearing in children. Trans Am Acad Ophthalmol Otolaryngol 76:340–342, 1971

Kanner L: Autistic disturbances of affective contact. Nerv Child 2:217–250, 1943

Kapur YP: panel discussion in Jazbi B (ed): Pediatric Otorhinolaryngology. Otolaryngol Clin North Am 10(1):248–252, 1977

Kates S, Yudin L, Tiffany R: Concept attainment by deaf and hearing adolescents. J Educ Psychol 53:119–126, 1962

Keating LW, Ruhm HB: Some observations on the effects of attention to stimuli on the amplitude of the acoustically evoked response. Audiology 10:177–184, 1971

Keith R: Impedance audiometry with neonates. Arch Otolaryngol 97:465–467, 1973

Keith R: The use of impedance measurements in infant hearing programs. *In* Mencher GT (ed): Early Identification of Hearing Loss. Basel, Karger, 1976

Kent G, Rosanoff A: A study of association in insanity. Am J Insanity 67:37–96, 317–390, 1910

Khechinashvili SN, Kevanishvili ZS: Experiences in computer audiometry (ECoG and ERA). Audiology 13:391–402, 1974

Khechinashvili SN, Kevanishvili ZS, Kajaia OA: Amplitude and latency studies of the averaged auditory evoked responses to tones of different intensities. Acta Oto-Laryngol (Stockh) Suppl 76:395–401, 1973

Khechinashvili SN, Kevanishvili ZS, Khachjdze OA, et al: Electrocochleographical studies in humans. Br J Audiol 8:6–13, 1974

Kish GB: Studies of sensory reinforcement. *In* Honig WK (ed): Operant Behavior: Areas of Research and Application. New York, Appleton, 1966

Klima E, Bellugi U: Syntactic regularities in the speech of children. *In* Lyons J, Wales R (eds): Psycholinguistic Papers. Edinburgh, Edinburgh Univ Press, 1966

Klockhoff I: Middle ear muscle reflexes in man. Acta Oto-Laryngol (Stockh) Suppl 164:1–92, 1961

Klockhoff I: Clinical use of ear impedance measurements. J Laryngol Otol 85:243–254, 1971

Koegel RL, Covert A: The relationship of self-stimulation to learning in autistic children. J Appl Behav Anal 5:381–387, 1972

Koegel RL, Firestone PB, Kramme KW, et al: Increasing spontaneous play by suppressing self-stimulation in autistic children. J Appl Behav Anal 7:521–528, 1974

Koegel RL, Schreibman L: Identification of consistent responding to auditory stimuli by a functionally "deaf" autistic child. J Aut Child Schizophr 6:147–156, 1976

Konigsmark BW: Hereditary congenital severe deafness syndromes. Ann Otol Rhinol Laryngol 80:269–289, 1971

Konigsmark BW: Hereditary and congenital factors affecting newborn sensorineural hearing. *In* Cunningham GC (ed): Conference on Newborn Hearing Screening. Berkeley, California Dept of Health, 1971

Konigsmark BW: Syndromal approaches to the nosology of hereditary deafness. *In* Bergsma D (ed): The Clinical Delineation of Birth Defects: Part IX, Ear. Baltimore, Williams and Wilkins, for the National Foundation/March of Dimes, 1971

Konigsmark BW, McKusick VA: Hereditary deafness. Volta Rev 68:336–341, 380, 1966

Koplin J, Odom P, Blanton RL, et al: Word association test performance of deaf subjects. J Speech Hear Res 10:126–132, 1967

Krech D, Rosenzweig MR, Bennett E: Environmental impoverishment, social isolation and changes in brain chemistry and anatomy. Physiol Behav 1:99–104, 1966

Kroger WS, Freed SC: Psychosomatic Gynecology. Glencoe, IL, Free Press, 1956

Kubler-Ross E: On Death and Dying. New York, Macmillan, 1969

Kumpf W: Objective hearing test by delayed acoustic stimuli-coupling with breathing sounds. Arch Klin Exp Ohren-Nasen Kehlkopfheilkd 186:80–97, 1966

Kumpf W, Landwehr FJ: Integrated level diagrams of breathing sounds. A useful supplement to breath sound audiometry. Monatsschr Ohrenheilkd Laryngol-Rhinol 12:535–539, 1970

Kumpf W, Munster W: Determination of the hearing threshold beginning with the age of infancy by stimulus synchronous level diagrams of the breathing sound. Arch Klin Exp Ohren-Nasen Kehlkopfheilkd 191:593–597, 1968

Kupperman GL: Effects of three stimulus parameters on the early components of the averaged electroencephalic response. Unpublished doctoral dissertation, Univ Wisconsin, 1970

Kupperman GL, Mendel MI: Threshold of the early components of the averaged electroencephalic response determined with tone pips and clicks during drug-induced sleep. Audiology 13:379–390, 1974

Labov W: The Study of Nonstandard English, Washington, Center for Applied Linguistics, 1969

Lacey JI: The evaluation of autonomic responses: Toward a general solution. Ann NY Acad Sci 67:123–164, 1956

Lane RH, Kupperman GL, Goldstein R: Early components of the averaged electroencephalic response in relation to rise–decay time and duration of pure tones. J Speech Hear Res 14:408–415, 1971

Lane RH, Mendel MI, Kupperman GL, et al: Phase distortion of averaged electroencephalic response. Arch Otolaryngol 99:428–432, 1974

Lehiste I: Suprasegmental features of speech. *In* Lass N (ed): Contemporary Issues in Experimental Phonetics. New York, Academic, 1976

Leiberman A, Sohmer H, Szabo G: Cochlear audiometry (electro-cochleography) during neonatal period. Dev Med Child Neurol 15:8–13, 1973a

Leiberman A, Sohmer H, Szabo G: Standard values of amplitude and latency of cochlear audiometry (electro-cochleography) responses in different age groups. Arch Klin Exp Ohren-Nasen Kehlkopfheilkd 203:267–273, 1973b

Lempert J, Meltzer PE, Wever EG, et al: The cochleogram and its clinical applications. Concluding observations. Arch Otolaryngol 51:307–311, 1950

Lempert J, Wever EG, Lawrence M: The cochleogram and its clinical applications. A preliminary report. Arch Otolaryngol 45:61–67, 1947

Lenard H, von Bernuth H, Hutt SJ: Acoustic evoked responses in newborn infants: The influence of pitch and complexity of the stimulus. Electroencephalogr Clin Neurophysiol 27:121–127, 1969

Lenneberg EH: The natural history of language. *In* Smith F, Miller GA (eds): The Genesis of Language. Cambridge, MIT Press, 1966

Lenneberg EH: Biological Foundations of Language. New York, Wiley, 1967

Lenneberg EH, Rebelsky FG, Nichols IA: The vocalizations of infants born to deaf and hearing parents. Human Dev 8:23–27, 1965

Lentz WE, McCandless GA: Averaged electroencephalic audiometry in infants. J Speech Hear Dis 36:19–28, 1971

Letein W, Bess F: Acoustic reflex relaxation in sensorineural hearing loss. Arch Otolaryngol 101:617–621, 1975

Lev A, Sohmer H: Sources of averaged neural responses recorded in animal and human subjects during cochlear audiometry. Arch Klin Exp Ohren-Nasen Kehlkopfheilkd 201:79–90, 1972

Lewis M: A developmental study of the cardiac response to stimulus onset and offset during the first year of life. Psychophysiology 8:689–698, 1971

Lewis M, Bartels B, Goldberg S: State as a determinant of infants' heart rate response to stimulation. Science 155:486–488, 1967

Lewis M, Freedle R: Mother–Infant Dyad: The Cradle of Meaning. Bethesda, ERIC Document Repro Service, ED 067 149, 1972

Lilly D: Acoustic impedance at the tympanic membrane: an overview of clinical applications. *In* Rose D, Keating L (comps): Impedance Symposium. Chicago, Zenith Hearing Inst Corp, 1972

Lindsley D: Average evoked potentials—Achievements, failures, and prospects. *In* Donchin E, Lindsley D (eds): Average Evoked Potentials: Methods, Results, and Evaluations. Washington, National Aeronautics and Space Administration, 1969

Ling D, Ling AH, Doehring DG: Stimulus, response, and observer variables in the auditory screening of newborn infants. J Speech Hearing Res 13:9–18, 1970

Lipton EL, Steinschneider A, Richmond JB: Autonomic function in the neonate. Psychosom Med 22:57–65, 1960

Lloyd LL: Behavioral audiometry viewed as an operant procedure. J Speech Hearing Dis 31:128–135, 1966

Lloyd LL, Cox BP: Behavioral audiometry with children. *In* Glasscock ME III (ed): Sensorineural Hearing Loss in Children: Early Detection and Intervention. Otolaryngol Clin North Am 8(1):89–107, 1975

Lloyd LL, Spradlin JE, Reid MJ: An operant audiometric procedure for difficult-to-test patients. J Speech Hear Dis 33:236–245, 1968

Loomis A, Harvey E, Hobart G: Potential rhythms of the cerebral cortex during sleep. Science 81:597–598, 1935

Lovaas OI: Behavior therapy approach to the treatment of childhood schizophrenia. *In* Hill JP (ed): Minnesota Symposia on Child Development. Minneapolis, Univ Minnesota Press, 1967

Lovaas OI, Schreibman L, Koegel RL, et al: Selective responding by autistic children to multiple sensory impact. J Abnorm Psychol 77:211–222, 1971

Lovaas OI, Simmons JQ: Manipulation of self-destruction in three retarded children. J Appl Behav Anal 2:143–157, 1969

Lowell EL, Troffer C, Warburton E, et al: Temporal evannation: A new approach in diagnostic audiology. J Speech Hearing Dis 25:340–345, 1960

Lowell EL, Williams CT, Ballinger RM, et al: Measurement of auditory threshold with a special purpose analog computer. J Speech Hear Res 4:105–112, 1961

Lunde A: The sociology of the deaf. *In* Stokoe W (ed): Studies in Linguistics. Buffalo, Univ Buffalo, 1960

MacGinitie W: Ability of deaf children to use different word classes. J Speech Hear Res 7:141–150, 1964

Madell JR, Goldstein R: Relation between loudness and the amplitude of the early components of the averaged electroencephalic response. J Speech Hear Res 15:134–141, 1972

Mahoney T: Personal communication, 1977

Marcus RE, Gibbs EL, Gibbs FA: Electroencephalography in diagnosis of hearing loss in the very young child. Dis Nerv Syst 10:170–173, 1949

Margolis R, Popelka RJ: Static and dynamic acoustic impedance measurements in infant ears. J Speech Hearing Res 18:435–443, 1975

Markowicz H: Some sociological considerations of American sign language. Sign Lang Stud 2:15–37, 1972

Marquis DP: Can conditioned responses be conditioned in the newborn infant? J Genet Psychol 39:479–492, 1931

Marsh JT, Brown WS, Smith JC: Farfield recorded frequency-following responses: correlates of low pitch auditory perception in humans. Electroencephalogr Clin Neurophysiol 38:113–120, 1975

Martin JL, Coats AC: Short-latency auditory evoked responses recorded from human nasopharynx. Brain Res 60:496–502, 1973

Mast TE: Short-latency human evoked responses to clicks. J Appl Physiol

20:725–730, 1965

McCandless GA: Clinical applications of evoked response audiometry. J Speech Hear Res 10:468–478, 1967

McCandless GA: Electroencephalic audiometry. *In* Rose D (ed): Audiological Assessment. Englewood Cliffs, NJ, Prentice–Hall, 1971

McCandless GA: Reflex measurement related to diagnosis. *In* Rose D, Keating L (comps): Impedance Symposium. Chicago, Zenith Hearing Instrument Corp, 1972

McCandless GA, Best L: Summed evoked responses using pure-tone stimuli. J Speech Hear Res 9:256–262, 1966

McCandless GA, Rose DE: Evoked cortical responses to stimulus change. J Speech Hear Res 13:624–634, 1970

McFarland W, Vivion M, Goldstein R: Middle components of the AER as a response index of threshold audiometry on normal and pathologic subjects. Annual convention, American Speech and Hearing Assn, Las Vegas, 1974

McFarland W, Vivion MC, Wolf KE, et al: Reexamination of effects of stimulus rate and number on the middle components of the averaged electroencephalic response. Audiology 14:456–465, 1975

McGettigen J, Rosenstein J: The influence of associative strength on identification of word meanings. *In* Rosenstein J, MacGinitie W (eds): Verbal Behavior of the Deaf Child. New York, Teachers College Pr, 1969

McNeill D: The creation of language by children. *In* Lyons J, Wales R (eds): Psycholinguistic Papers, Edinburgh, Edinburgh Univ Press, 1966

McRandle CC, Smith MA, Goldstein R: Early averaged electroencephalic responses to clicks in neonates. Ann Otol Rhinol Laryngol 83:695–702, 1974

Meadow K: Early manual communication in relation to the deaf child's intellectual, social and communicative functioning. Am Ann Deaf 113:29–41, 1968

Mencher GT: The University of Nebraska neonatal hearing project. Eleventh International Congress of Audiology, Budapest, 1972

Mencher GT: Report of a visit to Israel and Yugoslavia. Lincoln, Univ of Nebraska, 1972

Mencher GT: A program for neonatal hearing screening. Audiology 13:495–500, 1974

Mencher GT (ed): Early Identification of Hearing Loss. Basel, Karger, 1976

Mencher GT: Perinatal hearing assessment. *In* Jazbi B (ed): Pediatric Otorhinolaryngology. Otolaryngol Clin North Am 10(1):177–182, 1977

Mendel MI: Influence of stimulus level and sleep stage on the early components of the averaged electroencephalic response to clicks during all-night sleep. J Speech Hear Res 17:5–17, 1974

Mendel MI, Adkinson CD, Harker LA: Middle components of the auditory evoked potentials in infants. Ann Otol Rhinol Laryngol 86:293–299, 1977

Mendel MI, Goldstein R: The effect of test conditions on the early components of the averaged electroencephalic response. J Speech Hear Res 12:344–350, 1969a

Mendel MI, Goldstein R: Stability of the early components of the averaged electroencephalic response. J Speech Hear Res 12:351–361, 1969b

Mendel MI, Goldstein R: Early components of the averaged electroencephalic response to constant level clicks during all-night sleep. J Speech Hear Res 14:829–840, 1971

Mendel MI, Hosick EC: Effects of secobarbitol on the early components of the auditory evoked potentials. Rev Laryngol 96:178–184, 1975

Mendel MI, Hosick EC, Adkinson C: Effects of diazepam on the middle components of the auditory evoked potentials: A preliminary report. Combined meeting, Western Electroencephalography Society and Central Association of Electroencephalographers, Denver, 1974

Mendel MI, Hosick EC, Windman TR, et al: Audiometric comparison of the middle and late components of the adult auditory evoked potentials awake and asleep. Electroencephalogr Clin Neurophysiol 38:27–33, 1975

Mendel MI, Kupperman GL: Early components of the averaged electroencephalic response to constant level clicks during rapid eye movement sleep. Audiology 13:23–32, 1974

Mendel MI, Pals L. Harker LA: Two years' clinical experience with the middle components of the auditory evoked potentials. Annual convention, American Speech and Hearing Association, Houston, 1976

Menyuk P: The Development of Speech. Indianapolis, Bobbs–Merrill, 1972

Metz O: Threshold of reflex contractions of muscles of middle ear and recruitment of loudness. Arch Otolaryngol 55:536–543, 1952

Meyer DH, Wolfe VI: Use of a high-risk register in newborn hearing screening. J Speech Hear Dis 40:493–498, 1975

Miyazaki K: Teddy-bear screening audiometry for infants and mentally retarded children. Tenth International Congress of Audiology, Dallas, 1970

Mokotoff BL, Schulman-Galambos CA, Galambos R: Brain stem auditory evoked responses in children. Arch Otolaryngol 103:38–43, 1977

Møller A: The middle ear. *In* Tobias J (ed): Foundations of Modern Auditory Theory, Vol 2. New York, Academic, 1972

Møller K, Blegvad B: Brainstem responses in patients with sensorineural hearing loss: monaural versus binaural stimulation. The significance of the audiogram configuration. Scand Audiol 5:115–127, 1976

Monod N, Garma L: Auditory responsitivity in the human premature. Biol Neonate 17:292–316, 1971

Monsen RB: Durational aspects of selected consonant–vowel combinations in the speech of deaf and normally hearing children. J Speech Hear Res 17:386–398, 1974

Monsen RB: Normal and reduced phonological space: The production of English vowels by deaf adolescents. J Phonetics 4:189–198, 1976

Monsen RB: Second formant transitions of selected consonant–vowel combinations in the speech of deaf and normal-hearing children. J Speech Hear Res 19:279–289, 1976

Monsen RB, Engebertson AM, Fisher WM: Some characteristics of the glottal sound source of deaf children. J Acoust Soc Am 56:561A, 1974

Montandon PB, Megill ND, Kahn AR, et al: Recording auditory-nerve potentials as an office procedure. Ann Otol Rhinol Laryngol 84:2–10, 1975

Montandon PB, Shepard NT, Marr EM, et al: Auditory-nerve potentials from ear canals of patients with otologic problems. Ann Otol Rhinol Laryngol 84:164–173, 1975

Montgomery G: The relationship of oral skills to manual communication in profoundly deaf students. Am Ann Deaf 111:557–565, 1966

Moore EJ: Human cochlear microphonics and auditory nerve action potentials from surface electrodes. Unpublished doctoral dissertation, Univ Wisconsin, 1971

Moore EJ, Rose DE: Variability of latency and amplitude of acoustically evoked responses to pure tones of moderate to high intensities. Int Audiol 8:172–181, 1969

Moores D: Psycholinguistics and deafness. Am Ann Deaf 115:37–48, 1970

Moreau T, Birch HG, Turkewitz G: Ease of habituation to repeated auditory and somesthetic stimulation in the human newborn. J Exp Child Psychol 9:193–207, 1970

Morgon A, Charachon D, Gerin P: Electro-encephalographic audiometry for young children. Arch Klin Exp Ohren-Nasen Kehlkopfheilkd 198:144–150, 1971

Mouney DF, Cullen JK, Gondra MI, et al: Tone burst electrocochleography in humans. Trans Am Acad Ophthalmol Otolaryngol 82:348–355, 1976

Moushegian G, Rupert AL, Stillman RD: Scalp-recorded early responses in man to frequencies in the speech range. Electroencephalogr Clin Neurophysiol 35:665–667, 1973

Myers EN, Stool SE: Cytomegalic inclusion disease of the inner ear. Laryngoscope 78:1904–1915, 1968

Myklebust HR: Auditory Disorders in Children. New York, Grune & Stratton, 1954

Myklebust HR: Psychological effects of deafness. Am Ann Deaf 105:372–385, 1960

Myklebust HR: The Psychology of Deafness (2nd ed). New York, Grune & Stratton, 1964

Myklebust HR: Development and Disorders of Written Language. New York, Grune & Stratton, 1967

Nance WE, Setleff R, McLeod A, et al: X-linked mixed deafness with congenital fixation of the stapedial footplate and perilymphatic gusher. *In* Bergsma D (ed): The Clinical Delineation of Birth Defects: Part IX, Ear. Baltimore, Williams and Wilkins, for the National Foundation/March of Dimes, 1971

Nance WE, Sweeney A: Genetic factors in deafness of early life. *In* Glasscock ME III (ed): Sensorineural Hearing Loss in Children: Early Detection and Intervention. Otolaryngol Clin North Am 8(1):19–48, 1975

Nash J: Cues or signs: A case study in language acquisition. Sign Lang Stud 8:79–91, 1975

Naunton RF, Zerlin S: Basis and some diagnostic implications of electrocochleography. Laryngoscope 86:475–482, 1976a

Naunton RF, Zerlin S: Human whole-nerve response to clicks of various frequency. Audiology 15:1–9, 1976b

Neergaard E, Rasmussen P: Latency of the stapedius muscle reflex in man. Arch Otolaryngol 84:173–180, 1966

Nelson DA, Lassman FM: Effects of intersignal interval on the human auditory evoked response. J Acoust Soc Am 44:1529–1532, 1968

Nelson WE: Pediatrics (6th ed). Philadelphia, Saunders, 1962

Nelson WE: Pediatrics (9th ed). Philadelphia, Saunders, 1965

Newby HA: Audiology (2nd ed). New York, Appleton, 1964

Newman MH Jr: Hearing loss. *In* Strome M (ed): Differential Diagnosis in Pediatric Otolaryngology. Boston, Little, Brown, 1975

Neyhus A, Myklebust H: Early-life deafness and mental development. *In* McConnell F, Ward PH (eds): Deafness in Childhood. Nashville, Vanderbilt Univ Press, 1967

Norkus FJ, Derbyshire AJ, Mills PJ, et al: Frequency measure of the EEG. J Acoust Soc Am 32:1147–1150, 1960

Norris T, Stelmachowicz P, Taylor D: Acoustic reflex relaxation to identify sensorineural hearing impairment. Arch Otolaryngol 99:194–197, 1974

Northern JL, Downs MP: Hearing in Children. Baltimore, Williams and Wilkins, 1974

Nunnally J, Blanton RL: Patterns of word association in the deaf. Psychol Rep 18:86–92, 1966

Odenthal DW, Eggermont JJ: Clinical electrocochlcography. *In* Eggermont JJ, Odenthal DW, Schmidt PH, et al (eds): Electrocochleography, Basic Principles and Clinical Application. Acta Oto-Laryngol (Stockh) Suppl 316:62–74, 1974

Odenthal DW, Eggermont JJ: Electrocochleographic study of Ménière's disease and pontine angle neurinoma. *In* Ruben RJ, Elberling C, Salomon G (eds): Electrocochleography. Baltimore, University Park, 1976

Odenthal DW, Eggermont JJ, Hermans J: Diagnosis by electrocochleography. Rev Laryngol 95:481–488, 1974

Odom P, Blanton RL, Nunnally J: Some ''Cloze'' technique studies of language capability in the deaf. J Speech Hear Res 10:816–827, 1967

Odom RD: Effects of auditory and visual stimulus deprivation and satiation on children's performance in an operant task. J Exp Child Psychol 1:16–25, 1964

Ohlrich ES, Barnet AB: Auditory evoked responses during the first year of life. Electroencephalogr Clin Neurophysiol 32:161–169, 1972

O'Neill JJ, Oyer HJ: Applied Audiometry. New York, Dodd, Mead, 1966

Onishi S, Davis H: Effects of duration and rise time of tone bursts on evoked ''V'' potentials. J Acoust Soc Am 44:582–591, 1968

Ormerod FC: The pathology of congenital deafness. J Laryngol Otol 74:923–926, 1960

Ornitz EM: The modulation of sensory input and motor output in autistic children. *In* Schopler E, Reichler RJ (eds): Psychopathology and Child Development. New York, Plenum, 1976

Ornitz EM, Ritvo ER: Perceptual inconstance in early infantile autism. Arch Gen Psychiatry 18:76–98, 1968

Ornitz EM, Ritvo ER, Carr EM, et al: The variability of the auditory averaged evoked response during sleep and dreaming in children and adults. Electroencephalogr Clin Neurophysiol 22:514–524, 1967

Ornitz EM, Walter DO: The effect of sound pressure waveform on human brain stem auditory evoked responses. Brain Res 92:490–498, 1975

Osterhammel PA, Davis H, Wier CC, et al: Adult auditory evoked vertex potentials in sleep. Audiology 12:116–128, 1973

Paddison RM, Moossy J, Derbes VJ: Cockayne's syndrome. Dermatol Trop Ecol

Geogr 2:195–203, 1963

Paparella MM, Capps MJ: Sensorineural deafness in children—nongenetic. *In* Paparella MM, Shumrick DA (eds): Otolaryngology. Philadelphia, Saunders, 1973

Parmelee AH Jr: Sleep cycles in infants. Dev Med Child Neurol 11:794–795, 1969

Perl ER, Galambos R, Glorig A: The estimation of hearing threshold by electroencephalography. Electroencephalogr Clin Neurophysiol 5:501–512, 1953

Perlman MB, Case TJ: Electrical phenomena of the cochlea in man. Arch Otolaryngol 34:710–718, 1941

Peters JF, Mendel MI: Early components of the averaged electroencephalic response to monaural and binaural stimulation. Audiology 13:195–204, 1974

Peterson SJ: Speech pathology in craniofacial malformations other than cleft lip and palate. *In* Wertz RT (ed): Orofacial Anomalies: Clinical and Research Implications, ASHA Report No 8. Washington, American Speech and Hearing Assn, 1973

Piaget J: The Language and Thought of the Child. New York, Harcourt, 1926

Piaget J: The Language and Thought of the Child. New York, Meridian, 1955

Piaget J: Biology and Knowledge. Chicago, Univ Chicago Press, 1971

Pickett JM, Martin ES, Johnson D, et al: On patterns of speech feature reception by deaf listeners. *In* Fant G (ed): Proceedings of the International Symposium on Communication Ability in Profound Deafness, Stockholm, 1970. Washington, AG Bell Assn for the Deaf, 1972

Picton TW, Goodman WS, Bryce DP: Amplitude of evoked responses to tones of high intensity. Acta Oto-Laryngol (Stockh) 70:77–82, 1970

Picton TW, Hillyard SA: Human auditory evoked potentials. II: Effects of attention. Electroencephalogr Clin Neurophysiol 36:191–199, 1974

Picton TW, Hillyard SA, Krausz HI, et al: Human auditory evoked potentials. I. Evaluation of components. Electroencephalogr Clin Neurophysiol 36:179–190, 1974

Picton TW, Woods D, Baribeau-Braun J, et al: Evoked potential audiometry. J Otolaryngol 6:90–119, 1977

Pinter R, Paterson D: A measurement of the language ability of deaf children. Psychol Rev 23:413–426, 1916

Plantz R, Williston JS, Jewett DL: Spatio-temporal distribution of auditory-evoked farfield potentials in rat and cat. Brain Res 68:55–71, 1974

Poole R, Goetzinger CP, Rousey CA: A study of the effects of auditory stimulation on respiration. Acta Oto-Laryngol (Stockh) 61:143–152, 1966

Porges SW: Heart rate indices of newborn attentional responsivity. Merrill–Palmer Q Behav Dev 20:231–234, 1974

Portmann M, Aran JM: Electro-cochléographie sur le nourrisson et le jeune enfant. Acta Oto-Laryngol (Stockh) 71:253–261, 1971a

Portmann M, Aran JM: Electro-cochleography. Laryngoscope 81:899–910, 1971b

Portmann M, Aran JM: Relations entre ''Pattern'' electrocochléographique et pathologie retrolabyrinthique. Acta Oto-Laryngol (Stockh) 73:190–196, 1971c

Portmann M, Aran JM, LeBert G: Potentiels cochléaires obtenus chez l'homme et dehors de toute intervention chirurgicale. Note preliminaire. Rev Laryngol 88:157–164, 1967

Portmann M, Portmann C, Negrevergne M: Four years of clinical use of electrocochleography. Rev Laryngol Otol Rhinol 95:537–539, 1974

Potter RK, Kopp GA, Green HC: Visible Speech. New York, Van Nostrand, 1947

Powers D, Quigley S: Deaf children's acquisition of the passive voice. J Speech Hear Res 16:5–11, 1973

Pratt KC: The effects of repeated auditory stimulation upon the general activity of newborn infants. J Genet Psychol 44:96–116, 1934

Pratt KC, Nelson AK, Sun KH: The Behavior of the Newborn Infant. Columbus, Ohio St Univ Press, 1930

Prechtl HFR: The behavioral states of the newborn infant (a review). Brain Res 76:185–212, 1974

Price LL: Evoked response audiometry. *In* Fulton R, Lloyd LL (eds): Auditory Assessment of the Difficult-to-Test. Baltimore, Williams and Wilkins, 1975

Price LL, Goldstein R: Averaged evoked responses for measuring auditory sensitivity in children. J Speech Hear Dis 31:248–256, 1966.

Price LL, Rosenblut B, Goldstein R, et al: The averaged evoked response to auditory stimulation. J Speech Hear Res 9:361–370, 1966

Proctor CA, Proctor B: Understanding hereditary nerve deafness. Arch Otolaryngol 85:23–40, 1967

Pugh G: Summaries from appraisal of the silent reading abilities of acoustically handicapped children. Am Ann Deaf 91:331–349, 1946

Purves MJ: Initiation of respiration. *In* deReuch AVS, Porter R (eds): Ciba Foundation Symposium: Development of the Lungs. Boston, Little, Brown, 1965

Quigley, S: The influence of fingerspelling on the development of language, communication, and educational achievement in deaf children. Report of research grant RD 12996. Washington. Rehabilitation Services Administration, HEW, 1969.

Quigley S, Frisina DR: Institutionalized and psychoeducational development of deaf children. Council for Exceptional Children Research Monograph Series A, No 3, 1961

Quigley S, Smith N, Wilbur R: Comprehension of relativized sentences by deaf students. J Speech Hear Res 17:325–341, 1974

Quigley S, Wilbur R, Montanelli D: Question-formation in the language of deaf students. J Speech Hear Res 17:699–713, 1974

Rapin I, Bergman M: Auditory evoked responses in uncertain diagnoses. Arch Otolaryngol 90:307–314, 1969

Rapin I, Graziani LJ: Auditory-evoked responses in normal, brain damaged, and deaf infants. Neurology 17:881–894, 1967

Rapin I, Ruben RJ, Lyttle M: Diagnosis of hearing loss in infants using auditory evoked responses. Laryngoscope 80:712–722, 1970

Rapin I, Schimmel H, Cohen MM: Reliability in detecting the auditory evoked response (AER) for audiometry in sleeping subjects. Electroencephalogr Clin Neurophysiol 32:521–528, 1972

Reese HW, Lipsitt LP: Experimental Child Psychology. New York, Academic, 1970

Regan D: Evoked Potentials in Psychology, Sensory Physiology and Clinical Medicine. New York, Wiley, 1972

Reid L: The embryology of the lung. *In* DeReuch AVS, Porter R (eds): Ciba Foundation Symposium: Development of the Lungs. Boston, Little, Brown, 1965

Reneau J, Hnatiow GZ: Evoked Response Audiometry: A Topical and Historical Review. Baltimore, Univ Park, 1975

Restaino L: Word association of deaf and hearing child. *In* Rosenstein J, MacGinitie W (eds): Verbal Behavior of the Deaf Child. New York, Teachers Coll Press, 1969

Riesen AH: Sensory deprivation. *In* Stellar E, Sprague JM (eds): Progress in Physiological Psychology. New York, Academic, 1966

Rimland B: Infantile Autism. New York, Appleton, 1964

Rincover A, Newsom C, Carr T: Studies in motivation: Sensory stimulation as reinforcement. Annual convention, Western Psychological Association, San Francisco, 1974

Ritvo ER, Ornitz EM, Walter RD: Clinical application of the auditory averaged evoked response at sleep onset in the diagnosis of deafness. Pediatrics 40:1003–1008, 1967

Roberts B, Campbell D: Activity in newborns and the sound of a human heart. Psychon Sci 9:339–340, 1967

Robertson E, Peterson J, Lamb L: Relative impedance measurements in young children. Arch Otolaryngol 88:162–168, 1968

Roeser RJ, Price LL, Hnatiow GZ: Evoked response audiometry: Psychiatric patients. Arch Otolaryngol 94:208–213, 1971

Ronis BJ: Cochlear potentials in otosclerosis. Laryngoscope 73:212–231, 1966

Rose DE, Keating LW, Hedgecock LD, et al: Aspects of acoustically evoked responses: Interjudge and intrajudge reliability. Arch Otolaryngol 94:347–350, 1971

Rose DE, Keating LW, Hedgecock LD, et al: A comparison of evoked response audiometry and routine clinical audiometry. Audiology 11:238–243, 1972

Rosenstein J: Cognitive abilities of deaf children. J Speech Hear Res 3:108–119, 1960

Rosenzweig MR: Effects of environment on brain and behavior in animals. *In* Schopler E, Reichler RJ (eds): Psychopathology and Child Development. New York, Plenum, 1976

Ross B, Hormann H: The attainment of formal operations. Genet Psychol Monogr 91:61–119, 1975

Rossi P, Guidotti E: Problems associated with the early diagnosis of deafness in newborn babies. *In* Mencher GT (ed): Early Identification of Hearing Loss. Basel, Karger, 1976

Rothman HB: An acoustic and electromyographic investigation of consonant-vowel transitions in the speech of deaf adults. J Acoust Soc Am 52:159A, 1972

Rothman HH: Effects of high frequencies and intersubject variability on the auditory-evoked cortical response. J Acoust Soc Am 47:569–473, 1970

Rousey CL, Snyder C, Rousey CG: Changes in respiration as a function of auditory stimuli. J Aud Res 4:107–114, 1964

Ruben RJ: Cochlear potentials as a diagnostic test in deafness. *In* Graham AB (ed): Sensorineural Hearing Processes and Disorders. Boston, Little, Brown, 1967

Ruben RJ, Bordley JE, Lieberman AT: Cochlear potentials in man. Laryngoscope 71:1141–1164, 1961

Ruben RJ, Elberling C, Salomon G (eds): Electrocochleography. Baltimore, Univ Park Press, 1976

Ruben RJ, Knickerbocker GG, Sekula J, et al: Cochlear microphonics in man: A preliminary report. Laryngoscope 69:665–671, 1959

Ruben RJ, Lieberman AT, Bordley JE: Some observations on cochlear potentials and nerve action potentials in children. Laryngoscope 72:545–554, 1962

Ruben RJ, Sekula J, Bordley JE, et al: Human cochlear responses to sound stimuli. Ann Otol Rhinol Laryngol 69:459–479, 1960

Ruben RJ, Walker AE: The VIIIth nerve action potential in Ménière's disease. Laryngoscope 73:1456–1461, 1963

Rudmose W: Audiometric screening of the newborn. J Acoust Soc Am 41:868, 1967

Ruhm HB, Jansen JW: Rate of stimulus change and the evoked response: 1. Signal rise-time. J Aud Res 3:211–216, 1969

Ruhm HB, Walker E, Flanigin H: Acoustically-evoked potentials in man: mediation of early components. Laryngoscope 77:806–822, 1967

Sajwaj T, Twardosz S, Burke M: Side effects of extinction procedures in a remedial preschool. J Appl Behav Anal 5:163–176, 1972

Salamy A, McKean CM: Postnatal development of human brainstem potentials during the first year of life. Electroencephalogr Clin Neurophysiol 40:418–426, 1976

Salamy A, McKean CM: Habituation and dishabituation of cortical and brainstem evoked potentials. Int J Neurosci (in press)

Salamy A, McKean CM, Buda FB: Maturational changes in auditory transmission as reflected in human brain stem potentials. Brain Res 96:361–366, 1975

Salk L: The effects of the normal heartbeat sound on the behavior of the newborn infant: Implications for mental health. World Mental Health 12:168–175, 1960

Salk L: The importance of heartbeat rhythm to human nature: Theoretical, clinical, and experimental observations. Proc Third World Cong Psychiatry. Montreal, McGill Univ Press, 1961

Salk L: Mother's heartbeat as an imprinting stimulus. Trans NY Acad Sci 24:753–763, 1962

Salomon G: Middle ear muscle activity. Proc Royal Soc Med 54:966–971, 1966

Salomon G: On the continuous control of the middle ear muscle activity in cat. Acta Oto-Laryngol (Stockh) Suppl 224:218–219, 1967

Salomon G, Elberling C: Cochlear nerve potentials recorded from the ear canal in man. Acta Oto-Laryngol (Stockh) 71:319–325, 1971

Saul LJ, Davis H: Action currents in the central nervous system: I. Action currents of the auditory tracts. Arch Neurol Psychiatr 28:1104–1116, 1932

Schachter J, Williams TA, Khachaturian Z, et al: Heart rate responses to auditory clicks in neonates. Psychophysiology 8:163–179, 1971

Schein J: Word association conformity on deaf and hearing college students. Annual meeting, American Psychological Assn, New York, 1961

Scherer P: An open letter to educators of the deaf. Am Ann Deaf 116:404–407, 1971

Schimmel H, Rapin I, Cohen MM: Improving evoked response audiometry. Results of normative studies for machine scoring. Audiology 14:466–479, 1975

Schlesinger H: Language acquisition in four deaf children. *In* Schlesinger H, Meadow

K (eds): Deafness and Mental Health: A Developmental Approach. San Francisco, Langley Porter Inst. 1971

Schlesinger H, Meadow K: Sound and Sign: Childhood Deafness and Mental Health. Berkeley, Univ Calif Press, 1972

Schmitt P: Language instruction for the deaf. Volta Rev 68:85–108, 1966

Schmitt P: Deaf children's comprehension and production of sentence transformations and verb tenses. Unpublished doctoral dissertation, Univ Illinois, Urbana-Champaign, 1968

Schoenberg BS: Richard Caton and the electrical activity of the brain. Mayo Clin Proc 49:474–481, 1974

Schopler E: Infantile autism and the receptor processes. Arch Gen Psychol 13:327–335, 1965

Schucknecht HF: Pathology of sensorineural deafness of genetic origin. *In* McConnell F, Ward PH (eds): Deafness in Childhood. Nashville, Vanderbilt Univ Press, 1967

Schulman CA: Heart rate response habituation in high-risk premature infants. Psychophysiology 6:690–694, 1970

Schulman CA: Heart rate audiometry. Part II: The relationship between heart rate change threshold and audiometric threshold in hearing-impaired children. Neuropädiatrie 5:19–27, 1974

Schulman CA, Kreiter R: The contribution of heart-rate audiometry in the early identification of hearing impairment. Annual meeting, California Speech and Hearing Association, Los Angeles, 1971

Schulman CA, Smith CR, Weisinger M, et al: The use of heart rate in the audiological evaluation of nonverbal children. Part I. Evaluation of children at risk for hearing impairment. Neuropädiatrie 2:187–196, 1970

Schulman-Galambos CA, Galambos R: Brain stem auditory-evoked responses in premature infants. J Speech Hear Res 18:456–465, 1975

Schulze G: An evaluation of vocabulary development by thirty-two deaf children over a three year period. Am Ann Deaf 110:424–435, 1965

Scott TD: A psychophysiological investigation of cortical audiometry during human sleep. Unpublished doctoral dissertation, Univ Calif, Santa Cruz, 1973

Seitz S, Marcus S: Mother–child interations: A foundation for language development. Except Child 42:445–449, 1976

Shagass C: Evoked Brain Potentials in Psychiatry. New York, Plenum, 1972

Shock NW, Schlatter MJ: Pulse rate response of adolescents to auditory stimuli. J Exp Psychol 30:414–425, 1942

Silverman SR: Rehabilitative audiology. *In* Paparella MM, Shumrick DA (eds): Otolaryngology. Philadelphia, Saunders, 1973

Simmons A: A comparison of the type-token ratio of spoken and written language of deaf and hearing children. Volta Rev 64:417–421, 1962

Simmons FB: Binaural summation of the acoustic reflex. J Acoust Soc Am 37:834–836, 1965

Simmons FB: Perceptual theories of middle ear muscle function. Ann Otol Rhinol Laryngol 73:724–740, 1964

Simmons FB: Electrocochleography. Ann Otol Rhinol Laryngol 83:312–313, 1974

Simmons FB: Human auditory nerve responses: A comparison of three commonly used recording sites. Laryngoscope 85:1564–1581, 1975

Simmons FB, Glattke T: Electrocochleography. *In* Bradford LJ (ed): Physiological Measures of the Audio-Vestibular System. New York, Academic, 1975

Sinclair-de-Zwart H: Language acquisition and cognitive development. *In* Moore T (ed): Cognitive Development and the Acquisition of Language. New York, Academic, 1973

Skarakis EA: Early communication: Semantic functions and communicative intentions in the communication of the preschool child with impaired hearing. Unpublished master's thesis, Univ Calif, Santa Barbara, 1976

Skinner PH, Antinoro F: The effect of signal rise time and duration on the early components of the auditory evoked cortical response. J Speech Hear Res 14:552–558, 1971

Skinner PH, Glattke T: Electrophysiologic response audiometry: State of the art. J Speech Hear Dis 42:179–198, 1977

Skinner PH, Jones HC: Effects of signal duration and rise time on the auditory evoked potential. J Speech Hear Res 11:301–306, 1968

Skinner PH, Shimota J: A comparison of the effects of sedatives on the auditory evoked cortical response. J Am Audiol Soc 1:71–78, 1975

Slobin D: Grammatical transformations in childhood and adulthood. J Verbal Learning Verbal Behav 5:219–227, 1966

Slobin D: Developmental psycholinguistics. *In* Dingwall W (ed): A survey of Linguistic Science. College Park, MD, College Park Press, 1971

Smith JC, Marsh JT, Brown WS: Far-field recorded frequency-following responses: evidence for the locus of brainstem sources. Electroencephalogr Clin Neurophysiol 39:465–472, 1975

Sohmer H, Feinmesser M: Cochlear action potentials recorded from the external ear in man. Ann Otol Rhinol Laryngol 76:427–435, 1967

Sohmer H, Feinmesser M: Cochlear and cortical audiometry: Conveniently recorded in the same subject. Isr J Med Sci 6:219–223, 1970

Sohmer H, Feinmesser M: Routine use of electrocochleography (cochlear audiometry) in human subjects. Audiology 12:167–173, 1973

Sohmer H, Feinmesser M: Electrocochleography in clinical-audiological diagnosis. Arch Otolaryngol 206:91–102, 1974

Sohmer H, Feinmesser M, Bauberger-Tell L, et al: Routine use of cochlear audiometry in infants with uncertain diagnosis. Ann Otol Rhinol Laryngol 81:72–75, 1972

Sohmer H, Pratt H: Recording of the cochlear microphonic potential with surface electrodes. Electroencephalogr Clin Neurophysiol 40:253–260, 1976

Sohmer H, Pratt H, Feinmesser M: Electrocochleography or evoked cortical responses: Which is preferable in diagnosis of hearing loss? Rev Laryngol 95:515–522, 1974

Spradlin JE, Lloyd LL: Operant conditioning audiometry with low level retardates: A preliminary report. *In* Lloyd LL, Frisina DR (eds): The Audiological Assessment of the Mentally Retarded: Proceedings of a National Conference. Parsons, KS, Parsons State Hospital and Training Center, 1965

Stark RE: Some features of the vocalizations of young deaf children. *In* Bosma JE (ed): Third Symposium on Oral Sensation and Perception: The Mouth of the

Infant. Springfield, IL, Thomas, 1972
Starr A: Auditory brainstem responses in brain death. Brain 99:543–554, 1976
Starr A, Achor J: Auditory brainstem responses in neurological disease. Arch Neurol 32:761–768, 1975
Starr A, Amlie R, Martin WH, et al: Development of auditory function in newborn infants revealed by auditory brainstem potentials. Pediatrics (in press)
Starr A, Hamilton A: Correlations between confirmed sites of neurological lesions and abnormalities of far-field auditory brainstem responses. Electroencephalogr Clin Neurophysiol 41:595–608, 1976
Stein L: Clinical study of brainstem evoked response (BER) with untestable and high risk children. Annual convention, American Speech and Hearing Association, Washington, 1975
Steinschneider A, Lipton EL, Richmond JB: Auditory sensitivity in infant: effect of intensity on cardiac and motor responsitivity. Child Dev 37:233–251, 1966
Stensland-Junker K: BOEL—A child welfare program for early screening of communication abilities. *In* Mencher GT (ed): Early Identification of Hearing Loss. Basel, Karger, 1976
Stevens KN, Nickerson RS, Boothroyd A, et al: Assessment of nasalization in the speech of deaf children. J Speech Hear Res 19:393–416, 1976
Stewart J: High risk screening. Meeting of the Western Society for Pediatric Research, Carmel, 1974
Stillman RD, Moushegian G, Rupert AL: Early tone-evoked responses in normal and hearing impaired subjects. Audiology 15:10–22, 1976
Stokoe W: Sign language structure. *In* Stokoe W (ed): Studies in Linguistics. Buffalo, Univ Buffalo, 1960
Stool SE: The identification of hearing loss in children. Annual convention, American Speech and Hearing Association, Washington, 1975
Stubbs EM: The effect of factors of duration, intensity and pitch of sound stimuli on the responses of newborn infants. Univ Iowa Stud Child Welfare 9:77–134, 1934
Stuckless E, Birch J: The influence of early manual communication on the linguistic development of deaf children. Am Ann Deaf 111:452–460, 499–504, 1966
Sudaka J, Chaperon C: Notre experience d'électrocochléographie dans le service d'O-R-L des enfants malades. Ann Oto-Laryngol 89:699–706, 1972
Suter CM, Glaser EM, Goldberg A, et al: Auditory brainstem electric response to click trains and continuous tones. J Acoust Soc Am 60(Suppl #1):516, 1976
Suzuki T, Asawa I: Evoked potential of waking human brain to acoustic stimuli. Acta Oto-Laryngol (Stockh) 48:508–515, 1957
Suzuki T, Kamijo Y, Kuichi W: Auditory test of newborn infants. Ann Otol Rhinol Laryngol 73:914–923, 1964
Suzuki T, Ogiba Y: A technique of pure tone audiometry for children under three years of age. Conditioned orienting reflex (C.O.R.) audiometry. Rev Laryngol 81:33–43, 1960
Suzuki T, Ogiba Y: Conditioned orientation reflex audiometry. Arch Otolaryngol 74:192–198, 1961
Suzuki T, Ogiba Y, Takei T: Basic properties of conditioned orientation reflex audiometry. Minerva Oto-Laryngol 22:181–186, 1972

Suzuki T, Origuchi K: Averaged evoked response audiometry in young children during sleep. Acta Oto-Laryngol (Stockh) Suppl 252:19–28, 1969

Suzuki T, Taguchi K: Cerebral evoked response to auditory stimuli in young children during sleep. Ann Otol Rhinol Laryngol 77:102–110, 1968

Taft LT, Cohen HJ: Neonatal and infant reflexology. *In* Hellmuth J (ed): Exceptional Infant. Vol I: The Normal Infant. New York, Brunner/Mazel, 1967

Taguchi K, Goodman WS, Brummitt WM: Evoked response audiometry in mentally retarded children. Acta Oto-Laryngol (Stockh) 70:190–196, 1970

Taguchi K, Picton T, Orpin J, et al: Evoked response audiometry in newborn infants. Acta Oto-Laryngol (Stockh) Suppl 252:5–17, 1969

Tanaka Y, Arayama T: Fetal responses to acoustic stimuli. Prac Oto-Rhinolaryngol 31:269–273, 1969

Tanguay PE, Lee JCM, Ornitz EM: A detailed analysis of the auditory evoked response waveform in children during REM and stage 2 sleep. Electroencephalogr Clin Neurophysiol 35:241–248, 1973

Tanguay PE, Ornitz EM, Forsythe AB, et al: Basic rest–activity cycle rhythms in the human auditory evoked response. Electroencephalogr Clin Neurophysiol 34:593–603, 1973

Teas DC, Eldredge DH, Davis H: Cochlear responses to acoustic transients: An interpretation of whole-nerve action potentials. J Acoust Soc Am 34:1438–1459, 1962

Teel J, Winston MA, Aspinall K, et al: Thresholds of hearing by respiration using a polygraph. Arch Otolaryngol 86:172–174, 1967

Terkildsen K, Osterhammel P, Huis in't Veld F: Electrocochleography with a far field technique. Scand Audiol 2:141–148, 1973

Terkildsen K, Osterhammel P, Huis in't Veld F: Far field electrocochleography. Electrode positions. Scand Audiol 3:123–129, 1974

Terkildsen K, Osterhammel P, Huis in't Veld F: Far-field electrocochleography. Adaptation. Scand Audiol 4:215–220, 1975a

Terkildsen K, Osterhammel P, Huis in't Veld F: Far field electrocochleography. Frequency specificity of the response. Scand Audiol 4:167–172, 1975b

Thompson D: Influence of selective attention on the averaged electroencephalic response. Unpublished doctoral dissertation, Univ Wisconsin, 1972

Thornton A: The effects of stimulus frequency and intensity on the middle components of the auditory averaged electroencephalic response. Unpublished doctoral dissertation, Univ Iowa, 1975

Thornton A, Mendel MI, Anderson C: Effects of stimulus frequency and intensity on the middle components of the averaged auditory electroencephalic response. J Speech Hear Res 20:81–94, 1977

Thornton ARD: The diagnostic potential of surface recorded electrocochleography. Br J Audiol 9:7–13, 1975a

Thornton ARD: The measurement of surface-recorded electrocochleographic responses. Scand Audiol 4:51–58, 1975b

Thornton ARD: Statistical properties of surface-recorded electrocochleographic responses. Scand Audiol 4:91–102, 1975c

Thornton ARD: Electrophysiological studies of the auditory system. Audiology

15:23–38, 1976

Thornton ARD, Coleman MJ: The adaptation of cochlear and brainstem auditory evoked potentials in humans. Electroencephalogr Clin Neurophysiol 39:399–406, 1975

Tomlinson-Keasey O, Kelly R: The development of thought processes in deaf children. Am Ann Deaf 119:693–699, 1974

Toscher M, Rupp R: The psychological implications of deafness; the human factor. Mich Speech Hear Assn J 10:60–67, 1974

Turkewitz G, Birch HG, Cooper KK: Patterns of response to different auditory stimuli in the human newborn. Dev Med Child Neurol 14:487–491, 1972

Tweney R, Holmann H: The development of semantic associations in profoundly deaf children. J Speech Hear Res 16:309–318, 1973

Tyberghein J, Forrez G: Objective (ERA) and subjective (COR) audiometry in the infant. Acta Oto-Laryngol (Stockh) 71:249–252, 1971

Välimäki I: Postnatal alterations of cardiac rhythm. Clin Pediatr 9:652–655, 1970

Valverde F: Apical dendritic spines of the visual cortex and light deprivation in the mouse. Exp Brain Res 3:337–352, 1967

Valverde F: Rate and extent of recovery from dark rearing in the visual cortex of the mouse. Brain Res 33:1–11, 1971

Vandenberg D: The Written Language of Deaf Children. New York, Whitcombe and Tombs, 1971

Vasiliu DI: L'enfant est prêt a entendre même dans la vie intrauterine. Contributions sur l'embryogenese de l'orielle et la pneumatisation de la mastoide et du rocher. Int Audiol 7:181–185, 1968

Vaughn HG, Ritter W: The sources of auditory evoked responses recorded from the human scalp. Electroencephalogr Clin Neurophysiol 28:360–367, 1970

Velmans M: Effects of frequency recoding on the articulation learning of perceptively deaf children. Lang Speech 18:180–193, 1975

Vernon M: Sociological and psychological factors associated with hearing loss. J Speech Hear Res 12:541–563, 1969

Vernon M: Total communication. Talk 78:10–15, 1975–6

Vernon M, Koh S: Effects of manual communication on deaf children's educational achievement, linguistic competence, oral skills and psychological development. Am Ann Deaf 115:527–536, 1970

Vivion MC, Goldstein R, Wolf KE, et al: Middle components of human auditory AER: Waveform variation during averaging. Audiology 16:21–37, 1977

Waardenburg PJ: A new syndrome combining developmental anomalies of the eyelids, eyebrows and nose root with pigmentary defects of the iris and head hair and with congenital deafness. Am J Human Genet 3:195–253, 1951

Wahler RG, Sperling KA, Thomas MR, et al: The modification of childhood stuttering: some response–response relationships. J Exp Child Psychol 9:411–428, 1970

Walk RD, Gibson EJ: A comparative and analytical study of visual depth perception. Psychol Monogr 75:1–44, 1961

Ward PH, Lindsay JR, Warner NE: Cytomegalic inclusion disease affecting the temporal bone. Laryngoscope 75:628–636, 1965

Wedenberg E: Auditory tests on new-born infants. Acta Oto-Laryngol (Stockh) 46:446–461, 1956

Weibel ER: Postnatal growth of the lung and pulmonary gas-exchange capacity. *In* DeReuch AVS, Porter R (eds): Ciba Foundation Symposium: Development of the Lungs. Boston, Little, Brown, 1965

Weir RH: Some questions on the child's learning of phonology. *In* Smith F, Miller G (eds): The Genesis of Language. Cambridge, MIT Press, 1966

Weiss H, Mundie J, Cashin J, et al: The normal human intra-aural muscle reflex in response to sound. Acta Oto-Laryngol (Stockh) 55:505–515, 1962

Weitzman E, Fishbein W, Graziani LJ: Auditory evoked responses obtained from the scalp electroencephalogram of the full-term human neonate during sleep. Pediatrics 35:458–462, 1965

Weitzman E, Graziani LJ: Maturation and topography of the auditory evoked response of the prematurely born infant. Dev Psychobiol 1:79–89, 1968

Weitzman E, Kremen H: Auditory evoked responses during different stages of sleep in man. Electroencephalogr Clin Neurophysiol 18:65–70, 1965

Wever EG, Bray CW: Auditory nerve impulses. Science 71:215, 1930

Whetnall E, Fry DB: The Deaf Child. London, Heinemans, 1971

Wiesel TN, Hubel DH: Comparison of the effects of unilateral and bilateral eye closure on cortical unit responses in kittens. J Neurophysiol 28:1029–1040, 1965

Wilber L: Use of absolute and relative impedance in defining the nature of middle ear lesions in children. *In* Rose D, Keating L (comps): Impedance Symposium. Chicago, Zenith Hearing Instrument Corp, 1972

Wilbur R, Quigley S, Montanelli D: Conjoined structures in the language of deaf students. J Speech Hear Res 18:319–335, 1975

Wilder J: The law of initial values. Psychosom Med 12:393, 1950

Williams HL, Tepas DI, Morlock HC: Evoked responses to clicks and electroencephalographic stages of sleep in man. Science 138:685–686, 1962

Wilson WR, Moore JM, Thompson G: Sound-field auditory thresholds of infants utilizing visual reinforcement audiometry. Annual convention, American Speech and Hearing Assn, Houston, 1976

Winer BJ: Statistical Principles in Experimental Design. New York, McGraw–Hill, 1962

Withrow FB Jr, Goldstein R: An electrophysiologic procedure for determination of auditory threshold in children. Laryngoscope 68:1674–1699, 1958

Wright L: The theoretical and research base for a program of early stimulation care and training of premature infants. *In* Hellmuth J (ed): Exceptional Infant. Vol 2, Studies in Abnormalities. New York, Brunner/Mazel, 1971

Wright MJ: The Pathology of Deafness. Manchester, University Press, 1971

Yamada O, Yagi T, Yamane H, et al: Clinical evaluation of the auditory evoked brainstem response. Auris-Nasus-Larynx 2:92–105, 1975

Yanz JL: Frequency specificity of the auditory compound action potential. Unpublished master's thesis, Univ Iowa, 1976

Yoshie N: Auditory nerve action potential responses to clicks in man. Laryngoscope 78:198–215, 1968

Yoshie N: Clinical cochlear response audiometry by means of an average response computer: nonsurgical technique and clinical use. Rev Laryngol Suppl 92:646–672, 1971

Yoshie N: Diagnostic significance of the elctrocochleogram in clinical audiometry. Audiology 12:504–539, 1973

Yoshie N, Ohashi T: Clinical use of cochlear nerve action potential responses in man for differential diagnosis of hearing losses. Acta Oto-Laryngol (Stockh) Suppl 252:71–87, 1969

Yoshie N, Ohashi T: Abnormal adaptation of human cochlear nerve action potential responses—clinical observations by nonsurgical recording. Rev Laryngol 92:673–690, 1971

Yoshie N, Ohashi T, Suzuki T: Nonsurgical recording of auditory nerve action potentials in man. Laryngoscope 77:76–85, 1967

Yoshie N, Okudaira T: Myogenic evoked potential responses to clicks in man. Acta Oto-Laryngol (Stockh) Suppl 252:89–103, 1969

Zemlin W: Speech and Hearing Science. Englewood Cliffs, NJ, Prentice–Hall, 1971

Zerlin S, Mowry HJ, Naunton RF: Effect of frequency and intensity on early components of the evoked cortical response. Annual convention, American Speech and Hearing Association, Chicago, 1971

Zerlin S, Naunton, RF: Early and late averaged electroencephalic responses at low sensation levels. Audiology 13:366–378, 1974

Zerlin S, Naunton RF, Mowry HJ: The early evoked cortical response to third octave clicks and tones. Audiology 12:242–249, 1973

Zink GD: Comprehensive programming for early detection and management of communication disorders. *In* Mencher GT (ed): Early Identification of Hearing Loss. Basel, Karger, 1976

Zöllner C, Karnahl T, Stange G: Input–output function and adaptation behavior of the five early potentials registered with the earlobe-vertex pick-up. Arch Otolaryngol 212:23–33, 1976

Zubek JP: Sensory Deprivation: Fifteen Years of Research. New York, Appleton, 1969

Zvonar M, Zvonar-Kuhndl B, Odenthal DW: Anesthesia and sedation for electrocochleography. *In* Eggermont JJ, Odenthal DW, Schmidt PH, et al (eds): Electrocochleography, Basic Principles and Clinical Application. Acta Oto-Laryngol (Stockh) Suppl: 316:37–38, 1974

Author Index

Subject Index

a b c d 7 e 8 f 9 g 0 h 1 i 8 2 j